Nightmare Factories

NIGHTMARE FACTORIES

THE ASYLUM IN THE AMERICAN IMAGINATION

Troy Rondinone

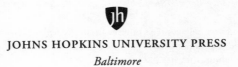

JOHNS HOPKINS UNIVERSITY PRESS

Baltimore

© 2019 Johns Hopkins University Press
All rights reserved. Published 2019
Printed in the United States of America on acid-free paper
9 8 7 6 5 4 3 2 1

Johns Hopkins University Press
2715 North Charles Street
Baltimore, Maryland 21218-4363
www.press.jhu.edu

Library of Congress Cataloging-in-Publication Data

Names: Rondinone, Troy, 1973– author.
Title: Nightmare factories : the asylum in the American imagination /
    Troy Rondinone.
Description: Baltimore : Johns Hopkins University Press, 2019. | Includes
    bibliographical references and index.
Identifiers: LCCN 2018059343 | ISBN 9781421432670 (hardcover : alk. paper) |
    ISBN 1421432676 (hardcover : alk. paper) | ISBN 9781421432687 (electronic) |
    ISBN 1421432684 (electronic)
Subjects: LCSH: Asylums—United States—History. | Psychiatric hospitals—
    United States—History.
Classification: LCC RC439 .R638 2019 | DDC 362.2/1—dc23
LC record available at https://lccn.loc.gov/2018059343

A catalog record for this book is available from the British Library.

*Special discounts are available for bulk purchases of this book. For more information,
please contact Special Sales at 410-516-6936 or specialsales@press.jhu.edu.*

Johns Hopkins University Press uses environmentally friendly book materials,
including recycled text paper that is composed of at least 30 percent post-
consumer waste, whenever possible.

In Memory of Alan G. Miller

CONTENTS

Nightmare Factories

INTRODUCTION

I t was, quite possibly, the strangest premiere in movie history. On Friday, December 19, 1975, an audience of mental patients, attendants, nurses, doctors, and Hollywood celebrities crowded into the historic Elsinore Theatre in Salem, Oregon, to watch a movie starring themselves. A quaint but dilapidated relic, the Elsinore rated as a second-run movie house, its creaky Gothic Tudor façade evoking Hamlet's castle. But, on this day, what mattered was not the look but the location. The Elsinore stood less than two miles from the Oregon State Hospital, where the movie had been shot. The emcee for the premiere was the institution's director, Dr. Dean Brooks. Brooks was no typical Hollywood player, but this was no typical Hollywood picture. *One Flew Over the Cuckoo's Nest* was a stark, realistic vision of life in an institution. The filmmakers not only had shot it in a working hospital but had also asked most of the actors to live on campus during the shoot. The actors followed patients around, even attended therapy sessions with them. It got so authentic that one performer, a young man from New Jersey named Danny DeVito, became convinced he was losing his mind. Dr. Brooks had to counsel him.

As the audience settled in, the Hollywood contingent hid out in the lobby. The celebrities were incredibly nervous. What would the patients think, seeing themselves and their home on screen? Would they feel mocked? Would it be confusing to them? Heaven knew that they keenly felt the stigma of their disease. America was not a safe place for the mentally ill, never had been. The very word "asylum" implied an unwelcome outside world. Now they were going to see their secluded domain lit up on the big screen. The Elsinore was about to host history.[1]

This rare event was owed to the personal efforts of Dr. Brooks. Scouring the Northwest for an institution like the one described in

Ken Kesey's source novel, the producers had been introduced to Brooks, who generously allowed them to shoot inside his hospital with the only caveat being that the patients be allowed to work on the production. As Brooks saw it, though "not without risk," the film could have "immense" "therapeutic value." The producers agreed. Strikingly, the patients would play the doctors as film extras, while hospital staff would play the patients. Brooks became intimately involved, even correcting the filmmakers on the portrayal of electroconvulsive therapy. Such particulars he might have expected; less anticipated was that the director would insist he play Dr. Spivey in the film.[2]

Dean Brooks had achieved minor celebrity once before. In 1972, he was featured in a *Life* magazine photo essay that showed him taking his troubled charges on a wilderness excursion. Images of young men and women rock climbing, whitewater rafting, and lounging in sunlit meadows could not have presented a starker contrast to popular portrayals of mental hospitals. Brooks told the reporter that the purpose of this two-week trip was "to break them out of the institutional mold." In an era of psychiatric mistrust and deinstitutionalization, Brooks was like a breath of fresh air. He had his patients call him by his first name. He replaced seclusion rooms with patient-run shops. He brought in a piano for them to play and had colorful murals painted on the walls. Nobody wore uniforms, except on the forensic, or criminal, unit.[3] But these efforts would be overshadowed by the film that made him and his workplace synonymous with institutional abuse. He would, until the end of his days, be associated with *One Flew Over the Cuckoo's Nest*.

Brooks had first encountered Ken Kesey's novel a decade earlier. He'd been getting calls from colleagues all over the country telling him that there was a new book set in the institution he was running. Intrigued, he got his hands on a copy of *One Flew Over the Cuckoo's Nest* and read it immediately. He hated it, seeing it as an attack on his profession. But when he later saw the stage play, in the words of his daughter Dennie, he realized that "it spoke a truth that needed to be told about institutions everywhere." He understood now. The asylum was a metaphor; Kesey was commenting about the ways that modern society imprisoned us. In an address to the American Psychiatric Association in 1976, Brooks explained that Kesey "is not an investigative reporter; he is a writer of fiction." His book did not "set psychiatry back 25 years," as some doctors believed. It was a work of art, as relevant as *Uncle Tom's Cabin* was in its day. Kesey had "exploded into consciousness the things we have refused to look at." Sure, it took place in a mental hospital, and yes, it did raise important issues of patients' rights. But it was, most emphatically, *not* a book about mental health. It was "an allegory of what happens in any institutional system that is created anywhere, any time."[4]

Director Milos Forman could not have agreed more. He'd fled Czechoslovakia in the wake of the failed Prague Spring revolt of 1968, and, in Kesey's novel, he saw a parable of his homeland. He knew about constant surveillance and the knowledge that one does not really possess anything. As Forman told reporters, "This is a movie about [a] society I just lived twenty years of my life [in]. You know, it's about everything I know. And I know how these people feel." The book also spoke to coproducer Michael Douglas. The young actor was part of the generation that saw Kesey's book as its "Bible." Like Kesey, Douglas had done a lot of LSD and had participated in experiments of alternative communal living. He, too, distrusted his father's generation. The unexpected twist in his case was that his father was a famous screen actor who had purchased the rights to Kesey's book. Michael acquired the property after Kirk Douglas had repeatedly failed to get the project greenlit for the screen. Michael was determined to make it happen. Yet he was nagged with apprehension. He felt "the weight of dealing" with this legendary book, assuaging himself by telling one reporter, "I don't think we can destroy whatever comments the book makes."[5]

The trip from Ken Kesey's typewriter to the Elsinore Theatre was a saga unto itself. Like many other famous fictions, *Cuckoo's Nest* has roots in reality. As a Stanford University graduate student, Kesey had worked nights as an attendant in the psych ward of the VA hospital in Palo Alto. Inspired by what he saw, he wrote most of the first draft of *Cuckoo's Nest* right there on the ward. The fourth book he'd written but the first to be published, *One Flew Over the Cuckoo's Nest* hit store shelves January 1962. Kirk Douglas had bought the rights after perusing a galley copy a producer friend sent to him. Once Michael got his hands on it, he secured funds with the help of coproducer Saul Zaentz. But it was going to be a low budget movie.

According to Michael, nobody expected *Cuckoo's Nest* to be a hit. Conventional wisdom held that asylum movies did not make money. This was odd, considering that there had been so many of them. The first, Georges Méliès's *Off to Bloomingdale Asylum*, appeared in 1901. It lasted one minute.[6] Since then, hundreds of filmmakers had dipped their toes in the mental hospital pool. Thomas Edison made one, as did D. W. Griffith and Alfred Hitchcock. Harry Houdini escaped from one in *The Man from Beyond*. Lon Chaney ruled one in *The Monster*. Boris Karloff, Edward G. Robinson, Bette Davis, Humphrey Bogart, Ingrid Bergman, Gregory Peck, Elizabeth Taylor, Katherine Hepburn, Montgomery Clift, Vincent Price, Anthony Perkins, Natalie Wood, Jerry Lewis, Olivia de Havilland, and Warren Beatty had all starred in celluloid asylums. Probably the most famous asylum movie at this point was 1948's *The Snake Pit*. It was such a sensation that it became an adjective—a "snake pit" was a synonym for a dismal state hospital. Critics used the term with frequency in the 1970s.

The filming of *Cuckoo's Nest* did not go smoothly. Dr. Brooks had to go to the governor personally to get approval, and many of his own staff fought him the whole time. Many actors turned down leading parts, and finding a giant Native American actor to play Chief Bromden was no small feat. The film budget bloomed from $1.5 million to $4.1 million (much of this going to star Jack Nicholson). Once primary shooting began, creative differences caused Forman to fire the first cinematographer. Filming in winter while trying to use natural light cut down the available shooting hours. Other problems piled up, including getting enough pot for the crew and finding "insane" looking extras, not to mention dealing with the mercurial Ken Kesey. Kesey's original script, commissioned and rejected by Douglas and Zaentz, was much more phantasmagorical than Forman could allow. Zaentz recalls reading about a massive Nurse Ratched with long claw-like nails walking down a narrow hallway, scraping the walls and making blood come out. Kesey also was not pleased with the actor who played his iconic hero. Instead of a big-shouldered, tattooed Irish rebel, they'd chosen Jack Nicholson, whom Kesey dubbed a "wimp." Kesey would later brag that he never watched the film. According to one legend, he was once channel surfing in the middle of the night and caught a few minutes of a flick about a madcap crew in an asylum. When he figured out it was *Cuckoo's Nest*, he changed the channel.[7]

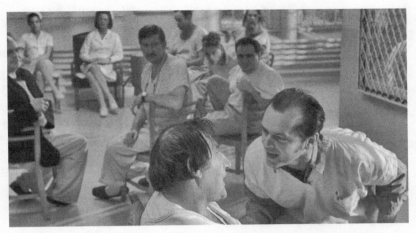

Jack Nicholson and the cast of *One Flew Over the Cuckoo's Nest* (1975) in the Oregon State Hospital

After eleven weeks of filming and six months of post-production, it was finally time to show the product. As part of a national rollout, in thanks for their support, the producers chose to premiere it to the patients and staff at the Elsinore Theatre. Much to everyone's relief, the audience loved it. Dennie Brooks recalls "the patients were hooting, laughing, and booing" at all the right times. Dr. Brooks remembered how the patients "roared. They loved, loved the movie." To Forman, it seemed that in the act of watching, the patients "felt like being liberated from themselves." Film liaison Kathleen Wilson recalls that the patients were absolutely silent following the closing credits, so enraptured were they. They communicated through a representative: "They had freed their brothers and sisters from the *stigmatism* of mental illness, and that God would reward the filmmakers and Dr. Dean Brooks for giving them a chance."[8]

One Flew Over the Cuckoo's Nest was a massive hit. It scored big in the box office and swept the Oscars, taking prizes for Best Picture, Best Director, Best Actor, Best Actress, and Best Adapted Screenplay. Like the book, it became a cultural phenomenon, profoundly influencing future asylum portrayals. In the view of many, it even influenced the law. According to Michael Douglas, thanks to the film, Florida revised its enforced commitment laws for the better. Electroconvulsive therapy, or ECT, also took a big hit. At least one study

(of one hundred Dublin factory workers) found that 66 percent of re-
spondents were "put-off" by ECT after watching the movie. The Royal
College of Psychiatrists grumbled that *Cuckoo's Nest* and similar films
"did for ECT what *Jaws* did for sharks."[9]

It is safe to say *Cuckoo's Nest* was a game changer. But it was also
something else: a link in a very long chain. As early as 1833, Robert
Fuller called his stay at the McLean Asylum for the Insane in Massachusetts incarceration in a "tyrannical Institution." Isaac Hunt's 1851
description of the Maine Insane Hospital told of a "most iniquitous,
villainous system of inhumanity, that would more than match the
bloodiest, darkest days of the Inquisition or the tragedies of the Bastille." Pioneering feminist Mary Wollstonecraft locked her protagonist up in an asylum with "dungeon-like apartments" in *Maria, or, the
Wrongs of Woman.* Here are the titles of some other early works: *The
Mysteries of Bedlam* (n.d.); *Dashington; Or, the Mysteries and Iniquities
of a Private Madhouse* (1855); *Great Disclosure of Spiritual Wickedness
in High Places: With an Appeal to the Government to Protect the Inalienable Rights of Married Women* (1865); *The Prisoners' Hidden Life, or,
Insane Asylums Unveiled* (1868); *Lunatic Asylums: Their Use and Abuse*
(1870); and *Behind the Bars* (1871). Going into the twentieth century,
one finds literally hundreds of narratives that tell us just how awful
these places are. Forman's film also owed much to movies, especially
The Snake Pit. In that film, a woman finds herself trapped in a hellish,
modern institution, replete with brutal nurses, horrifying ECT, and
prison-like walls. In sum, Forman, and Kesey, worked within an established cultural framework.[10]

This book tells the story of this tradition. While the history of real
institutions is referenced, my main focus is on the dubious watering
hole of mass entertainment, where most people gather information
about mental hospitals. Here treatments are tortures, attendants are
thugs, and psychiatrists are despots. This is not what most scholars
have in mind when they write about mental hospitals. This is the
"asylum."

My narrative flows chronologically and thematically. I set out in
chapter one discussing the paradox of total control in a climate of
rising democracy, examining select nineteenth-century writings that
illuminate worries of confinement, madness, and social disorder. In
chapter two, I track popular tales of asylum captivity and escape to

highlight gendered meanings, especially the growing sense that the home itself was becoming an asylum. In the Progressive Era, the topic of chapter three, I show how Darwinian models of hereditary horror intermingled with fears of new immigrants and science run amok to fill pop culture asylums with new monstrosities, notably Dracula. Freud enters the picture in chapter four. He would "rescue" the institutionalized via talk therapy, typified by heroic doctors who enter asylums to facilitate healing catharses. By the early Cold War years, the subject of chapter five, this "golden era" would be smothered by dark new referents, epitomized by postwar *noirs* and rising nuclear paranoias. In chapter six, I deal with the impact of the counterculture, as the asylum took on establishment overtones, and one treatment, lobotomy, looked especially insidious as a device for social control. Next, in chapter seven, I turn to influential works in the early years of Women's Liberation. Betty Friedan's *The Feminine Mystique* and Sylvia Plath's *The Bell Jar* reached back to the nineteenth-century asylum despot to facilitate bold, new methods of patriarchal escape. Chapter eight takes us through the beginnings of deinstitutionalization, when the state hospitals collapsed under the weight of a broken social contract, new drug therapies, and antipsychiatry critiques. In the wake of this process, a new figure emerged: the escaped maniac. Chapter nine covers the advent of the mechanical, murderous psychotics who erupted from failing mental institutions in films like *Halloween*. By this point, cinema asylums had become standardized. In chapter ten, I examine this, summarizing common film referents that made it easy for directors to relate nightmares of institutionalization. I close my narrative in chapter eleven by exploring the resurgence of gothic themes in the wake of deinstitutionalization. As old and abandoned hospitals rotted away, a new flock of films, TV shows, and books recreated and flattened out the history of psychiatry, rendering it into a seamless past of horrors and tortures.

Before commencing, a few caveats. This narrative covers the asylum in pop culture from the nineteenth century through today. As there are far too many primary sources to discuss meaningfully, I have had to do a good bit of winnowing. Having surveyed hundreds of films, books, and articles, not to mention taking personal tours of mental hospitals both functioning and defunct, I've endeavored to balance thoroughness with cohesion. I focus mainly on the most influential works—occasionally exploring other, lesser known pieces—that shed telling light on specific cultural currents. Some works I explore deeply, while others I reference only briefly. Though most of my subjects take place in asylums, a few reflect the power of the asylum metaphorically, such as *Star Wars* and *Moby-Dick*. I hope the reader will be tolerant of my ambition—with a wide enough lens, a fascinating, new landscape can be revealed.

I build my study on a mountain of scholarship, which I cite as I go. This includes landmark works by Gerald Grob, David Rothman, Nancy Tomes, Elaine Showalter, and Roy Porter, not to mention recent sociological efforts and disability studies. Last, the towering influence of Michel Foucault must be acknowledged. His theories of the structure of psychiatric knowledge and of the role of asylums cannot be ignored by any student of mental institutions. Though few academics agree with all of his findings, and some find his work preposterous, his key argument—that madness presents a problem of historicity and an arena for social control—is very valuable.

Since Foucault, few argue that the history of the mental hospital is a simple one of linear progress. While every social stratum has been institutionalized, treatments are often class specific and problematic, and popular narratives strongly privilege middle-class whiteness. African Americans, ethnic minorities, and Native Americans are not the heroes of the vast majority of these stories. They are pushed into the background, made into caricatures, or rendered entirely invisible. This is significant, because the "nightmare" of (white) mental incarceration in pop culture often caricatures the real nightmares of slavery, imprisonment, and surveillance that minorities are subjected to historically. To situate the asylum in American culture, then, one must always endeavor to keep in mind structures of power, as Foucault argued. That said, I agree with the current medical consensus that mental illness is a real and lived phenomenon, and that it often has a biological basis. In this study, I mainly avoid the medical debates, focusing instead on the words and concepts that informed social meaning. If one thing is certain, it is that, despite constant efforts at destigmatizing mental health, our society mistreats and misrepresents people suffering from mental illness.[11]

A final word about nomenclature. I use the word "asylum" in the cultural sense. I fully understand that this is a stigmatizing, and not a medical, term. Psychiatrists began shucking it in the late nineteenth century, as it had already acquired too many negative connotations. However, the term remains quite popular in fiction and film. This raises the question: *Why has a word that is inherently positive come to mean something so negative?* In the pages ahead, I hope to answer this.

CHAPTER 1

THE ENCHANTER'S CASTLE

> He can be but little conversant with Lunatic Asylums . . . who
> does not know, that the prejudice against such institutions is very
> great—that they are regarded by a large part of the unenlightened
> portion of the community, as prisons and dungeons, where men
> and women are confined in cells, chained and abused.
>
> —Letter to the Editors of *The American Journal
> of Insanity*, October 1845

The story goes like this: A man is strolling along a French country road with an acquaintance when it occurs to him that there
is an insane asylum nearby. His pulse quickens. "Medical friends" in
Paris have told him about the place, and he does not want to miss an
opportunity to visit. His associate is not so sure. He is in a hurry and,
besides, he has "a very usual horror at the sight of a lunatic." Nonetheless, he amiably agrees to introduce the man to the superintendent,
whom he personally knows. A by-path takes them through two miles
of "dank and gloomy wood." Then he sees "a fantastic *château*, much
dilapidated, and indeed scarcely tenantable through age and neglect.
Its aspect inspired me with absolute dread, and, checking my horse,
I half resolved to turn back. I soon, however, grew ashamed of my
weakness, and proceeded." Once introductions are made, the companion departs, leaving the man to enter alone. He will learn to his
horror that the lunatics have taken over the asylum.[1]

This is the plot of Edgar Allan Poe's short story, "The System of Dr.
Tarr and Prof. Fether." Published in *Graham's Magazine* in July 1845,
Poe's tale presents a place where all is not as it seems. The Maison
de Santé is an upside-down kingdom of craziness, lorded over by

a lunatic and his demented court. Unlike the warped characters of some of his more famous stories, here the protagonist is a simple-minded, decent fellow. He naively follows the superintendent, Monsieur Maillard, as he discourses on his "system of soothing." Maillard's system is a progressive treatment, avoiding all punishments and locking up only the "raging maniac" who "is usually removed to the public hospitals." The hallmark of his method is to indulge the fantasies of the mad. If they believe themselves to be chickens, they get chicken feed. The absurd fulfillment of delusions gently coaxes patients back to reality. "In this manner," the doctor explains, "a little corn and gravel . . . perform wonders." Then Maillard says that his method has since been replaced. After dinner, he promises to show the visitor his *new* system, "which," he touts, "in my opinion, and in that of every one who has witnessed its operation, is incomparably the most effectual as yet devised."[2]

Things get weird at dinner. The thirty or so guests, "apparently, people of rank—certainly of high breeding," are overdressed to the point of absurdity. A band plays a cacophonic sound "intended for music," and the guests behave bizarrely. Not content to merely discuss the idiosyncrasies of the patients, they act out the behaviors themselves. One tells of an inmate who believes himself to be a champagne bottle and then commences a several-minute-long impression of an uncorked bottle. Another relates a frog delusion and then croaks away with abandon. In response to the narrator's growing unease, Monsieur Maillard launches into an unnerving laughing fit.[3]

Maillard then gathers himself, quieting down a lady pretending to be a chicken. An attractive woman describes a patient who feels compelled to undress and starts to demonstrate on herself. When the others try to stop her from disrobing, a wave of terrifying howls erupts from underneath the mansion. The dinner party grows silent. Monsieur Maillard quells the narrator's jangled nerves by explaining that the patients occasionally get to screaming but then settle down. Further, he soothes, the bizarre behavior of the dinner guests is nothing to worry about. They are all perfectly sane attendants and friends.

By this point, Poe has the absurdity spread on pretty thick. We know that everyone here, including the doctor, is mad, and that the narrator is a fool. Poe raises the stakes by having Maillard note that his new technique owes something to the "learned Doctor Tarr" and "the celebrated Professor Fether." This system, he says, came into being after a disobedient patient led a revolt and had the attendants locked away. The narrator asks how long it took for the neighbors and visitors to catch on. "There you are out," replies Maillard. "The head rebel was too cunning for that. He admitted no visitors at all—with the exception, one day, of a very stupid-looking young gentleman of whom he had no reason to be afraid. He let him in to see the place— just by way of variety—to have a little fun with him. As soon as he had gammoned him sufficiently, he let him out, and sent him about his business." The oblivious narrator has no clue that Maillard is talking about himself.[4]

Shortly, the "lunatics" (the imprisoned attendants) escape their cells. They beat down the dining room door and tear apart the shutters, crashing their way through the hall. The band finally plays something in unison: "Yankee Doodle Dandy." The deranged attendants resemble "Chimpanzees, Ourang-Outangs, or big black baboons of the Cape of Good Hope." The "system" of Dr. Tarr and Professor Fether, the shocked visitor now realizes, is tarring and feathering, plus a daily dousing of water. Maillard, who had indeed once been the superintendent, went insane and became a patient, after which he led a revolt and threw the attendants in cells. Reduced to barbarity, the attendants finally succeed in their own rebellion. The narrator survives the battle to report that he has since searched "every library in Europe" to find the work of the renowned Dr. Tarr and Professor Fether. Sadly, he has come up short.[5]

Poe's dark comedy is a good place to start our exploration of the pop culture asylum. Future asylum themes are found here. The Maison de Santé is isolated and forbidding and ruled by a mad genius. It has the appearance of orderliness and medical prudence but is instead a hell where treatments are tortures and despotism reigns. Other minor notes are here too: the beautiful (white) waif, the reduction of sanity to insanity, the bizarre collection of residents, the inmate rebellion, and the differences between the aristocratic, private sanitarium versus the "warehouse" public institution. Perhaps most significantly, Poe's asylum is metaphorical.

A number of scholars have argued that "The System of Dr. Tarr and Prof. Fether" is an allegory. The Maison de Santé could be a stand-in for the chaotic young republic, or perhaps it represents white fears of slave revolt. Some believe that Poe is jeering reformers, tut-tutting the failed promises of modern institutions. Benjamin Reiss's argument, that the social breakdown of the Maison de Santé represents popular concerns about revolutionary inheritances, seems most apropos. Poe is tarring and feathering the utopian fever sweeping his young country. This asylum does not work. Perhaps neither does American democracy.[6]

Though the events in "Tarr and Fether" are set in France, Poe is telling an explicitly *American* story. France symbolized a mix of good and bad for antebellum Americans: overturned authority, intellectualism, "dangerous" ideas infecting the Blacks of Haiti, social reform, and malignant populist violence were common signifiers. Poe also likely knew that one Stanislas-Marie Maillard had stormed the Bastille and served as people's prosecutor in the bloody days of the French Revolution. Other American cues abound. Tarring and feathering was a tactic used by angry colonists; the story is set in a rural and backwoods "south;" the band plays the theme song of the American Revolution; the insane put on airs of respectability that flatten out rank and highlight their ignorance of true distinction; and the dangerous mob at the end is shown to be (literally) dark-skinned.

In Poe's prototypical pop culture asylum, misguided reforms create anarchy and spark racialized revolt. His story speaks to the concerns of a country coming to grips with a revolution and with unsettling upheavals accompanying the rise of market capitalism. "The System of Dr. Tarr and Prof. Fether," like the works discussed in the pages ahead, needs to be understood both as an exemplar of its own time and as an expression of a distinct narrative genre. Places both real and allegorical, asylums gathered about them nightmare threats to the Republic prior to the Civil War.

THE HORRORS OF DEMOCRACY

When Poe was found near death in a tavern armchair in Baltimore's gritty Fourth Ward in 1849, his city embodied the best and worst of the transformations rocking the country. On the plus side of the ledger, Baltimore was, in the words of an English visitor, "a flourishing city" of some 125,000 souls, with "very regular, clean, broad, and straight"

streets, "upwards of one hundred churches," and "several fine monu-
ments." The nation's first railroad, the Baltimore and Ohio (B&O), had
arrived in 1830, as did some early steamboat lines. The port boasted
a fine shipbuilding industry, and Baltimore Clippers were especially
popular. But the city also endured horrendous crimes, overcrowded
almshouses (filled with a "swarm of foreign beggars . . . who infest our
streets" according to civic leaders), racial unrest, and periodic epidemics. A meteor shower in the autumn of 1833 had convinced many
that the End Times were at hand.[7]

Baltimore's unplanned expedition to modernity accompanied a
disconcerting national revelation. Nobody seemed to be in charge.
How was one to know one's place when "everybody," according to
Charles Dickens in *American Notes* (1842), "is a merchant." Describing a steamboat trip from New Haven to New York, the famed British
author observed, "You wonder for a long time how she goes on, for
there seems to be nobody in charge of her; and when another of these
dull machines comes splashing by, you feel quite indignant with it, as
a sullen cumbrous, ungraceful, unshiplike leviathan: quite forgetting
that the vessel you are on board of, is its very counterpart."[8] Dickens
might have been describing the nation as a whole. The leviathan was
on the move but to where and at whose hands?

Visiting French aristocrat Alexis de Tocqueville offered a more
nuanced and less censorious judgment. Tocqueville meditated on the
ironies of liberty and the chimeras of abundance. In his epochal *Democracy in America*, he writes, freedom "circumscribes their powers
on every side, while it gives freer scope to their desires . . . [T]his constant strife between the propensities springing from the equality of
conditions and the means it supplies to satisfy them harasses and
wearies the mind." The paradox of limits in a land of unlimited promise did more than weary the mind: It birthed the American asylum. It
came down to a simple question: How can an open, market-driven,
democratic society create order amid economic and social incoher-
ence? Underneath this lurked a more worrying query: Are the two
connected? America's earliest master of horror, Charles Brockden
Brown, tapped into this concern. He worried that democracy not only
obliterated "superstition" and "prejudice," but that it had also torn
down "the props which uphold human society, [to] annihilate not
merely the chains of false religion but the foundations of morality."

The revolution, in other words, had loosed forces that might consume us before we could reap its benefits. Writing decades before Poe, Brockden Brown's novels featured religious fanaticism, incest, mesmerism, hallucinations, ventriloquism, insanity, and murder. Democracy could be a Pandora's Box.[9]

But Americans did not throw in the towel and beg for monarchy. Thoughtful reformers had a variety of novel plans to establish lasting order. The key was to build structures that nurtured our best selves. Public schools and universities, correctional facilities, and public insane asylums could be constructed so as to produce virtuous minds and robust bodies. The mercurial and brooding Poe was not impressed. The ludicrous title of his asylum story says it all. And he would dismiss reformers as *"Believers in everything Odd."*[10]

Leading medical authorities agreed that madness was a by-product of the American experiment. The esteemed Dr. Benjamin Rush cautioned back in 1788 that Americans were

> wholly unprepared for their new situation. The excess of the passion for liberty, inflamed by the successful issue of the war, produced, in many people, opinions and conduct which could not be removed by reason nor restrained by government. For a while, they threatened to render abortive the goodness of heaven to the United States, in delivering them from the evils of slavery and war. The extensive influence which these opinions had upon the understandings, passions and morals of many of the citizens of the United States, constituted a species of insanity, which I shall take the liberty of distinguishing by the name of *Anarchia.*

Avoiding *Anarchia* meant cultivating moderation and rationality. Rush promoted temperance, abolition, public education, and meritocracy. He opposed chains and basement strong rooms and argued that insanity was a treatable medical condition. But he fought a strong current. Religious explanations for madness were still very popular; God was never far off when it came to diagnosing lunacy, "touching" some people to show the rest of us His mysterious ways. Prayer and repentance were common lay prescriptions for mental health. Rush and other Enlightened public intellectuals pushed back against eschatological conventions.[11]

Lest we situate this as a story of Progress versus Backwardness, it's good to remember that Rush also believed that bleeding was sound treatment. He developed a "gyrator" that spun patients around at terrific speeds, and he approved of near-drowning, arguing in *Medical Inquiries and Observations upon the Diseases of the Mind* (1812), "Terror acts powerfully upon the body, through the medium of the mind, and should be employed to cure madness." Asylum doctors such as Charles Caldwell, Isaac Ray, and Pliny Earle followed Rush for good or ill, consciously evoking his spirit in their treatments and theories. While taking much from Europe, American alienists proved much more likely to employ Rush's "heroic" methods. This amounted to an offensive that included bleeding, emetics, purgatives, restraints, opiates, strong rooms, humiliation, and hydrotherapy. A farcical 1834 poem begins:

> Soon as the man is growing mad,
> Send for a doctor, have him bled:
> Take from his arm two quarts at least,
> Nearly as much as kills a beast.

The poem goes on to describe blistering, hot and cold cures, and calomel treatment. It ends with a call for yet more bleeding.[12]

Products of their times, asylum doctors veered between physical and "moral" etiological models. As alienist Amariah Brigham argued in *Remarks on the Influence of Mental Cultivation*, "insanity is a disease of the brain, and whatever excites this organ may so derange its action as to produce derangement of the mind. Sometimes this disease is occasioned by *blows* or *falls* upon the head, at other times by inflammation or fevers, which produce an unusual determination of blood to the brain. But far oftener this disease is occasioned by moral causes." Moral causes included gambling, drinking, religious fervor, "doubtful business speculations," and the always-devastating scourge of masturbation. For women, insanity might result from spousal abuse, "disappointments in love," and poor health, most of these being "womb-related." One asylum doctor included both "Mormonism" and "meningitis" in his summary of that year's intakes. African Americans were separately believed to have their own insanities. According to a New Orleans doctor, slaves were prone to "drapetomania," or the urge to escape. This was caused by masters who either "made themselves too familiar with them, treating them as equals" or who "treated them cruelly." When the Census of 1840 seemed to indicate higher rates of insanity among free African Americans, much medical discussion ensued regarding their fitness for freedom. While heritable factors tended to predominate by the end of the century, cultural preconceptions of race, religion, rationality, and social trauma always informed diagnoses and commitments.[13]

Regardless, psychiatry did not steer the insanity conversation in the marketplace of antebellum ideas. This was a do-it-yourself time. Phrenology, the "science" of the skull, drew many adherents eager to understand how the bumps on one's head indicated one's proclivity toward drink, sex, or whatever else seemed problematical. Poe, who prided himself on his scientific acumen, proclaimed that phrenology "has assumed the majesty of a science; and as a science, ranks among the most important which can engage the attention of thinking beings." Phrenology also hit the mark with some asylum superintendents, one of whom having commissioned a "phrenological hat" built to take skull measurements.[14]

Phrenology circulated in a nation awash with psychological ideas. Titillating court dramas in newspapers spread the concept of criminal insanity. Gothic novels and short stories told tales of derangement and homicide. Then there was "monomania," a nineteenth-century staple and catchall for a panoply of lunatic behaviors. It had been deployed as early as the writings of Benjamin Rush, and it derived from the common psychiatric diagnosis of "mania" (as opposed to "melancholia"). By the 1840s, monomania was a word in widespread circulation, typically referencing a form of derangement characterized by extreme fixation on a single object. Monomaniacs were otherwise functional people who could not resist atrocious behaviors. In a society reliant on self-control, the inability to master one's own behavior seemed especially dangerous.[15]

Poe did his part to bring mad-talk to lay readers. Terms such as "monomania," "epilepsy," "deranged," *mania a potu*," "morbid irrationality," "raving maniac," "strait jacket," "hypochondriac," "hysteria," "cataleptic disorder," and "nervous agitation" set the tone of many of his tales, buttressed by references gleaned from "medical friends" and "medical books." Isaac Ray's influential *A Treatise on the Medical*

Jurisprudence of Insanity (1838) seems to be referred to in Poe's work. In "Tarr and Fether," Poe references moral treatment, strong rooms, hydrotherapy, psychology, and even what later generations would call occupational therapy.[16]

THE ASYLUM CRAZE

Poe's tales suited an age entranced by the asylum. By the eve of the Civil War, nearly every state legislature had funded one. Affirming the reformist ethos of the day, public asylums were investments in social engineering, places where patients were sorted by gender and race, and often by wealth and ethnicity, before undergoing "moral treatment." They were to get fresh air, healthful activity, simple food, and space. A healthy body was considered not only necessary for a healthy mind, but also a prerequisite for democratic citizenship. Tonics for the nervous, laudanum for the restless, and opium and morphine for the violent were *de rigueur*. Hydrotherapies were also necessary, in the form of warm baths, cold baths, cold showers, and so on. Add to this bleeding and blistering and sometimes even hypnotism. More horrifically, a few doctors performed clitoridectomies to combat female masturbation. But patients were not merely subjects acted upon. Doctors believed that they must participate in their own cures. Historical occupational therapy included farming, sewing, making handicrafts, and doing other tasks based on gender and class position.[17]

Architecture reinforced the program. Buildings communicated the power of psychiatry, the godliness of rational order, the influence of environment, and the isolation necessary for healing. They were often laid out symmetrically, with elements of surveillance and control similar to those found in the burgeoning textile and shoe factories. As David Rothman argues, all of these places participated in the same reform impulse. The most expensive public structures, at the time, were prisons and asylums. Most Americans probably considered it money well spent.[18]

The unspoken motive behind asylum investment was the fear that unrestricted democracy provided too many opportunities for extravagance and immorality. For many middle-class reformers, social stability occasionally required a kind of enlightened despotism. Breaking the will of the institutionalized was part of the care that asylums advanced. Yet this very control triggered the sorts of fears that American soil also nurtured—fears of conspiracy, of tyranny, of lost independence. Twisted into this conversation was the vexed concept of race. Reformers unconsciously applied techniques of surveillance and control already used daily on most African Americans. From slave patrols and passes to "lantern laws" in cities, race-based laws informed the content of American control and discipline. This, in turn, influenced the entire discourse of incarceration. The rhetoric of enslavement and racial degradation shaped the process that walled off the insane "different" from the "healthy" body politic. Poe's degenerate beasts in the cellar were racialized in terms familiar to his day, words like "orangutan" and "chimpanzee" being commonly employed to denote blackness and subjection. Understanding the racial overtones of incarceration helps us grasp why total control was so troubling to a white psyche nurtured on myths of racial superiority. It explains why so many asylum narratives begin with facetious descriptions of care and healing only to later inevitably reveal the horrid enslavement beneath.[19]

Still, it would be a mistake to think that the asylum arrived and immediately went about casting a frightful shadow over the countryside. In Poe's day, asylums were very much celebrated. Dickens eagerly visited mental hospitals in Massachusetts, New York, and Connecticut. In *American Notes*, he describes the Insane Asylum at Hartford as being "admirably conducted." At the Boston Lunatic Hospital, Dickens finds the lack of fetters and restraints refreshing; patients can "walk, run, fish, paint, read, and ride out to take the air in carriages provided for the purpose." This place embodies "enlightened principles of conciliation and kindness."[20]

Dickens's sanitarium tour correlates with a trend of antebellum vacationing—the visit to the madhouse. Beginning with the early, zoo-like exhibitions of patients for a nominal fee in Benjamin Rush's day, by Dickens's visit, a large number of tourists traveled long distances to see asylums. Visitors to New York City, for instance, commonly took the ferry over to Blackwell's Island to view the insane. Any understanding of the asylum in popular culture should recognize the fact that these tourists often came away with happy memories and postcards.[21]

Asylum doctors purposely cultivated the public. They had to, being dependent upon families to send their loved ones out of the home (where the mad were typically cared for), and also counting upon the public to vote tax dollars toward costly constructions and lengthy rehabilitations. Awareness and education were key to institutional survival, hence the eagerness to let the curious in. An 1846 broadside intended to attract people to the Eastern Lunatic Asylum of Virginia tried to reconcile concerns and gently dismiss them: "Institutions for the insane were formerly little more than mere places of confinement . . . [however] the humane principles which modern science has revealed are now more fully and entirely established." Pastoral, serene settings, coupled with well-placed articles and tourist materials, were thought to showcase the reformist spirit at the heart of the asylum.[22]

But problems were still evident, even to the sympathetic. When Dickens visited Blackwell's Island (he confusingly described it as being "on Long Island or Rhode Island"), he saw a different scene than he had in Hartford.

> I saw nothing of that salutary system which had impressed me so favourably elsewhere; and everything had a lounging, listless, madhouse air, which was very painful. The moping idiot, cowering down with long dishevelled hair; the gibbering maniac, with his hideous laugh and pointed finger; the vacant eye, the fierce wild face, the gloomy picking of the hands and lips, and munching of the nails: there they were all, without disguise, in naked ugliness and horror.

Worse, this place was run by politics not charity. He asked the reader, "Will it be believed that the governor of such a house as this, is appointed, and deposed, and changed perpetually, as Parties fluctuate and vary, and as their despicable weathercocks are blown this way or that?"[23] What goes unnoticed is that the wealthier clientele of the Hartford Asylum had it better, less by dint of politics than of personal means. A class-based system was beginning to take shape. What Dickens did capture, however, and perhaps without meaning to, is that the horror asylum is related to the tragedy of mental health care. In America, asylums depended less upon state laws than upon public relations and political connections. This meant that they had to advertise, and once the failings of their promises came to light, they were viewed with suspicion. The birth of asylum horror—the daunting hallways, the Hogarthian "snake pits" of the gibbering mad, the secret torture rooms—were as much products of underfunding and continuous scrabbling for resources as they were of aristocratic machinations. The horror began in the private asylum, but the salient features came as a result of public problems.

BASTILLE BY THE BAY

Situated in a magnificent mansion fringed by sturdy three-story wings for men and women and overlooking a tributary of the Charles River, McLean Asylum for the Insane was originally the estate of a wealthy merchant. Thanks to the opening of the public mental hospital at Worcester a few years later, McLean doffed any responsibility for curing the poor and quickly became the place to be for the rich and disturbed. It was also here that the horror of the asylum in American culture made its noisy debut.[24]

In 1833, an ex-patient named Robert Fuller published a sensational account of his confinement in McLean. In *An Account of the Imprisonment and Sufferings of Robert Fuller*, he implores the reader not to be fooled:

> The McLean Asylum for the Insane possesses a large share of public favour. Its character is not known. Its location is pleasant, and its outward appearance delightful—and on that account more than from any other cause, it has acquired its present popularity... Every thing looks happy... But let him go with me within its walls: let him hear the groans of the distressed: let him see its inmates shut up with bars and bolts: let him see how deserted they are: how they are neglected and cruelly treated; how unfit so lonely an abode is for the disconsolate and melancholy—and his views of that Institution will change.

Fuller had been committed for reasons connected with the socioeconomic transformations twisting America. He had made bad investments, had fought with local elites, had argued religion. One day, a group of neighbors stopped by and told him to meet with a local physician. Fuller became excited and demanded that they leave, and he was forced onto a couch in a state of "great agitation." He finally permitted them to bring Dr. Walker, who escorted him to McLean (located conveniently two miles from his house). Here the nightmare begins.[25]

Taken to a place "where I could see the light of heaven only through iron grates," Fuller is ordered to take two pills, which he only pretends to swallow. Later that night, four men arrive. He flings a table at them, but they overpower him and carry him "through a long dark entry into a dark room or inner prison, where they lay me on a bed and literally robbed me." Whereas he had recently been "enjoying the blessings of freedom," now he was "confined within the walls of a dark gloomy prison." The asylum begins its evil work, making his "imagination [become] disordered." He tries to escape several times but is always caught. He finally grasps the dark logic of the place: "I understood that some persons had been kept in the Hospital from 3 to 14 years, and was told I must be easy in order to ever regain my liberty." Fuller learned to behave as expected, ultimately convincing his jailors that he was sane. He finally received his "emancipation" after two and a half months. Then came the insult added to the injury: the bill. At $199.45, "Was there ever such an instance of gross extortion?"[26]

Like many a muckraker since, Fuller set pen to paper to expose evil. The contradiction of a "secret institution" in a land of liberty is too much to countenance. Yes, insanity is indeed on the rise, he concedes. But this is not the answer. In the first place, it is far too easy to commit someone ("Witches were never convicted with less testimony than the insane now are"). Once inside the asylum, healing does not happen, despite all the advertising and the carefully manicured surroundings. "Instead of happiness, it gives distress: instead of health, sickness: instead of life, death: and instead of being an instrument of benevolence, it is made an instrument of extortion." This is a place of torture "worse than Spanish Inquisition." The question we must ask ourselves is "whether we shall live as freemen, or whether we shall pass through life in bondage through fear of being seized and shut up in insane hospitals . . . The liberty which we have enjoyed, and which the half-finished monument on Bunker Hill was intended to commemorate, has vanished."[27]

Importantly, Fuller does not deny that McLean should exist. What needs to happen is a concerted effort to "reform and purify this

Asylum—and make it no longer the abode of the persecuted, doomed to neglect and privation, but what its name imports, a place of safety and happiness for that unfortunate class of human beings, deprived of their reason." Unfortunately, the exposé did not lead to reform, though it did help establish certain pop culture asylum motifs: illegitimate incarceration, secret tortures, undemocratic power, and cruel attendants. The structure's description, an essentially gothic one, would resonate with a literate public, cuing well-worn references to decrepit and decadent Europe.[28]

On the heels of Fuller's exposé came other McLean tell-alls, including John Derby's odd *Scenes in a Mad-House* (1838) and Elizabeth Stone's *A Sketch of the Life of Elizabeth T. Stone, and of her Persecutions, with an Appendix of her Treatment and Sufferings While in the Charlestown McLean Assylum* [sic] *Where She was Confined under the Pretense of Insanity* (1842). In Stone's case, wrongful confinement stems from her family's misunderstanding of her religious conversion. She is duped by her brother into taking a carriage ride to a "young ladies' boarding place." After meeting with a physician (who clearly does not understand the meaning of her spiritual conversion), she begs to leave, but her brother compels her to remain. Next thing she knows, "a tall, black eyed, masculine looking female came and took me by the arm." Stone is led to a gallery filled with women when an "iron grate" meets her eyes. She cannot leave.[29]

As with "Tarr and Fether," the sense that something is wrong does not arrive suddenly but rather creeps up insidiously. When the bell rings to call the ladies to tea, Elizabeth notes, "The company presented a strange appearance . . . many things did not look right." She falsely concludes that this is a house of refuge for prostitutes. The next day, she is given medicine that sends her into painful convulsions. Finally, she asks someone where she is. "She then told me that I was in the Insane Assylum [sic]." The drugs and torture continue. She asks the reader, "Can you imagine what my sufferings were? No you cannot." She is kept drugged, her brain slowly becoming "a mineral substance." She's moved out to a cottage ("it might more properly be called a stone dungeon"), the humiliations escalating to the point where Stone envies the slave: "Oh, they do not know their happiness." Her trial finally ends upon her release some five months later.[30]

Stone's narrative, like Fuller's, ends in a reformist plea. The gist comes down to republican warnings: "If it was thought best to have

all the power put into the hands of one individual, then we should
have a King in this country, but it was not thought best." Democracy
could certainly bring justice to the asylum, Stone reasoned. It was just
a matter of introducing the light of public awareness to the dark corridors and dungeons. This was logical, even inevitable, once the people
became aware of the situation.[31]

Like Fuller, Stone does not question the need for the asylum.
These were places, after all, where reform was made manifest, evidence of the body politic taming the troubles of an unsettled country. Exposés would continue nibbling away at the edges but never
resolve the paradox at the core: freedom restored by way of total control. Phebe B. Davis understood this, explaining in her 1855 narrative
about her stay at Utica, "The great trouble in Lunatic Asylums is, they
want to cure them by rule . . . and their rules are enough to make a
rational person crazy."[32] Perhaps only Poe resolved the paradox, over-
turning Maillard's lunatic government in a revolution at once justified
and horrific.

GOTHIC MASTERS

The superintendent inhabited a precarious perch. He needed cus-
tomers, good press, and tax dollars to survive. His job required all the
demands of business manager, physician, and masterly patriarch. But
this was not the character that Americans encountered in memoirs,
novels, stories, and newspaper exposés. Rather, they learned about
autocratic lords of questionable domains. This perspective drew not
from medical journals and the minutes of professional organizations
but from a genre suitable for mystery, mastery, and madness: the
gothic.[33]

Gothic stories provided a formula of darkness: sinister, decay-
ing structures; past secrets come to wreak havoc on the present; a
woman in peril trapped in a castle that gets worse the deeper you get;
minute, floorplan-style details about said structure; dissolute, aristocratic family lines; disturbing behaviors that might include murder,
incest, rape, even cannibalism; and a villainous mastermind oversee-
ing it all. Gothicism might seem to be more apropos to Europe than
to the New World, and indeed there it began, but it was a style easily
transposed. *Uncle Tom's Cabin*, for instance, is a gothic tale centered

on, in the words of Edmund Wilson, "the nightmare plantation of Simon Legree." James Fenimore Cooper's *The Last of the Mohicans* has gloomy woods, strange sounds, labyrinthine caves, and layers of insecurity and fear. Nathaniel Hawthorne's "Young Goodman Brown" reveals a conclave of devil-worshippers hidden in the New England forest. Leslie Fiedler famously places the gothic at the heart of American literature, it being fueled by "certain special guilts" such as "the slaughter of the Indians" and "the abominations of the slave trade."[34]

The gothic style flourished in Jacksonian America. This was an unsettled society, shot through with fears of riots and slave revolts, worried by urban disorders and political intrigue, and haunted with the conspiratorial fear of evil aristocrats. Gothic tropes helped Americans accommodate changes that did not easily fit within the framework of a Protestant-republican morality. Popular "city mystery" novels, for instance, banked on fears of begrimed alleys, swarthy races, houses of sin, and crimes too abhorrent to mention but too titillating to ignore. These horrors drew from the promises and perils of American freedoms. The pursuit of happiness did not come with a rulebook.[35]

Buildings rooted the gothic to the world of letters. Isaac Mitchell's 1804 *The Asylum, or Alonzo and Melissa* (which is not about a madhouse) includes a castle in Connecticut inhabited by bloody specters and secret places. Poe's "The Fall of the House of Usher" (1839) gives us a mansion with "bleak walls" and "vacant eye-like windows," surrounded by "a few white trunks of decayed trees." Prospero's abbey in Poe's "The Masque of the Red Death" (1842) is a frightening construction, with suites containing "sharp" turns at intervals of "twenty or thirty yards," replete with "delirious fancies such as the madman fashions." Factories could be gothic too. In "The Paradise of Bachelors and the Tartarus of the Maids" (1855), Herman Melville presents a paper mill as a forbidding "high-gabled . . . edifice" that converts women into zombies. Inside, one could witness "rows of blank-looking counters" with "rows of blank-looking girls, with blank, white folders in the blank hands, all blankly folding blank paper." The machines that symbolized progress are here not as our servants but as our masters, whom the employees serve "mutely and cringingly as the slave serves the Sultan."[36]

The asylum was the ultimate gothic locale. In a country without castles, these massive, stone and brick structures sequestered citizens and placed them under the control of a single master. The New York State Lunatic Asylum at Utica (completed in 1843), for instance, presented a massive 550-foot-long Greek Revival structure, one of the biggest and most expensive in the country. Despite tours, postcards, an inmate publication, and behavioral codes, Utica could not shake its gothic-ness. It would become famous mainly for the Utica Crib, an adult-sized restraint cage reminiscent of a coffin. Lamented a resident physician in 1881, the Utica Asylum resembled "the castle of an enchanter, whose dread power can only be dissipated by tearing down its walls." For the public, the enchanter—the superintendent—derived his power from the building itself.[37]

The superintendent was a tailor-made gothic villain. In a society that treasured face-to-face exchanges but was increasingly buffeted by unseen economic forces, these powerful and mysterious figures could introduce evil into the paradise of democracy. They might be supernaturally hypnotic, superior geniuses, or merely ruthless blackguards. Elizabeth Stone likened Dr. Bell of McLean to Torquemada. Isaac H. Hunt, in his shocker *Astounding Disclosures! Three Years in a Mad-House* (1852), described the Maine Mental Hospital's Dr. Isaac Ray in no uncertain terms: "Not even the Spanish Inquisition ever produced the superior of Dr. Ray as a horrid, barbarous, cruel and vindictive Inquisitor!" Hiram Chase's exposé of Utica compared the powers of his superintendent to the "Sultan's of Turkey." The term "Bastille" comes up a lot in these narratives.[38]

Limited by certain realities, asylum memoirs emphasized how the superintendent was foreign and monarchical in *behavior*. In fiction, however, authors were not so constrained. Brockden Brown's villains were often elitist European immigrants, possessed of dark powers and malicious intent. Popular "convent escape" stories, like *The Awful Disclosures of Maria Monk* (1836), presented French-speaking nuns and monks who degraded innocent women in hidden, labyrinthine spaces under forbidding stone structures. Hawthorne's Giacomo Rappaccini ("Rappaccini's Daughter") is a demented Italian scientist who makes his beguiling daughter into a poisonous creature. The gothic villain was the ultimate "moral monster," a creature (in the words of Karen Halttunen) fundamentally "deviant." Unlike the rest of us, the moral monster had no ethical center.[39]

George Lippard introduced a vicious and alien superintendent in his blockbuster novel *The Quaker City, or The Monks of Monk Hall:*

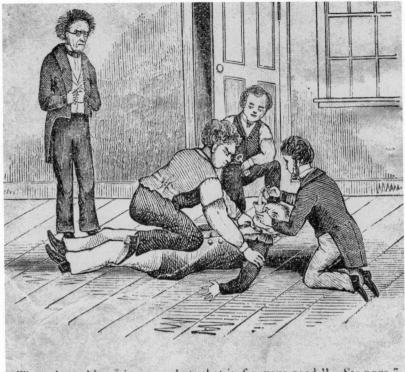

" There is nothing given you but what is for your good." *See page* 7.

Asylum treatment in Isaac H. Hunt, *Astounding Disclosures! Three Years in a Mad-House*
(1852)

A Romance of Philadelphia Life, Mystery, and Crime. Lippard's masterpiece of mayhem provides a definitive early popular example of
the evil gothic superintendent. Published the same year as Poe's
"Tarr and Fether," *The Quaker City* sold some sixty thousand copies
in twelve months.[40] Like Harriet Beecher Stowe—whose *Uncle Tom's
Cabin* would prove an even bigger hit—Lippard sought to awaken
Americans to the evils infesting the land. Also like Stowe, he used
gothic settings to shock and upset readers into agitation for change.
But Lippard was much more extreme. He included every variant of
deviancy: dissolute clergymen, grasping merchants, old world aristocrats, selfish bank presidents, philanderers, pimps, madams, and
cruel henchmen. Unlike Stowe's high-minded cries to evangelical
purity, Lippard seemed much more eager to plumb the depths and

even to revel in the muck. In his America, nothing is what it seems. It is much, much worse.

Lippard's story was ripped from the headlines. In 1843, a Philadelphian named Singleton Mercer shot and killed Mahlon Hutchinson Heberton, a man who had seduced his sister by luring her into a brothel, duplicitously promising her marriage. Both men were respectable upper-class citizens, and their story shocked the reading public. Lippard's novel contains a version of this: a man brags to his friend about how he will seduce a woman, and the woman ends up being the sister of the other man. The seducer is eventually murdered by the angry brother. But this is only the barest skeleton of Lippard's tale. What happens over the course of some five hundred pages is a carnival of evil and hypocrisy.[41]

The main villain of *The Quaker City* is Devil-Bug, a ferocious, demented pimp. His face is "one loathsome grimace," with a single eye, matted hair, a "flat nose and pointed chin," and "long rows of bristling teeth." Even his soul is "hideous." He presides over Monk Hall, a den of vice, gambling, and prostitution, "originally erected by a wealthy foreigner, sometime previous to the Revolution." Devil-Bug has no compunctions about killing and is subject to hallucinations from his murderous past that only reinforce his "deviance." His evil is explained in environmental terms. He was born in a brothel, "No mother had ever spoken words of kindness to him; no father had ever held him in his arms." He never knew love, nor even received a Christian name. He is an elemental result of the evils of urban life.[42]

The other villain featured in the story is something else entirely. Ravoni is an aristocratic immigrant equipped with wondrous, frightening powers.

> He arrived in the city almost a year ago, coming from god knows whence, and going the devil knows where. Well, this Italian or Frenchman, or Turk or Jew, no sooner puts his foot on the soil of the Quaker City, than he astonishes the Faculty; strikes science dumb; plucks Theology by the beard, and in fact walks over everybody's notions on everything.

Ravoni is a "Mad-Doctor" who rules a "Mad-House." Unlike Monk Hall, Ravoni's sanitarium appears respectable on the outside, a place where wealthy parents can send their troubled daughters. Ravoni has no need to lure victims into his mansion. Like Maillard, Ravoni's medical status makes him alluring to gullible people. His "reputation for skill in all cases of Insanity, was without a parallel."[43]

Ravoni looks and acts the part of the classic gothic villain. He has a "sallow face," wears "dark robes," and possesses a "deep sepulchral voice." He is a "Sorcerer" who can apparently raise the dead and has conquered death himself, being centuries old by his own account. His lair evokes enigmatic Eastern lands. It has marble floors, columns, incense, fountains, and strange flowers from Africa and Persia. Ravoni garbs himself in a "lustrous coat of dark satin" that is "adorned with rich embroidery of golden lace" with diamonds where buttons should be. His "red-heeled shoes," we are told, were "worn by the French nobility previous to the Revolution." His face, with its "wide, massive" brow, phrenologically connotes unnatural intelligence. He is the ultimate anti-democrat.[44]

When Devil-Bug confronts Ravoni, he is no match. He cowers like a "spaniel," obeying his new "master." Lippard editorializes, this is "The triumph of an Intellect, over the Brute and the Savage!" Yet Devil-Bug's base nature briefly overcomes his subservience, and he plunges a knife into the Sorcerer's back. Playing the gothic villain to the hilt, Ravoni takes several pages to die, offering up a variety of suitably evil prophecies, including directions for his own cremation and predictions of his imminent resurrection.[45]

Like any good reformer, Lippard wants to uplift, and his editorial asides sometimes overcome both his narrative and good sense. Never mind the prurient descriptions of rape, murder, incest, theft, lying, and flights of half-clad women through darkened streets. Lippard wants us to realize his higher ambitions. This is a warning. There are real Monk Halls. The rich do control and degrade the poor. Prostitution is a problem. And Ravoni is real.

Let me point your vision, to the grim cells of that Legal Mad-House, where a reckless Charlaton [sic] administers his brutal rule . . . When you have taken in the full details of the picture, when you have impressed on your mind the fact, that this Quack and his Mad-House are both the creatures of your Statute-Books, that sane men have been dragged into their clutches, by designing relatives, and kept chained and lashed, until insanity came to their relief, followed by sudden death; then quarrel with the Madhouse of the Sorcerer![46]

Importantly, Ravoni, like Monsieur Maillard, rules a *private* madhouse. Although the massive public asylums generated their share of concern, in the world of fiction the private asylum beat the public institutions to the punch. The key is that gothic horror associated evil with aristocracy and mystery, and the private madhouse knitted these fears together in the unsettling vision of the stately house with barred windows.[47] George Thompson describes one of these places in *Dashington, Or the Mysteries of a Private Mad House* (ca. 1855):

> [Locals] invested it with a character of mystery and terror. The midnight traveler quickened as he passed it; and little children were frightened by foolish mothers into good behavior, when threatened with being given over to the tender mercies of "Monk, the Mad Doctor." Occasionally, persons would be tempted by curiosity to approach the house, and then they beheld pale, melancholy and anxious faces peering out through the barred windows. Sometimes they heard the most heart-rending wails of anguish, and shrieks that made their blood run cold.

Thompson's potboiler offers up all of the major notes to a public attuned to gothic fears of subversion, aristocracy, and enslavement. The book starts by following the evil exploits of a rogue going by the name of Captain Dashington. He is first seen disheveled, bearded, matted, and wearing a "worn out and very unclean" suit. He fools a local public house owner into thinking he's a captain, and then conducts a catalogue of infamies including the murder of a visiting minister and the assumption of the unfortunate man's identity. Cleaned up and well attired, Dashington is betrayed by his "dark eyes, which were strongly indicative of a bad heart." He worms his way into the embrace of the local minister's family, fooling them into believing he is the murdered clergyman. As the story unfolds, Dashington's past catches up with him, and he finds he cannot continue the charade without murdering a visiting Bishop who could reveal his true identity. When the homeowner's somnambulist daughter Almira stumbles in just after the slaying, Dashington and his partner-in-crime place the murder weapon in her hand. Startled awake by the family, Almira believes that she has committed murder and promptly loses her mind.[48]

Almira is taken to a private madhouse by the family physician. Here lives Dr. Monk who convinces the family that their daughter will be well cared for. Once left to Monk and his sinful family (his wife affects to read a Bible while company is over, but then quickly resorts back to her "loose French novel"), Almira is promptly locked away in a dungeon-like room, her hair shorn for added humiliation.[49]

Dr. Monk's madhouse is a "den of horrors" masquerading as a place of healing. When Almira's father hesitates to send his daughter "to a *Lunatic Asylum*," he is corrected by the family physician who tells him that this is not a "common Insane Hospital" but rather a place for the "gentle and harmless." The "raving, dangerous maniacs and madmen [Monk] will have nothing to do with." Presumably, these people go to public hospitals.[50]

Dr. Monk is a stereotypical gothic villain, albeit not a foreigner (though the name Monk evokes the "foreign" religion of Roman Catholicism). He and his clan are, as the book's chapter XV announces, "A Family of Hypocrites." He presents an air of intelligence and respectability and fools families into sending their children to his asylum, where he tortures and dehumanizes them. In high melodramatic style, Monk soliloquizes, "How little do people suspect that within these walls are daily and nightly enacted scenes that would cause the blood of weak-hearted fools to run cold with horror!" Some of his patients are here by dint of self-interested family members. One, a massive figure kept chained up in the basement, was once the respectable Dr. Maxwell, but his adulterous wife paid Monk to shut him away. Dr. Monk's professional jealousy (deriving from a "quarrel about some matters connected with the medical profession") causes him to treat Maxwell with "ten times more cruelty" than the other patients, which is saying something. This treatment has made Maxwell insane. At the book's end, while he is being tortured with a hot iron by Monk's cruel son, Maxwell breaks free and tortures and then murders the boy. Roaming through the house, axe in one hand and lantern in the other, Maxwell finds and butchers the remaining Monks. He then releases Almira, sets the place aflame, and dances on the roof until it caves in, killing him and all the remaining patients. The tale ends with the other villains meeting appropriately bad ends and the girl marrying her beau. He goes on to build a "humane" asylum where people are actually healed.[51]

Dashington rehearses the key elements of gothic horror. The asylum's description as "a den of horror, cruelty and oppression" captures republican fears of abuse and enslavement. Inside, the sane are "converted" to insanity via torture, a beautiful woman is locked away and degraded. The superintendent is malevolent, intelligent, duplicitous, and aristocratic. The inmates break free and wreak havoc. As with other asylum stories, there are variations on themes. In this instance the burly, abusive attendant is really a kind soul who helps patients (appealing to the target working-class audience), the superintendent is not himself insane or supernatural, and the asylum, though destroyed, is later reformed under a healthful guise.[52]

SEA ASYLUMS

Antebellum asylums served as metaphors for larger social concerns, typically having to do with reform and power, often with racialized, gendered, and class tonalities. They emerged in the context of democratic turbulence and dug deeply into the paradox of electorally approved total control. The river that nurtured them was fed by many tributaries. One was the sea tale. This genre tapped the same anxieties, shedding light on the substructure of the pop culture asylum.

Ships at sea were total institutions: isolated, autocratic places ruled by fiat. They were designed for productive purposes, even to the point of "reforming" rough crews by instilling self-control and cooperation. Works by Charles Frederick Briggs, Richard Henry Dana, and Herman Melville served up high adventure, social allegory, reformist pleadings, and philosophical speculation. Dana's popular *Two Years before the Mast* describes a place captained by a "lord paramount" who "is accountable to no one, and must be obeyed in everything, without a question." His ship is more stifling than a penitentiary. "In no state prison are the convicts more regularly set to work, and more closely watched." After one brutal flogging, the captain rants to the crew, "You see your condition! You see where I've got you all, and you know what to expect! . . . I'll make you toe the mark, every soul of you, or I'll flog you all, fore and aft, from the boy, up!"—"You've got a driver over you! Yes, a slave-driver,—a nigger driver!" Ultimately, Dana does not stand in judgment of the system, explaining that as "a parent may correct moderately his child, and the master his apprentice . . . the captain may inflict moderate corporal chastisement, for a reasonable cause." Like the asylum exposés, Dana's book questions not the institutional idea but rather particular abuses within it. Dana's "superintendent" is merely a bully. It would be up to another writer to provide a gothic captain worthy of a Ravoni or a Monk.[53]

In 1851, Herman Melville gave us *Moby-Dick*. Considered a failure at the time, it grew in stature to make prophetic a contemporary who called it the "Whaliad." Like other sea narratives, this tale is open to multiple allegorical readings. The gothic asylum is one. Lest one finds this a stretch, I quote the main character of Melville's sea novel *White-Jacket*: "The navy is the asylum for the perverse, the home of the unfortunate." (Conversely, the national organization of asylum superintendents compared the running of an asylum to that of a military vessel at an annual meeting in the 1860s). The *Pequod* is gothic, no doubt about it:

> A cannibal of a craft, tricking herself forth in the chased bones of her enemies. All round, her unpanelled, open bulwarks were garnished like one continuous jaw, with the long sharp teeth of the sperm whale, inserted there for pins, to fasten her old hempen thews and tendons to . . . Scorning a turnstile wheel at her reverend helm, she sported there a tiller; and that tiller was in one mass, curiously carved from the long narrow lower jaw of her hereditary foe. The helmsman who steered by that tiller in a tempest, felt like the Tartar, when he holds back his fiery steed by clutching its jaw. A noble craft, but somehow a most melancholy!

On deck is a crew in need of improvement, all working on an infernal processing facility (described, as her try-works melt the blubber through the night, as "freighted with savages, and laden with fire, and burning a corpse, and plunging into that blackness of darkness"), under the control of an autocrat.[54]

In *Moby-Dick*, an insane captain converts an otherwise sane crew into fellow lunatics. In a shocking inversion of the purpose of their mission, they sail not to mine the seas for sperm whales but rather to kill a single animal at the risk of their own lives. At one point, first mate Starbuck tells Captain Ahab that the oil casks are leaking, and that they must be hoisted and examined. Ahab explodes: "Let it leak! I'm all aleak myself." When Starbuck mentions the financial interests of the owners, Ahab replies, "What cares Ahab? Owners, owners?" The situation escalates until the captain seizes a loaded musket and points it at Starbuck, roaring, "There is one God that is Lord over the earth, and one Captain that is lord over the Pequod.—On deck!" Though Ahab does indeed search for the leak, it is clear that his interest is not financial, but monomaniacal, in origin. Like Monsieur Maillard, Ahab is God-like and demented, the mad ruler of a ship of fools destined for the depths.[55]

Melville's book makes plentiful references to the discourse of madness. Ahab is physically disfigured by both an enormous vertical scar on his face and by a leg made of whalebone. His madness springs from this disfigurement. Chasing the white whale on a previous voyage, Ahab's limb had been sheared off "as a mower a blade of grass in the field." Though insanity did not immediately set in, it gestated on the trip home. While isolated and straitjacketed, Ahab gained the superhuman power to dominate others. Writes Melville,

> . . . his torn body and gashed soul bled into one another; and so interfusing, made him mad. That it was only then . . . that the final monomania seized him, seems all but certain from the fact that, at intervals during the passage, he was a raving lunatic; and, though unlimbed of a leg, yet such vital strength yet lurked in his Egyptian chest, and was moreover intensified by his delirium, that his mates were forced to lace him fast, even there, as he sailed, raving in his hammock. In a strait-jacket, he swung to the mad rockings of the gales. And, when running into more sufferable latitudes, the ship, with mild stun'sails spread, floated across the tranquil tropics, and, to all appearances, the old man's delirium seemed left behind him with the Cape Horn swells, and he came forth from his dark den into the blessed light and air . . . even then, Ahab, in his hidden self, raved on. Human madness is oftentimes a cunning and most feline thing.

Ahab's madness is of a peculiar nineteenth-century sort, a "special lunacy" that transformed his intellect from "living agent" to "living instrument." His madness makes him powerful. "[F]ar from having lost his strength, Ahab, to that one end, did now possess a thousand fold more potency than ever he had sanely brought to bear upon any one reasonable object." Laments Starbuck, "My soul is more than matched; she's overmanned; and by a madman! Insufferable sting, that sanity should ground arms on such a field! But he drilled deep down, and blasted all my reason out of me! I think I see his impious end; but feel that I must help him to it."[56]

Beyond the plot and characters, the book itself seems a monomaniacal exercise. (One critic called the book "maniacal—mad as a March hare—mowing, gibbering, screaming, like an incurable Bedlamite.") Ahab's fixation on the whale is mirrored by the author's own. *Moby-Dick* opens with page after page of quotes about whales. There are also entire individual chapters dedicated to ruminations on the color, head, tail, skeleton, spout, fat, ambergris, and oil of the whale, not to mention a chapter outlining a brand-new scheme of whale classification.[57]

Ahab is the greatest monomaniac in all of the American letters, a suitable model for monstrous asylum superintendents to come. His authoritative, lunatic voice distills the gothic fear of a secret, malevolent agency at work undermining a fragile social order. Like the asylum master, Ahab is a tyrant in the service of his own agenda. His special authority is reinforced by his racialized "attendants," a group of Asiatics that emerges from the hold to man his personal boat. Among them is Fedallah, an exotic, turbaned, "muffled mystery," who might even have "authority" over Ahab himself.[58]

Like many a fictional superintendent, Ahab's dismasted sanity bestows upon him an uncanny vision. In his most famous rant, he lets slip the disastrous knowledge that even masters are but inmates of a larger, cosmic institution. "All visible objects," he exclaims, are "but as pasteboard masks. But in each event . . . some unknown but still reasoning thing puts forth the mouldings of its features from behind the unreasoning mask. If man will strike, strike through the mask! How can the prisoner reach outside except by thrusting through the wall?" Ahab's tragedy is that he is a master and slave both, ruling one total institution only to be locked inside another. This mimics the self-flagellating exhortations of reformers to police ourselves in order to become perfect democratic citizens. Ahab's dark fear of a captain-less

universe similarly exercises the unconscious worry of antebellum
zealots in their quests for mastery. The critique culminates in Ahab's
drinking of his institution's power too deeply, inverting its stated goal
of *production* and creating instead a conflagratory *consumption* of all
aboard. Well, nearly all. Like Poe's narrator in "Tarr and Fether," Ish-
mael lives on to tell the tale, a babe in the teeth of a machine he does
not comprehend.[59]

The *Pequod* ships the same cultural cargo as the fictional, antebellum asylum. It is a total institution, run by a crazed master and his attendants, carrying its inmates toward a purpose that undermines the
agenda of those who finance it. Ahab's gothic asylum-ship correlates
with popular fears of the insane hospital as an ironic nightmare, a
funhouse mirror of the open, yet untamable, world bequeathed by
the American Revolution.

CHAPTER 2

WOMAN IN WHITE, ANGEL IN BLACK

"Hark!" said Ruth, with a quick, terrified look, "what's that?"

"Oh, nothing," replied the matron, "only a crazy woman in that room yonder, screaming for her child. Her husband ran away from her and carried off her child with him, to spite her, and now she fancies every footstep she hears is his. Visitors always thinks she screams awful. She can't harm you, ma'am," said the matron, mistaking the cause of Ruth's shudder, "for she is chained. She went to law about the child, and the law, you see, as it generally is, was on the man's side; and it just upset her. She's a sight of trouble to manage. If she was to catch sight of your little girl out there in the garden, she'd spring at her through them bars like a panther; but we don't have to whip her *very* often."

—Fanny Fern, *Ruth Hall* (1854)

America loves a story about capture and escape, especially, but not always, when it involves white women. Beginning with Mary Rowlandson's best-selling tale of suffering and release from the Wampanoag Indians in the late 1600s, the captivity narrative has held our attention. Asylums provided a tantalizing setting. They were isolated, enclosed, and ruled by tyrants. From Elizabeth Stone's 1841 tale of persecution at the McLean Asylum through Clarissa Lathrop's account of the "secret institution" in 1890, asylums proved enduring locales for confinement and arenas for moral redemption. The most influential of these narratives, Elizabeth Packard's chronicle of her stay at the Jacksonville State Hospital for the Insane, inspired changes in state laws in favor of women's rights.

As capitalist relations allocated the middle-class man into the "sphere" of work, homes became centers of consumption, schools of virtue, and "havens" from the bustle of salaried life. Yet they also could be stifling prisons ruled by cruel patriarchs. As superintendents pushed the idea that asylums mimicked the home, the links between the two grew insidious. Americans well knew that looks could be deceiving.[1]

Two images guide this chapter. The first is the Woman in White, captured strikingly in Wilkie Collins's 1860 novel of the same name. This ghostly figure is a solitary waif who is lured into an asylum for nefarious reasons and serves to relate dark messages of domestic peril. Her garments summon both the grave and the virginal marriage bed, drawing upon conflicted cultural ideals of "the angel in the house." Sandra M. Gilbert and Susan Gubar wrote, "It is surely significant that doomed, magical, half-mad, or despairing women ranging from Hawthorne's snow-image to Tennyson's Lady of Shalott, Dickens's Miss Havisham, and Collins's Anne Catherick all wear white." The second image is the Angel in Black. She is the crusader for Christ, the religiously inspired reformer who understands America's millennial mission. Dressed in serious black and personified by reformer Dorothea Dix, the Angel in Black manifests the woman's role as caretaker and moral guardian. Both images are archetypes, two sides of a rubric of femininity that simultaneously empowered and smothered the nineteenth-century female.[2]

To contextualize these images, it is necessary to briefly summarize what historians call the "cult of true womanhood." This ideological vision exalted the home and praised feminine submissiveness and piety. Women were to be lovely and pure, covered in layers of clothes that shielded them from sex while simultaneously exaggerated their womanly curves. They were instructed to purchase the right goods and to raise their children to value hard work. The cult of true womanhood instilled women with moral power, emphasizing their role as nurturers and builders of democracy-loving, future citizens. Yet it also kept them, according to Barbara Welter, "hostage" to the home. This is important. To escape from the asylum was, in a sense, to attempt an exit from a woman's place.[3]

THE WOMAN IN WHITE

It is night on a country road. The moon is full, illuminating a "dark blue starless sky." A man makes his way, walking stick in hand, blissfully imagining his new job as a tutor for a wealthy family. He is alone. Suddenly, a hand touches his shoulder. He grips his stick and whirls about. Before him stands "the figure of a solitary Woman, dressed from head to toe in white garments." Yet this "extraordinary apparition" is corporeal. She explains that she has been in an accident and needs to get to London. The man construes that she has been mistreated, and she concedes that she's been "cruelly used and cruelly wronged." After a short walk, the man puts the woman into a carriage and sends her off. Ten minutes later, two men in a carriage fly along the road, stopping in front of a police officer nearby. The man overhears them asking the officer if he has seen a woman dressed in white. The policeman says no, asking if there was something she has done. "Done!" replies one, "She has escaped from my Asylum. Don't forget; a woman in white. Drive on."[4]

This scene is from *The Woman in White* by Wilkie Collins. Though composed by an Englishman, the novel was a huge hit in the States, selling some 126,000 copies following its serialization in *Harper's Weekly*.[5] Briefly told, the novel is about an art teacher named Walter Hartright who falls in love with his student, Laura Farlie, but is forced away because she is betrothed to another. Her fiancé, Sir Percival Glyde, is a greedy, dissolute aristocrat who aims for Laura's money with the aid of the mysterious Count Fosco. The woman dressed in white is Anne Catherick. She is Laura's illegitimate half-sister, sent off to an asylum to keep her silent about a "secret" she knows in regards to Glyde. She will later serve as a corpse body-double (when she dies of heart failure, Percival and Fosco switch her identity with Laura, placing the false "Anne Catherick" in an asylum and the real one in the grave). After all secrets are revealed, Walter is able to set things right. Percival is exposed as false gentry and dies horribly by fire; Fosco meets an untimely demise; and Walter and Laura live happily ever after.

What stays with the reader is the haunting image of a solitary waif escaped from an asylum, here to let dangerous truths out. This imagery had good company. In Sir Walter Scott's *The Bride of Lammermoor*

(1819), Lucy Ashton is prevented from marrying her true love and goes insane, stabbing her imposed groom on her wedding night. She is found raving in her "night-clothes." In Edgar Allan Poe's "The Fall of the House of Usher," Madeline Usher, who suffers from a "partially cataleptical" ailment, emerges from her premature burial "lofty and enshrouded" in bloodstained "white robes." The reality of her horror literally brings down the house. Harriet Beecher Stowe's *Uncle Tom's Cabin* includes an escape scene of two female slaves from an attic hiding place via a white sheet and a believable ghost story. Miss Havisham (from Dickens's *Great Expectations*, published in *Harper's Weekly* starting in November 1860) dons a decomposing, white wedding dress daily. Then there was the ever-popular Ophelia, who graced countless nineteenth-century productions of *Hamlet*. She is quite mad, typically dressed in white, with her hair down and mussed. Some stagings included putting straw in her hair, evoking popular imagery of lunatics sleeping on dungeon floors. In *The Woman in White*, Anne Catherick wears a white frock that, while not an undergarment, is outlandish in its way—it is akin to a child's dress.[6]

Anne Catherick's torment involved what was commonly known as *railroading*, a process by which a person is tricked or unjustly forced into the asylum. While in reality, nineteenth-century asylums were mainly filled with people committed by their families or by themselves voluntarily, popular narratives typically featured duplicity and malignant motives. In *Ruth Hall* (1854), for instance, the protagonist's friend Mary Leon is sent off to an asylum "for her health" by a wealthy, uncaring husband who has no further need of her. She deteriorates and dies under the watch of a cruel matron. In the British novel *Hard Cash*, which found a wide American audience, young Alfred Hardie is committed by his father for fear of his son making public his embezzlements (the "hard cash" of the title).[7]

Louisa May Alcott offers a classic railroading event in "A Whisper in the Dark," a short story published pseudonymously in *Frank Leslie's Illustrated Newspaper* in 1863. It concerns an orphan named Sybil who learns that her uncle intends to marry her off to her cousin in an effort to inherit her fortune. After she discovers that her father's will allows her the right of refusal, she tries to turn the tables by playing the two men off each other. Her scheme fails, and her unscrupulous uncle, with the help of evil Dr. Karnac, commits her to a private madhouse. She is drugged and awakens in a strange, sparse room with grated windows. The doctor gets to work undermining her sanity via more drugs and solitary confinement. In her room, Sybil finds a hidden message warning her, "If you are not already mad, you will be, I suspect you were sent here to be made so; for the air is poison, the solitude fatal, and Karnac remorseless in his mania for prying into the mysteries of the human mind." Upstairs, she hears a person constantly pacing. The pacing, the drugs, and the loss of liberty soon reduce her to "a melancholy wreck of my former self."[8]

Alcott's story plays many of the notes of asylum horror: a person enters the asylum without even knowing it; the asylum makes one deranged; it is run by a powerful foreign genius (in this case, "a stealthy, sallow-faced Spaniard" who possesses "a magnetic power"); and the treatments are suspect. But the true horror of Alcott's story rests in the derangement of a *home*. The protagonist begins the tale in control of a large inheritance and much property. Then, thanks to an unscrupulous, male relative and an evil mind doctor (and, though only implied, the law as well), she loses everything and lands in a new "home." This home is a fortress of tyranny ruled by a gothic villain. Early on, Alcott emphasizes Sybil's headstrong independence, an independence that gets thoroughly punished. Although Alcott delivers a happy ending, an undeniable indictment of a social system that indoctrinates female dependency lurks beneath the surface.[9]

Both Alcott and Fern were influenced by British author Charlotte Brontë, whose popular book, *Jane Eyre*, provided a horrifying Woman in White archetype. In Brontë's novel, the titular character's romance with the brooding Mr. Rochester is upended by the revelation that he is still married. His wife, Bertha, is a "lunatic" whom he keeps locked away in the uppermost floor of his mansion. Bertha keeps trying to burn down the house, and she eventually succeeds, after which she hurls herself to her doom.[10]

Bertha has been much examined by scholars. Some see her as the embodiment of female rebellion, perhaps Brontë's defiant "double." It is important to note that she was conceived and represented as a direful example, in Brontë's words, of "moral madness, in which all that is good or even human seems to disappear from the mind and a fiend-nature replaces it." Indeed, Brontë worried that instead of fostering "profound pity" for her creation, she had "erred in making *horror* too prominent." Considering that the novel's power resides in the gothic world of buried secrets, this "error" comes across less as a misstep than a motor.[11]

Bertha is a fearsome creation indeed. She enters the story as a disembodied laugh, "distinct, formal, mirthless." Later, the laugh takes on darker properties, "a demoniac laugh—low, suppressed, and deep . . ." When Bertha emerges from the attic, she is monstrous, rending a visitor (whom we later learn is her brother) with a knife—and her teeth. Recalls the victim, "She sucked my blood: she said she'd drain my heart." Later, Jane describes "it" to Mr. Rochester as "a woman, tall and large, with thick and dark hair hanging long down her back. I know not what dress she had on: it was white and straight; but whether gown, sheet, or shroud, I cannot tell." When Mr. Rochester tries to convince Jane that she merely saw an apparition, she retorts that it more resembled "the foul German spectre—the Vampyre."[12]

Brontë's madwoman provides a literary template for the escaped, female lunatic. She is ghostlike yet ghoulishly corporeal. Her hair is wild and her manner carnally suggestive; her dress is a "white gown." She is incarcerated in a mansion that evokes the creepiest asylum. Thornfield Hall is "this accursed place," a "vault, offering the ghastliness of living death to the light of the open sky—this narrow stone hell, with its one real fiend, worse than a legion of such as we may imagine." She is maintained in her "cell" by Grace Poole who, like the brutal female attendants and nurses to come, is unwomanly, boorish, and prone to drink.[13]

Bertha's madness speaks to a culture brimming with warnings about diabolical femininity. Women's "purity" was portrayed as a fragile bulwark against a dangerous, sexual interior. Popular author and physician Oliver Wendell Holmes, Sr. called a hysterical woman "a vampire who sucks the blood out of the healthy people about her." Karen Halttunen observes, "The new medical field of obstetrics and gynecology thus generated its own Gothic language of female sexuality. Female sexuality, the new specialists affirmed, was a matter of mystery, with its 'strange and secret influences,' its dark interiority focused on its central organ, the womb (which Gardner associated with those quintessentially Gothic institutions, the prison and the mental asylum)."[14]

Reinforcing this criminal-medico discourse was the oppressive weight of a culture that demanded that women know and accept their place. Indeed, nineteenth-century physicians seemed bent on medi-calizing women's bodies. Specialists rooted any number of psycholog-ical ailments in the reproductive organs. One gynecologist specialized in treating madness by removing healthy ovaries. It almost didn't matter if the patient died. As he explained, "An insane woman is no more a member of the body politic than a criminal . . . her death is always a relief to her dearest friends." Dr. Silas Weir Mitchell, a famous neurologist, made his fortune by treating what he called "the large and troublesome class of thin-blooded emotional women." Mitchell treated such influential persons as Jane Addams and Edith Wharton. He recognized that middle-class women seemed stifled; his answer was confinement and immobility.[15]

No wonder the asylum became a tool of discipline in the gothic world of sentimental fiction. The first instance of this seems to be Mary Wollstonecraft's *Maria: or, the Wrongs of Woman* (published posthumously in 1798). A sequel of sorts to her earth-shaking *A Vin-dication of the Rights of Woman* (1792), *Maria* provides a lesson in so-ciety's mistreatment of women. Significantly, Wollstonecraft chose the asylum as the ultimate metaphor for the sequestration and deg-radation of females. The tale begins with a spectacularly dismal de-scription of a woman entombed in a madhouse. "Abodes of horror have frequently been described, and castles, filled with spectres and chimeras, conjured up by the magic spell of genius to harrow the soul, and absorb the wondering mind. But, formed of such stuff as dreams are made of, what were they to the mansion of despair, in one corner of which Maria sat, endeavoring to recall her scattered thoughts!" The horror of this story is that dungeon asylums are *real* places, and that the reduction of women to childlike-slavery within their own homes is just as real.[16]

Maria suffers in a "private madhouse," left to listen to "groans and shrieks" through the wall, rotting away in a "dreary cell," "blotted out of existence." The superintendent is almost nonexistent, though he is described as responding to Maria's pleas with a "malignant smile." The story unfolds as a series of recollections; Maria, her attendant Jemima, and her asylum love-interest Darnford all share their sto-ries of abuse and injustice. Wollstonecraft's novel remained unfin-ished; she died due to complications giving birth to her daughter Mary (who would herself create a character of interest to the asylum, *Frankenstein*). Like future heroines, Maria is "buried alive" and made to feel insane, getting sent away because a brutal male uses the law to impose control. Later theorists such as Phyllis Chesler would argue that women were routinely sent away to asylums in this period in order to silence them for expressing unpopular views or as a means of removal for adulterous purposes. This view is articulated in *Maria* and forcefully seconded in other works. In 1861, feminist Elizabeth Cady Stanton wrote, "Could the dark secrets of those insane asylums be brought to light . . . we would be shocked to know the countless number of rebellious wives, sisters and daughters that are thus annually sacrificed to false customs and conventionalisms, and barbarous laws made by men for women." A bit later Lydia Smith laid out the strategy in her memoir: "It is a very fashionable and easy thing now to make a person out to be insane. If a man tires from his wife . . . it is not a very difficult matter to get her in an institution . . . Belladonna and chloroform will give her the appearance of being crazy enough, and after the asylum doors have closed upon her, adieu to the beautiful world and all home associations."[17]

Yet asylum narratives were not always so straightforward. What if the person sent away really *is* mad and dangerous? (Anne Catherick, Collins made clear, was a monomaniac.[18]) Even scarier, what if the incarcerated is not really sure? This is the plot of Harriet Prescott Spofford's short tale, "Her Story." Published in *Lippincott's* in 1872 and narrated in a confessional Poe style, this is a tale of a woman on the edge. With the asylum as looming backdrop, Spofford captures effectively the dilemmas of Victorian womanhood.

"Her Story" begins with the protagonist writing to a friend from the confines of an asylum. She does not know whether she is mad or not, nor whether the events that led to her commitment were real or imagined. She despairs, "I can't make out, sometimes, whether I am really beside myself or not; for it seems that whether I was crazed or sane, if it was true, they would put me out of sight and hearing—bury me alive, as they have done, in this Retreat." The author then relates her tragic story, in which she falls love and marries a man of the cloth, has two children by him, and then loses everything to a seductress who also happens to be her husband's uncle's stepchild. This other woman is "dark as an Egyptian" with "perfect features." The narrator's descent begins upon her rival's coming to stay with them. Not only is the intruder gorgeous, she demonstrates an unearthly hold over those around her. The protagonist's husband is entranced, and her children are enticed into "witch-dances." Most unsettlingly, the seductress builds a "little altar" in her room and has bizarre beliefs. The protagonist tries to warn her husband, telling him, "Her very gifts are unnatural in their abundance. There must be a scrofula there, to keep such a fire in the blood and sting in the brain to such action: she will die in a madhouse, depend upon it." But by this point, the narrator is completely unhinged. She imagines hanging herself, then fantasizes about killing her husband with chloroform. "Spirits" begin talking to her day and night. She sees them flying in and out of the seductress's mouth. Most horrifyingly, the spirits suggest that she kill her children. When she finds her husband and the seductress in a passionate embrace in the music room, she collapses, only to awaken in an asylum.[19]

The madhouse in "Her Story" is a bit different. It detains but with justifiable cause. The protagonist is clearly tormented by her own mind. There is no tyrant, though after an unsuccessful escape attempt, she is made "a prisoner" and kept on indefinitely. "Medicines and books and work" are afforded to her, standard therapeutics of contemporary asylums. But like in *Maria*, this asylum serves as metaphor for contained and violated womanhood, highlighting the power of males to dictate the lives of female dependents. Still, the question of reality budges in. Is she imagining things? What is real? All we know is that this woman's version of events, literally, "Her Story," inspires dread.[20]

THE WOMAN IN THE WALL

The asylum was a hopeless place to be avoided if at all possible. In Lillie Devereux Blake's *Southwold* (1859) the heroine drinks poison because she fears insanity and doesn't want to end up in a "lunatic asylum" like her paternal grandmother. Even *thinking* too much can get you locked away. Physician Edward Clarke, in his popular *Sex in Education* (1873), warned that girls studying too hard were liable to lose their minds. He helpfully provided the example of a young woman of good breeding and intelligence who, by emulating the boys' rigorous study program, gradually lost both her menstrual cycle and her energy. Sadly, explained Clarke, "I was finally obliged to consign her to an asylum."[21]

Once institutionalized, women had to police themselves at the strictest level. Resistance—that most American of behaviors—became evidence of insanity. As Phebe Davis notes in her 1855 Utica exposé, "When I was in the Asylum, I saw a concentration of evils in condensed form; and when I said anything to the Doctors about the wrongs of the house, they would tell me that was my insanity. I told them that a fact was no less a fact because it was told by a crazy person." Once inside, the logic of the institution inverts right and wrong. Enslavement under the superintendent is the only road to freedom.[22]

Dr. Silas Weir Mitchell's suffocating, infantilizing treatment of strong-minded women caused one of his patients, Charlotte Perkins Gilman, to respond with a horror story for the ages. *The Yellow Wallpaper* (1892) is about a woman who has a nervous breakdown after the birth of her baby. Her husband, a well-respected physician, puts her on "the rest cure" in the attic-nursery of the old, spooky house they are summering in. He then fills her with "cod liver oil and lots of tonics and things" and threatens to send her to Dr. Mitchell. Soon the descent begins. The wallpaper comes alive.[23]

The Yellow Wallpaper captures the Victorian household-as-asylum trope in the clearest manner. This house is *literally* the asylum. It is lorded over by an all-powerful patriarch who sequesters his female patient and subjects her to infantilizing, liberty-crushing treatments. Underlining the boast that asylums are homes away from homes, Gilman contends that this is indeed, horrifically, true. In *The Yellow Wallpaper*, control is the beating heart of domesticity, clearly revealed when resistance inspires greater levels of patriarchal correction. In real life, Gilman had suffered postpartum depression and had been treated by Dr. Mitchell. His prescriptions of total rest and abstinence from all writing drove her to a point where she felt divorce was the only way out. "It was not a choice between going and staying, but between going, sane, and staying, insane." In her 1913 essay, "Why I Wrote *The Yellow Wallpaper*," she notes that she sent a copy of the story to "the physician who so nearly drove me mad." Years later, she heard that Mitchell had subsequently changed his treatment methods. If this was the case, she mused in her autobiography, "I have not lived in vain."[24]

The spookiness of *The Yellow Wallpaper* lies in the protagonist's descent into a place where reality and fantasy blur, where home and hell commingle. Like Spofford, Gilman masterfully follows the per-spective of a protagonist whose grasp of the world is slipping. In her attic-nursery, she watches a woman in the wallpaper trying to break out, "all the time trying to climb through. But nobody could climb through that pattern—it strangles so . . ." Ultimately the woman in the wall escapes, "creeping" about outdoors where no one notices. The story ends after the narrator strips off the wallpaper. "You can't put me back!" she screams as she creeps along on the floor. Her husband faints, and so she creeps over his prostrate body. Tearing the paper is not an act of simple destruction; rather it is a breaking of prison walls. Fleeing from domestic tyranny takes an act of destruction.[25]

THE ANGEL IN BLACK

Nineteenth-century women were considered delicate, but they were also morally powerful, equipped by their gender to police honor and to correct sin. Feminine gentleness was thus intertwined with a so-cially acceptable firmness, and this power was commonly played up. Women like Clara Barton, Catherine Beecher, Florence Nightingale, Louisa May Alcott, Harriet Beecher Stowe and others maintained their feminine position while pushing into public, male realms. Ab-olitionism, temperance, and suffrage, along with school, prison, and asylum reform were all fair game for the brave, female moralist. Such crusaders managed to project domestic authority outwards.

Dorothea Dix was America's most influential asylum reformer. In her 1843 exposé/call to arms, *Memorial to the Massachusetts Legisla-ture*, she boldly takes to task the mistreatment of those suffering from mental illness. This remarkable document galvanized New England and would be the basis for Dix's lasting national influence.[26]

Dix spoke the language of Victorian Womanhood—particularly the ideal of the unerotic, aloof, moral guardian. She dressed in dark silk, wore no makeup and little jewelry, and kept her hair pulled back in a severe bun. Her bearing was stern, and her personal notebooks tell a story of one obsessed with discovering and conquering personal failings. As a school teacher, she was remembered by her students as a disciplinarian who did not spare "the whip." In her early twenties, Dix wrote religious poetry and cautionary fiction for youngsters. After experiencing a bout of depression and traveling to England to recover, she began to investigate the treatment of the indigent insane in America. Her findings appalled her and gave mission to her life.[27]

Dix's *Memorial* offers a tour of hell. It does not read like a narrative; it is more impressionistic. In Newburyport, for instance, she tells of hearing about a woman in a cellar. She is warned that this madwoman is "dangerous to be approached" and is "often naked." Dix persists, and the warden relents, escorting her down a staircase where "a strange, unnatural noise seemed to proceed from beneath our feet." The gothic tone is indelible. The horror lies beneath; we cannot resist learning dark secrets. The warden removes a padlock and they enter the cellar. Dix looks around the gloomy, dank, subterranean space. Then, to her "horror and amazement," a door is opened to a "closet *beneath* the *staircase*." Here, "in the imperfect light a female apparently wasted to a skeleton, partially wrapped in blankets, furnished for the narrow bed on which she was sitting." The prisoner "poured forth the wailings of despair," extending her arms and pleading, "Why am I consigned to hell?" The horror is crowned with a query: "Perhaps it will be inquired how long, how many days or hours, was she imprisoned in these confined limits? *For years!*"[28]

Notes Dix's biographer David Gollaher, the *Memorial* used the "conventions of gothicism" to "shape her incredible experiences, imposing on them a pattern that audiences understood." Dix addressed a readership accustomed to fictional horror to describe the sad and very real lives of the neglected and abused. We read of people shivering on the straw-strewn floors of unheated rooms, whipped, chained, and stuffed in cages. A shocking journalistic flourish meets with gothic sensibility to deliver punishing descriptions. Many have a frightening brevity: "*Lincoln.* A woman in a cage." That's all we read about the poor woman here. And that's enough.[29]

When Dix toured asylums, she wore mourning apparel in honor of her departed friend William Ellery Channing. Looking like an "angel of mercy dressed in black," she entered asylums, prisons, and almshouses and spoke tenderly with the troubled within, bravely ignoring warnings to keep her distance. At the Eastern Penitentiary of Pennsylvania, she found the most violent prisoner and helped to personally reform him by aiding in his education. Her work, she was told by an influential friend, was "angel work."[30]

Dix knew she was treading on dangerous ground. Women were

angels in the house, but did public institutions, however homelike, meet domestic criteria? The *Newburyport Herald* questioned her language, noting that the dark cellar where the lunatic woman was kept was not a dungeon but rather a "cellar-kitchen, not much worse than many kitchens of very genteel city mansions." This critique unconsciously reveals the problem men had with Dix. She was overstepping. Asylums should be left to be run by the proper authorities. What right had Dix to question them? Indeed, Dix's later memorials were less sensationalistic, perhaps the result of fending off criticism. Yet she proved to be incredibly influential. Her power grew from the same source as the "weakness" her critics focused on: her womanhood. For Dix, the cult of true womanhood served as both armor and motivator. It protected her from attacks and inspired her to heal the helpless. The advantages, and disadvantages, of her strategy are best summarized by her attempt to create a nationwide system of mental health providers. The so-called Ten-Million Acre Bill would have given some twelve million acres of federal lands for the benefit of the insane, blind, and deaf. Dix started making arguments before Congress in 1850, capitalizing on her publicized ability to get states to fund asylums. She almost succeeded. The bill passed through both houses before being vetoed by President Pierce. His rationale was that the federal government was not in the business of intruding on local responsibilities. But Congress had long used federal funds for public schools and internal improvements. The Ten-Million Acre Bill was, as a critic of Pierce phrased it, a piece of "sentimental legislation." Associated with nurturing womanhood, charity was not the responsibility of the manly federal government. Still, Dix gained enough traction to get a massive health-care bill all the way up to the top. Unfortunately, the top patriarch trumped her.[31]

MODERN PERSECUTION

If Dorothea Dix wanted people in better asylums, Elizabeth Packard was the Angel in Black who wanted to free the unjustly trapped within. After the two met, Packard wrote that Dix was "a Christian, although honestly and conscientiously wrong, in sustaining our present system of Insane Asylums."[32] Packard's perspective was informed by the fact that she was the most famous asylum victim of her day.

In 1860, Elizabeth Packard was involuntarily committed to the Illinois State Hospital for the Insane by her preacher husband The- ophilus. He committed her because, she said, she contradicted his strict Calvinist principles and because she refused to sign real estate deeds to allow him to sell her property. In other words, she rejected her husband's psychological and financial authority. She asserts, "the *subjection* of the wife was the cure [Theophilus] was seeking." Pack- ard spent the next three years in the state hospital and, afterwards, found herself imprisoned in her own home, trapped in a bedroom with nailed-shut windows. She finally freed herself, with the help of some friends, in the dramatic court case *Packard v. Packard* (1864). She went on to write extensively about her experiences and to argue for women's rights. Her captivity narratives sold well and helped pro- duce change in the world.[33]

When Packard was shipped off—literally "railroaded" by train— the law was on her husband's side. She quotes a statute in *The Pris- oners' Hidden Life, or Insane Asylums Unveiled*: "Married women and infants, who, in the judgment of the medical superintendent (mean- ing the Superintendent of the Illinois State Hospital for the Insane) are evidently insane or distracted, may be entered or detained in the hospital on the request of the husband of the woman or the guardian of the infant, without the evidence of insanity required in other cases." This law aimed to "protect" women from the public humiliation of a trial. It was in line with the enshrined codes of coverture that posi- tioned married women as wards of their husbands. As abolitionist William Lloyd Garrison put it, "The Common Law, by giving to the husband the custody of his wife's person, does virtually place her on a level with criminals, lunatics and fools, since these are the only classes of adult persons over whom the law-makers have thought it necessary to place keepers." Packard's husband had the right to send her off with little due process, merely his own "request." In fact, The- ophilus spent much time carefully building his case, gathering sig- natures and accruing allies. This complication does not intrude on Packard's narrative. Hers is a tale of male domination, virtue tram- pled, and redemption.[34]

Packard's battle to prove her sanity and attain her release might have made scarcely a mark were it not for her marvelous publicizing skills. In 1868, she published her first asylum narrative, *The Prisoners'*

Hidden Life, or Insane Asylums Unveiled. This book, printed at her own expense, sold briskly. In 1873, she published a two-volume work. The first volume, *Modern Persecution, or Insane Asylums Unveiled*, is basically a reprint of the earlier book (with some modifications). The second, *Modern Persecution, or Married Woman's Liabilities, as Demonstrated by the Action of the Illinois Legislature*, details Packard's court battles. At this point, she was traveling the country, fighting for new laws to protect women asylum inmates and, more importantly, revise marriage statutes.[35]

Packard's is a story in the sentimental mode. Her institutionalization was due to her husband's nefarious doings. In *The Prisoners' Hidden Life*, she sets the stage: "Mr. Packard had for some time been trying to induce me to sign a deed, so that he could sell some real estate, and I had objected, unless he should give me some equivalent for what he had already unjustly taken from me. This he would not do. He therefore went to Esquire La Brie, and took an oath that his wife was insane, so that he could sell the property without my signature." But she is also committed for confronting her Calvinist husband with the religious truth that contradicted his false teachings. She notes that the "pivot on which my reputation for sanity was suspended" was that "I could not be made to confess that God made a bad or sinful article when He made human nature; but on the contrary, I claimed that all which God made was 'good.'" In other words, her husband wanted her money *and* her soul. He wanted to suffocate her revealed knowledge of God's love.[36]

In line with captivity narratives, which borrowed from nun escapes and slave narratives, Packard's tale begins with her being "kidnapped." She chooses to emphasize this over the less titillating "involuntarily committed" description. In an episode that oddly predicts *The Shining*, she locks the door to her bedroom, and her husband comes through the window with an axe. She dashes under the bedcovers, because she is undressed. It is an "untimely, unexpected, unmanly, even outrageous entrance into her private sleeping room." The naked female flees but is caught by the villain.[37]

A heart-wrenching scene of a seven-year-old child chasing his mom's train down the tracks (yelling, "I will get my dear Mamma out of prison!") is followed by Packard being "forcibly entombed" in the Jacksonville asylum. The superintendent, Dr. Andrew McFarland, comes across as a more complex tyrant than in other asylum stories. He shows concern, but, alas, he's only interested in control and submission. Packard's relationship with McFarland unfolds in a series of letters and conversations, made yet more complicated by her admitted early attraction to him. He would later argue that Packard fixated on him; she would say that he made sexual advances on her. Ultimately, her writings condemned McFarland in the strongest manner. He does not heal; he does just the opposite. As she notes in a letter to him reprinted in *Modern Persecution,* "It is my honest opinion that the principles upon which you treat the inmates of this institution, are contrary to reason, to justice, to humanity. They are treated in a very insane manner—in a manner the best calculated to make maniacs that human ingenuity could devise. No human being can be subjected to the process to which you subject them here, without being in great danger of becoming insane; especially, if their physical or mental constitution is in the least degree impaired."[38]

Working for McFarland are brutal attendants. Most frightful is Miss Elizabeth "Lizzie" Bonner who is described as "a large, coarse, stout Irish woman, stronger than most men; of quick temper, very easily thrown off its balance, when, for the time being, she would be a perfect demon, lost to all traces of humanity. Her manners were very coarse and masculine, a loud and boisterous talker, and a great liar, with no education, and could neither read nor write."

Bonner brutalizes those who challenge her authority. In the case of one resistant woman, she "choked, pounded, kicked, and plunged underwater, until well nigh strangled to death." The woman eventually kills herself, and Packard cannot blame her. When another woman insults Bonner, she's bound and her head is beaten against solid bars, "each blow inflicting a deep gash into her head—so that every blow was followed with blood splashing in every direction, besmearing the floor and walls, our clothes, and a pie I had in my hand, with human gore." A graphic illustration accompanies the description.[39]

To make sense of the horror in Packard's tale, we must return to the Victorian home. These were places ostensibly managed by republican mothers, but, like asylums, were dependent upon the moral leadership of patriarchs. When run by a tyrant, the legal weakness of a woman's position became apparent. The blood-spattered pie in Packard's hand offers the ultimate image of imperiled womanhood.

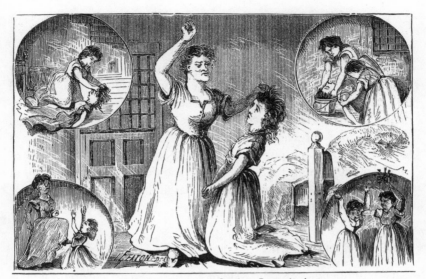

Popular Mode of Curing Insanity!
Lizzie Bonner punishing Miss Hodson, on suspicion of taking her key. See page 336.

Lizzie Bonner in Elizabeth Packard's *Modern Persecution, or Insane Asylums Unveiled* (1873)

Packard emphasizes this weakness to unleash her devastating critique. The laws that support the superstructure of marriage must change. For this, she is rightly viewed as a feminist pioneer.

But Packard's critique of patriarchy is embedded in a Victorian sensibility that makes her experiences difficult for the modern reader to relate to. Her battle was a nineteenth-century battle; she wanted to improve the marital relation, not revolutionize it. As she explains in *Modern Persecution, or Married Woman's Liabilities*, "We do not want the man's rights, but simply our own, natural, womanly rights. There are man's rights and woman's rights. Both different, yet both equally inalienable. There must be a head in every firm; and the head in the Marriage Firm or Union is the man, as the Bible and nature both plainly teach." Her contribution to the pop culture asylum is unmistakable. She takes the captivity narrative, which by mid-century was suffused with gothic elements and aligned with asylum stories, and constructs a horror tale that "asylumizes" the home. Just as her husband has alienated her from domesticity, so does the asylum strip away her natural rights. The inevitable solution is to go back to the drawing board and redefine the parameters of the gender relationship.[40]

Packard's battle was with more than commitment laws, though it was here that she made her greatest impact. She fought a society that encouraged women to medicate their emotions and to take full responsibility for the heaviness they felt on their shoulders. If unsatisfied with domestic power structures, common wisdom went, women should figure out what was wrong *with them*. An entire industry of advice manuals and popular medical texts reinforced this. Packard made the argument that, despite her incarceration, she was *not* at fault. It was the social order that was at fault. Packard was a soldier in a battle yet unfinished.[41]

"THE PRETTY CRAZY GIRL"

On September 25, 1887, the *New York Sun* ran an article about a mysterious and enchanting young creature being examined at Bellevue Hospital. Titled "Who Is This Insane Girl," the piece described a "modest, comely, well-dressed girl of 19" who was "probably suffering from hysterical mania." The *New York Times* similarly portrayed this "mysterious waif" as having a "manner of good breeding" and a "comely appearance." They suggested she was probably afflicted with "melancholia."[42]

Several days earlier, this "waif" had walked into the *New York World*'s managing editor's office and demanded a hearing. She was a reporter named Nellie Bly (a *nom de plume*; it was unseemly for female reporters to use their own names) and she had loads of ideas. Perhaps she could go undercover as an immigrant and ship over from Europe in steerage? If the editor was not interested, she curtly informed him, she'd be happy to shop her ideas to the competition. He wisely chose to keep her on retainer. Soon came her break. Bly would feign insanity and get sent to Blackwell's Island.

A narrow, two-mile strip of land situated in New York's East River, Blackwell's Island housed a clutch of buildings for New York's impoverished, criminals, diseased, and insane. It had been purchased by the Department of Charities and Corrections in 1828, mainly because its surrounding tidal currents made escape difficult. It would go on to generate a long, infamous history. Dickens, as we have seen, visited in the 1840s and was not impressed. In 1870, the *New York Times* described "an amount of discomfort quite sufficient to drive a patient mad, even should he happen to have entered sane." Bly would call it a "human rat-trap."[43]

Bly started her journey to Blackwell's by discarding all forms of identification and practicing looking "crazy" in front of a mirror. "I remembered all I had read of the doings of crazy people, how first of all they have staring eyes, and so I opened mine as wide as possible and stared unblinkingly at my own reflection." She then checked into the Temporary Home for Women on Second Avenue as "Nellie Brown." Her erratic behavior convinced a worried fellow-boarder to spend the night with her in her room. By morning, two policemen escorted her to the station house. Here, a judge proposed putting her away where she could be "taken care of." A policeman suggested "the Island." The assistant matron of the Temporary Home protested, "Don't! She is a lady and it would kill her to be put on the Island." Nellie worried to herself, "To think the Island was just the place I wanted to reach and here she was trying to keep me from going there!"[44]

After Bellevue, where she easily fooled a doctor into thinking she was insane, she was finally shipped over to Blackwell's Island. Nellie Bly's account contains many of the hallmarks of asylum narratives. There's the isolated fortress; the brutal and coarse matrons; the stripping of liberty and dignity; the "chattering" inmates; the atrocious food; the physical and mental abuse; and the protests of sanity interpreted as *in*sanity. She had initially aimed to be placed on the violent ward but, after hearing the stories about its horrors, "decided not to risk my health."[45]

Bly's "escape" was effected when the *Sun* sent an attorney who claimed Nellie had friends who would "take charge" of her. Bly's resulting story broke big, thanks to the *World*'s owner Joseph Pulitzer, a publicity genius who reinvented news by being both watchdog and sensation-monger. Bly became a phenomenon. She had entered the abyss of madness and returned to shed light on the horrors. She had transformed herself from "waif" into avenging angel. She'd later claim responsibility for the $1 million in additional funds allocated for the care of the city's insane (the truth is a bit more complicated).[46]

Bly's undercover adventure inaugurated a new archetype—the female daredevil reporter. Her instantly released book *Ten Days in a*

Mad-House sold well, and her later circumnavigation of the world—inspired by Jules Verne's *Around the World in Eighty Days* (her book being titled *Around the World in 72 Days*)—was such a hit that she received a parade down Broadway.

It is significant that the pioneer female entrant into journalistic stardom involved an asylum trip. For a national audience weaned on captivity narratives launched on the Indian-haunted frontier and nurtured in dark excursions to nunneries, urban spaces, slave plantations, and asylums, Bly's tale resonated. Her success also tapped the creeping fear that the asylum mimicked the home and revealed the horrors of domesticity.

And Bly added something new. She was neither wife nor daughter betrayed. She was modern yet supremely aware of her social limitations. She recapitulated women's progress, entering the asylum as helpless waif only to emerge triumphantly as an independent voice of reform. Just as she later navigated the world, she navigated the asylum, playing multiple roles to her advantage: "crazy girl," adventurer, reformer. That she embodied the Woman in White and the Angel in Black both speaks to the dilemmas and opportunities for womanhood as America became an industrial powerhouse. Bly knew how to negotiate a society that offered ambitious women precious few opportunities.

Bly's triumph did not sound any death knells for the domestic prison. In the myriad asylum iterations to come, the Woman in White would persist, even through Second and Third Wave feminist insurgencies. One film that we would not call a madhouse movie in any universe captures its endurance. In this film, a waif in white is imprisoned by an evil master possessed of insidious mind powers (and vaguely British accent) and in command of legions of uniformed men. In one terrifying scene, he looms over her and administers a truth drug via a scary, hovering needle. The movie is *Star Wars*.

CHAPTER 3

MONSTERS OF THE ASYLUM

"I shall be patient, Master. It is coming—coming—coming!"
—Renfield's musings inside Seward's
"lunatic asylum," in Bram Stoker's *Dracula* (1897)

Superintendents started renaming their institutions "hospitals" at the end of the nineteenth century. The word "asylum" had simply become too negative. It was an unintentional act of irony, "asylum" originally being a replacement word for "madhouse." Sadly, Progressive Era mental institutions summoned forth new nightmares of warehousing, hereditary degeneracy, permanent categories like "idiot" and "moron," and back wards where anonymous, chronic patients rotted away. In his 1776 pamphlet *Common Sense*, Thomas Paine had used asylum as the ultimate juxtaposition: "This new World hath been the asylum for the persecuted lovers of civil and religious liberty from EVERY PART of Europe. Hither have they fled, not from the tender embraces of the mother, *but from the cruelty of the monster*." In a spectacular reversal of this dream, crowded asylums now produced monsters as inexorably as factories churned out stoves and hats. This was the new common sense.[1]

Progressive America witnessed sharp social changes only hinted at on Dickens's "leviathan" creeping down Long Island Sound. While a bright future beckoned, the journey left behind a twisted wreckage of lost dreams and lost souls. Some, deemed unequipped to navigate modernity, grew monstrous in massive state hospitals. Soon, asylums encased retrograde Darwinian abominations and mad scientist brain-exchangers. Both Dracula and Frankenstein would find homes within their walls.

OF MONSTERS AND MANAGERS

Karl Marx famously wrote that capitalism is born "dripping from head to toe, from every pore, with blood and dirt." Once it emerges from history, it feeds *Nosferatu* fashion, "dead labour which, vampire-like, lives only by sucking living labour, and lives the more, the more labour it sucks." Elsewhere Marx enhanced this imagery, saying, "the bourgeois order . . . sucks out [peasants'] blood and brains and throws them into the alchemist's cauldron." In Progressive America's capitalism, increasingly alienated wage earners regularly put in twelve-hour days and were monitored, timed, replaced, and switched about like mindless automata. Workers' compensation, weekends, vacations, and even retirement were more utopian ideals than facts of life.[2]

The asylum seemed to be changing for the worst as well. Gone was the dream of moral treatment in stately, home-like manors. It was clear that the cures were not working. In fact, as neurologists had been asserting for several decades, no empirical evidence yet existed that psychiatry cured anything. Overfilled wards, padded strong rooms, and heavy medications seemed to yield no results. Patients were becoming permanent residents. Prior to 1890, most asylum patients remained less than a year, and the old and senile were farmed out to local almshouses. But starting with a widely copied New York law that required the state to care for the deranged, the institutionalized tended to remain inside for longer periods. By 1923, over half of mental patients had been hospitalized for five or more years. Most of these were warehoused in massive hospitals containing over one thousand beds. The largest, the Georgia State Sanatorium in Milledgeville, housed over ten thousand by 1950. Residents typically experienced atrocious patient-to-doctor ratios, bombardments of high-octane opiates, and general human neglect. This was compounded by racism. "Colored" asylums had much lower budgets and fewer treatment options. Regardless, many people sent to asylums were already in a bad physical state. In New York State, some 20 percent of those admitted between 1910 and 1920 were in the final stages of syphilitic paresis. Eighty-seven percent of these people expired in the hospital, typically within four years.[3]

Undeath was becoming the new asylum reality. Poe is again a good place to start. As he writes in "The Premature Burial," "The boundaries which divide Life from Death are at best shadowy and vague. Who shall say where the one ends, and where the other begins?" To be trapped in-between, to be buried alive, is the worst of all "extremes." Freud agreed. In his influential 1919 essay "The Uncanny," he calls living burial "the most uncanny thing of all." Both Poe and Freud recognized the scariness of existing in a situation of existential uncertainty. In-between-ness seems to be at the core of much horror. Writes Noel Carroll, "Many monsters of the horror genre are interstitial," meaning that they transgress boundaries that clearly delineate ideas and give safe meaning to the world. Monsters emerge where there is a "breakdown of intelligibility." This terrifying uncertainty, which begets helplessness, is at the center of living burial horror. Obviously, there is the immediate threat of suffocation and agony, but there is also something else. There is the terror of being alive but also dead, unable to communicate with the world, exiled from one's friends and family, stifled. This was why calling asylums "living tombs" was calculated to produce rage, and why patient exposés commonly referenced being "buried alive."[4]

This sort of horror was familiar enough to Americans. In fact, it had a legal name: slavery. Both Frederick Douglass and Harriet Jacobs described their slave experiences as "living death," and David Walker simply noted, "in fact I am dead." Whites transposed well-known slavery horrors into asylum contexts to highlight their own sufferings. Elizabeth Stone wrote that McLean had "a system worse than slavery." Elizabeth Packard regularly compared commitment, and even marriage under current Illinois law, to slavery. In *A Plea for the Insane by Friends of the Living Dead*, Alice Bingham Russell explains, "At your commitment you are without lawful rights, for you are legally dead and without influential interference if maliciously committed it can be life long." Earlier still, William Hotchkiss in *Five Months in the New-York State Lunatic Asylum* (1849) spoke of his fellow inmates as "just risen from the dead," and one in particular as "an Egyptian mummy and incapable of motion." Even physicians saw fit to use undead imagery. In his devastating 1894 address to the American Medico-Psychological Association, famed neurologist Silas Weir Mitchell told a distinguished collection of superintendents that they reigned over massive collections of "living corpses," "silent, grewsome [*sic*] machines which eat and sleep, sleep and eat."[5]

The new Darwinian paradigm also "monsterized" the mentally ill. Though stigmatization extended back a long time, the new science helped rigidly cast certain persons into permanent, subhuman molds in order to excise them from the body politic. Certain behaviors, coupled with suspect physiognomies, unkempt clothing and hair, and degraded "blood" told of dangerous genetic inferiority. Heralded by such bright minds as Francis Galton (Darwin's half-cousin) and George Bernard Shaw, the neo-Darwinian "science" of eugenics put forth the argument that some humans were better than others, biologically. They couldn't help it. Now the mad could be efficiently categorized as nature's mistakes. State laws, academic authorities, and popular culture combined to promote the weeding out of the unfit. Much was made of the argument that madness and race were connected. Typically, the mentally "weak" races hailed from the global south or from non-English speaking European locales inhabited by people of non-Protestant extraction. (Though some, like the eponymous family in the bestseller *The Jukes*, came straight from the good-old USA; rural, damaged specimens of inequity.) The arguments all came together in over-generalizations that the biggest asylums had large, pauper, foreign-born populations. Solutions could steer toward the Final variety. Madison Grant, in his hugely influential *The Passing of the Great Race*, commented, "A rigid system of selection through the elimination of those who are weak and unfit—in other words social failures—would solve the whole question in one hundred years, as well as enable us to get rid of the undesirables who crowd our jails, hospitals, and insane asylums."[6]

The asylum also made monsters of those who managed them. It begins, perhaps, with Ravoni, the foreign, mystical aristocrat of *The Quaker City*. Ravoni might even be called the prototypical *anti*-American. He is unassimilable, lordly, secretive, and blasphemous. He uses undemocratic mind power to take control of beautiful, white women while performing hideous, secret acts in his "dissecting room." Ravoni capitalized on contemporary worries of immigration and the mysterious power granted to medical science. Doctors and foreigners could be scary, and hospitals were places where people went to die. Why not combine it all under one monstrous brow, under one gabled roof? Once eugenics took hold, the Ravonis gained new powers.[7]

The business of the monstrous superintendent was to *dis*assemble his victims. Mimicking the life-sucking alienation of industrial work, evil asylum managers created factories from hell. Here the sane went mad, bombarded with drugs or tied up to beds, monitored in a manner that would make management icon Frederick Taylor envious. As former patient Kate Lee described the Elgin Insane Asylum, "In the asylum the inmate becomes part of a great iron machine, which continues to revolve, carrying her with it." Writes Florence Seyler Thompson in her novel *A Thousand Faces* (1920), "an 'Institution' supposed to cure persons of diseased minds, and which instead, manufactured idiots, maniacs and corpses."[8] The asylum production of madness puts the superintendent in the role of monstrous boss. The very name "superintendent" consents to this interpretation. He lords a manufactory of the living dead.

Behold the greatest asylum superintendent of all time—Count Dracula.

Go back and re-read Bram Stoker's original and it's all there. Dracula is a supernatural, aristocratic, mind-controlling foreigner who commands the mad. He looks like a monster and actively recruits an underling from a sanitarium. Influenced by cutting-edge, evolutionary thinking, Stoker combines the evil genius trope with Darwinian horrors. An instructive contemporary referent is Svengali. Created by George Du Maurier in his novel *Trilby*, Svengali is a mysterious, mind-controlling Jew. He is "a tall man, deathly pale, with long black hair and beard," a "canine snarl" and mesmeric powers. He is racially foreign ("Hebrew-German") and he dominates a beautiful, white woman while being followed by a "doglike" minion named Gecko. Dracula has a similarly telling physiognomy. He has a "very strong" face, with a "thin nose and peculiarly domed forehead" and "massive eyebrows." His mouth is "fixed and rather cruel-looking, with particularly sharp teeth," his breath "rank." Weirdly, he has hairy palms. Later, he becomes even more Svengali-like. In London, he is described as being "a tall, thin man, with a beaky nose and a pointed beard." He too mind controls women and has a "slave" named Renfield. Dracula's plan is to invade England in an effort to infect and control stolid, Anglo-Saxon folk in what one scholar calls the "late-Victorian nightmare of reverse colonization."[9]

Madhouse gothicism informs Stoker's narrative. When Jonathan Harker is sent by his boss to the East to discuss a real estate deal with the Transylvanian count, he finds himself trapped and dominated, locked in a room, isolated from friends and family. Dracula controls Harker's correspondence and has his blood drained by assistant, female vampires. The Englishman slowly loses his mental faculties. He writes in his diary, "Whilst I live on here there is but one thing to hope for, that I may not go mad, if, indeed, I be not mad already." Like other superintendents, Dracula feigns a dignified air of rationality, answering Harker's questions and even earning his respect as the master of the domain. Like other asylum captives, Harker manages to flee. He returns to England to warn others about the foreign monster.[10]

In league with Jonathan Harker are a crew of bold men, including a superintendent, Dr. Seward, who manages a "private insane asylum" next to Carfax. Also on the team is Abraham Van Helsing, a Dutch doctor and all-around Renaissance Man, whose wife, we are told, is mad. Dracula's assault begins with wiping out the crew of the ship transporting him and then by going after the beautiful Lucy Westenra, a friend of Harker's fiancée Mina. Lucy is eventually killed by the Count, to return undead in the form of "The Woman in Black" (echoes of Wilkie Collins). She is a ghastly creature who preys on children and haunts the graveyard. Dracula also recruits a "homicidal maniac" from Seward's asylum named Renfield. Renfield spends his days eating flies and speaking longingly of his "Master." He eventually decides to break with Dracula and battle him, explaining, "I had heard that madmen have unnatural strength; and as I knew I was a madman—at times anyhow—I resolved to use my power. Ay, and He felt it too, for He had come out of the mist to struggle with me." Unfortunately, Renfield can't defeat the Count, who wounds and later kills him. Eventually, the team hunts down Dracula during his retreat back to his castle and dispatches him along with his vampire underlings.[11]

As the master of the mad and the commander of an asylum-like castle in the middle of nowhere, Dracula manifests multiple levels of asylum-inflected worries for industrial America. He acquires wealth and land by parasitically feeding off the populace, converting them in the process into his living dead servants. He has qualities of the factory manager, the robber-baron, the con-man, the degenerate immigrant, and the mind doctor. He is Marx's nightmare of alienation and expropriation made corporeal. He literally drips with "blood and dirt."[12]

The asylum locale gets emphasis in early film and stage adaptations of Stoker's book. The first Dracula movie, the now-lost Hungarian silent *Dracula's Death* (1921), featured a woman visiting an insane asylum in which one of the patients claims to be the Count. Interestingly, the actor who played Dracula, Paul Askonas, had previously appeared as Svengali in a 1912 version of *Trilby*. Like future Draculas, Askonas was clean-shaven and less monstrous than Stoker's vivid description. In a popular 1924 stage play authorized by Stoker's widow, the action begins in the library of Seward's "sanatorium," described in the script as "medieval, the walls are stone with vaulted ceilings." In the version brought to Broadway in 1927 by Horace Liveright, a new performer took the role and made it his own. Hungarian actor Bela Lugosi's Dracula was aristocratic and seductive and, like Askonas, much less bestial than Stoker's character. In Lugosi's hands, the Count tilts away from Svengali and toward Ravoni. His would be the enduring version for popular culture. Lugosi's Dracula kept the villainous foreign aspects that made Stoker's creation so alarming to American readers. He is an aristocratic invader whose racialized otherness, deceptiveness, and lustfulness tag him as the enemy of liberty. At a time when financiers were regularly parodied as puffing about overdressed and pompous, Lugosi's characterization tapped both the silliness and fear beneath the American horror landscape. Ludicrous as he looked, Dracula was here to take what was ours—our wealth, our women, our liberty.[13]

It is ironic that the public was unaware that, in real life, there were worse asylum masters than Dracula. Investigating the New Jersey State Hospital in 1924, physician Dr. Phyllis Greenacre noticed that the patients spoke in a slurry, sloppy manner. On closer inspection, she discovered that they had no teeth. Dr. Henry Cotton, the superintendent, was pioneering a breakthrough treatment. His miraculous cure involved rooting out areas of "focal sepsis" where infectious bacteria lurked to poison the brain and instigate premature dementia. The sepsis was often located in the teeth. With the help of a team of dentists, Dr. Cotton extracted them. But the teeth were only one danger spot. Sepsis could also settle in the gut. Out came yards of bowels, sections of stomachs, parts of colons, lengths of urinary tracts. Eventually, he pulled out some of his own teeth and all of those of his wife and sons. In searching for the roots of one of his children's troubles, he performed an abdominal operation on him. Notably, Dr. Cotton did not work in secrecy. He loudly publicized his techniques and astonishing success rates (up to 85 percent) in curing the mad. He conceded that the mortality rates were not good. A third or more of the abdominal patients died. But death under these circumstances must be put in perspective, said Cotton. Expiry was "justified in chronic insane patients who would never leave the institution." In other words, these folks were already dead to begin with.

Dr. Cotton was a risk-taker and was praised by a number of luminaries, including John Kellogg of the famed Battle Creek Sanitarium and Hubert Work, president of the American Medical Association. A popular, progressive journal even reported that Cotton had finally replaced the old asylum with a modern hospital. He'd made a place complete with "young women nurses dressed in immaculate white, which harmonizes with the white interior, the snow-white bedding, the white iron beds and the other equipment. In place of the traditional dungeons or strong rooms and burly keepers, these nurses, with the aid of beams of sunlight which burst through the expansive windows, soothe, comfort, and win the excited newcomer back to a semblance of quietude."

Dr. Cotton *had* replaced the old dungeon—with a nightmare factory. Fortunately for most patients, Cotton's methods were never widely copied.[14]

MONSTERS AND REFORMERS

By the 1920s, asylums held more inmates than all the almshouses, prisons, and reformatories combined. Some superintendents pushed for dramatic eugenic solutions, as when Dr. G. Alder Blumer called for outlawing marriage of people with a family history of insanity and alcoholism in his 1903 Presidential Address to the American Medico-Psychological Association. Though Dr. Blumer later backed away from this view, the concept became law. States started restricting marriage to the legally sane in 1895, and later laws required the forced sterilization of the insane and epileptic. Asylums were one step ahead of the trend, with some superintendents mass-sterilizing their patients before any laws were drafted. The apogee of eugenic legislation came in 1924 with an immigration law that severely restricted the entrance of the most "degraded" races from Asia and southern and eastern Europe, along with the mentally handicapped. Hitler would praise America for its "advanced" thinking.[15]

While some reformers urged legislation to "solve" the insanity problem, others dreamed of saving the lost souls languishing inside asylums. What the mental hospital needed was its own *Uncle Tom's Cabin*. This is what Clifford Whittingham Beers set out to do in *A Mind That Found Itself*. The book proved a sensation, marking a bold new entry into the mass market: a muckraking asylum exposé written by an admittedly mad patient and openly endorsed by some of the most respected reformers and physicians.[16]

Mr. Beers was not the first accurately diagnosed person to report on asylum experiences with reform in mind. Admittedly troubled people had been telling madhouse stories from an insider's perspective and calling for justice in America since the nineteenth century. But *A Mind That Found Itself* was the first to find a huge market and create real-life changes. To tell his story, Beers finds it appropriate to use horror conventions. He provides frightful descriptions of the "little demon" who tortures him, the bizarre sense that the blood of his relatives is being hidden in his food, hallucinations that include a gorilla metamorphosing "strictly in accordance with Darwin's theory," and his belief that his relatives are actually imposters. There is even an assistant physician he dubs "Dr. Jekyll" for his seeming personality change from good to evil.[17]

Unlike many earlier memoirs, Beers's institutions are more hospitals than dungeons. They are "clean" and well-lit, though the doors only open one way and the beds are screwed to the floor. This is not to say that the gothic is absent. The attendants are "burly keepers" of "the brute-force type," and, once consigned to the violent ward, he finds himself in a "hole" with little light and air and no furniture at all. Beers fights the institution at first, battling attendants and getting restrained, and then suffers periods of shocking neglect. In the last section, he describes his return as "one risen from the dead."[18]

Beers wrote his book in order to change the world. It is a peculiar construction: a memoir that includes a description of the writing and then the initial promotion of the book itself. His aim, he states, is to produce a new *Uncle Tom's Cabin*. He ponders, "Why cannot a book be written which will free the helpless slaves of all creeds and colors confined to-day [*sic*] in the asylums and sanitariums throughout the world? That is, free them from unnecessary abuses to which they are now subjected." Beers would elevate them all, not just to freedom but back to their full (white) humanity. At a time when reformers were busy addressing social problems such as filthy factories and "white slavery" and the genetically unfit, Beers hit the right Progressive tone.

Beers's book would go on to sell out multiple editions and be cited repeatedly (including in a popular textbook on psychiatry). Working with his newly cultivated allies, he launched the National Committee for Mental Hygiene in 1909. The purpose of this organization was to *prevent* asylum incarceration. It would do this by scrubbing clean sick minds. The word "hygiene" captures current ideals of sterility and sanitation. Remove the filth, purify the mind, and the monsters would vanish.[19]

Beers had his *Uncle Tom's Cabin*, and, although it did not lead to the freeing of "the helpless slaves" of the asylum, it did create awareness and inspire lasting reforms, including an organization that would grow into a national patients' rights and mental health movement. Other asylum writers wanted their own *The Jungle*. Upton Sinclair's landmark fictionalization of the plight of packinghouse workers was a beautiful, horrific tale, best remembered for its galling descriptions of the meat house floor. It influenced the passage of legislation and became a standard-bearer for Progressive idealism. In 1920, Florence Seyler Thompson hoped to repeat the feat for the incarcerated insane. As George W. Galvin, MD, writes in her book's Preface, *A Thousand Faces* might do for the mad what *The Jungle* did for the Beef Trust and *The Turn of the Balance* for prisoners. The plot revolves around the tribulations of Harold Fitzgerald, a young man who has invented a machine that can solve the world's energy needs. His nemesis is the dastardly Dr. Sydney Phillips, a mind doctor who connives to have Fitzgerald committed in order to steal his invention. With the help of a villainous crew that includes a corrupt ex-senator and a wealthy faux "philanthropist," Dr. Phillips has Harold sent off to Allendale Asylum. Eventually Harold is freed, thanks to the exertions of his reporter friend, a beautiful female asylum doctor, and a crusading physician.[20]

Appropriate to the times, physiognomy inscribes the destiny of the players. Harold is a combination of "Irish and Swede" with a "beautiful Greek head." The villain's face similarly telescopes his purpose. If at first glance Dr. Phillips looks like a handsome fellow, a close inspection reveals the truth. His "brilliant, restless, black eyes . . . were set under the high arch of his brow just an eighth of an inch too near each other," his nose "remarkably like those of many Egyptian mummies." At one point, his face changes: "A look stole momentarily into Phillips' face from some secret recess of nature darker than his visage; a look not good to see, in countenance of man or of woman. It was a writhe, seen by a lightning flash, of some strange, pre-Adamite, reptilian monster wallowing in ooze and slime." His retrograde nature shows itself in a look, in the width of his eyes, in his nose, even in his hairdo.[21]

Like Dr. Phillips, the Allendale Asylum initially hides its maleficence. "Everything most cunningly conspired to suggest the peace, the beauty, the cheerfulness that were not." This is a familiar theme in asylum literature. The "head deputy" attendant is a brutal man with a "sugar-loaf head" and abnormally long arms that "suggested an ape's when hanging in repose—'a reg'lar go-rillar' one admiring attendant styled him." He instructs Don, the reporter who poses as a fellow employee, to beat patients in order to "get . . . work out of them."[22]

Defeating Dr. Phillips's evil plan takes up the last part of the book. Don goes undercover in the hospital under the tutelage of the muckraking Dr. George, discovers Harold, and frees him while reforming the hospital thanks to his shocking exposé. Dr. George's personal crusade receives its due in a chapter aptly titled "Dr. George Rends the Veil." Harold witnesses the doctor speaking, aptly, at revolutionary Faneuil Hall in Boston. Dr. George exhorts the crowd to see that "there were even worse slaves than the wage-earners in Massachusetts; men and women in places fouler than prisons, fettered by iron circumstance, crying out to be freed, and dying hideous deaths whose causes were hushed up." Yes, some of these are chronically mad and deserve "the very kindest treatment." But others are suffering from "forms of lunacy" that are "easily curable, under proper conditions." Worst of all, there are those who are sane when they enter but are made mad "from their surroundings, from their loss of liberty, and possibly from a contagion or infection of insanity." Dr. George then steers his argument into bolder currents, if contradicting his earlier point, stating, "Insanity certainly is, and has been for a long time, curable." What holds all of this together is the hellish asylum. The cure is to be found somewhere, just not here. The fact that the story pivots on a brilliant inventor of sturdy racial pedigree is telling. The author seems to be saying that the asylum is a place where unscrupulous social parasites (an evil alienist and his capitalist cronies) waylay bright, young producers (he includes "philosophers adjudged insane for proclaiming advanced ideas" as likely inmates). The asylum is an un-American bastion of an evil, aristocratic order. Cleaning it out serves the same social function as ending slavery, reforming prisons, and busting the trusts.[23]

A Thousand Faces speaks to Progressive-era urges to reform. The main villain, beyond the cabal of mind doctors and associated fat cats, is the Allendale Asylum. Its attendants and coarse nurses are underpaid and overworked, brutal hirelings of a brutal system set up along tyrannical lines. Violence and deception are necessary in order to maintain the production line of maniacs. The tragedy, Thompson makes abundantly clear, is that, while insanity is curable, inside the asylum only derangement is produced. The sane become "befouled, slavering, cursing, howling creatures," in short, "manufactured" monsters. The factory metaphor is heavy and obvious. Like the capitalists and foremen who discipline while simultaneously sucking the lifeblood out of their employees, at Allendale the attendants and nurses brutalize their charges to get them to work, driving them insane to boot. Thus, the asylum not only extracts labor, it generates the broken minds needed to sustain its operations. To heal patients and treat them gently would be to limit profits. Not unlike the uplifting exhortation made by the Socialist Party speaker at the end of *The Jungle*, Harold makes it clear that he will not rest until the asylum system is completely overthrown.[24]

And there is more. As Poe made certain in the *Maison de Santé*, the Allendale Asylum works on *all* of its inhabitants. It makes patients mad while subtly deranging the minds of the management and staff as well. The male attendants of Allendale, for instance, "had come from the logging camps of the north country, where they had been under rigid and often cruel dominion. They were ignorant, vicious, bigoted, superstitious." Once at the asylum, "They gloried in their newly-acquired power and their uniforms . . . They ate enormously, and got drunk as often as they dared. Then they became bestial

demons, finding in the Asylum secure means of gratifying every instinct of brutality and lust." Elsewhere they are described as "fiends."
The women attendants and nurses are monstrous too. They are "large
of stature, well-built, very strong, and coarse." The ward manager of
a woman's section, Margaret King, is actually described *as* a "monster." She is "drunk, actually intoxicated, with a malignant hatred of
her sex."[25]

The fate of Margaret King melodramatically proves the point. An
old patient named Mrs. Jones drops her water glass right at the feet
of Ms. King. In a rage, "King grabbed the old woman by the hair and
almost lifted her from her feet." The battle is on, the two struggling
like "wild beasts." Eventually, King's shirtwaist is torn away, "laying
bare the nurse's breasts." Here Mrs. Jones sees a birthmark, crying out,
"Margaret—my Margaret!" just before dying on the floor. Realizing the
woman she just killed is her long-lost mother, Nurse King takes the
nearest knife and plunges it "to the hilt into her neck." She falls dead
on top of her mom. The hospital reports the deaths as natural, and
"Thus the grave finally hid another tragedy of Allendale—one more, of
God knows how many in that place of unspeakable horrors."[26]

MONSTER MACHINES

A new technology added yet another layer of monstrosity to
the asylum. Moving pictures came into their own in the 1890s, as
inventor-entrepreneurs like the Lumière brothers and Thomas Edison
developed successful means for rapidly stringing together images.
Almost from the start, madhouses showed up in film.

In April 1904, American Mutoscope and Biograph Company released *The Escaped Lunatic*, in which a maniac dressed as Napoleon
flees his confinement. The film was highly successful, spawning a
knockoff by Edison's company, *Maniac Chase*. In this near shot-by-
shot remake, Napoleon escapes, struggles with one attendant, and
tosses him off a bridge. Later, he goes back to his cell of his own
accord. In 1906, Biograph released *Dr. Dippy's Sanitarium*, a longer (a
little under fifteen minutes) movie about an attendant's first day on
the job. The experience is not a positive one. He's accosted by a band
of patients who proceed to break out and then chase him across the
countryside. They roll him down a hill in a barrel, then into a stream,

and finally tie him Christ-like to the side of a barracks before launching knives at him. Fortunately, Dippy and staff save the day, distracting the patients with a picnic lunch. In 1913, director D. W. Griffith took audiences inside the asylum in *House of Darkness*. Here a "lunatic" escapes, gets his hands on a gun, and enters the doctor's nearby house. The doctor's daughter uses her piano skills to soothe him and he's recaptured, to end up whiling away his days on the porch listening to piano music. This asylum is a stately mansion surrounded by shade-dappled paths and trees. The patients definitely belong here: there's the violent escapee, as well as the woman who fawns over a fake baby and assorted other "Poor Unfortunates." Collins's *The Woman in White* showed up in a full-length feature in 1917, re-released in 1920 as *The Unfortunate Marriage*. This film begins with a madwoman in a white gown fleeing an asylum. We see her exiting a massive iron gate, a wild look in her eyes, long, black hair disheveled. The asylum is shown only fleetingly, mainly in scenes of a big but regular-looking building, in interior shots that don't convey anything out of the bourgeois ordinary, and on a bench in a pleasant outdoor scene. There is one sequence that suggests the role of the institution as quarantine for dangerous secrets. When Marian helps her sister, Lady Glyde, escape from the asylum (a consequence of the plot to replace her with the dead Anne Catherick), an iris-in wipe reveals a huge, stone wall filling the screen. Lady Glyde rappels down the side on a rope, her sister on the ground helping her. This daring fortress escape affirms the castle of madness theme, if briefly.[27]

In 1920, German director Robert Wiene brought to life cinema's first diabolical superintendent. *The Cabinet of Dr. Caligari* (*Das Cabinet des Dr. Caligari*) is a masterpiece of expressionism. Stylized, exaggerated structures and shadows emphasize the distorted reality of the narrator, Francis, who tells his tale of woe to an old man after they watch a ghostly Woman in White stroll by. He explains that this is Jane, his fiancée, and that the trials they have endured are stranger than the "spirits" that the old man was just relating to him. In a flashback, we see Francis go to the fair with his friend Alan, where they watch a stage show in which Dr. Caligari presents Cesare, a ghastly somnambulist. Cesare lives in a coffin-like box and comes out to deliver prophecies at Caligari's command. The previous night the town clerk, who mocked Caligari, was murdered. Now, at the fair, when Alan asks Cesare how long he will live, Cesare responds, "'Til the break of dawn." Alan duly dies, and everyone believes Cesare responsible. Hot on the trail of Cesare and Caligari, Francis and Jane become targets themselves, with Cesare breaking into Jane's room with a knife and carrying her off, leading the townsfolk on a wild chase before he releases her and then collapses. Dr. Caligari flees to a nearby insane asylum. Francis enters and is shown into the office of the director, who turns out to be none other than Caligari himself. While Caligari sleeps that night, Francis and the doctors break into his office and discover a secret shelf containing a book relating the story of an eighteenth-century Italian magician also named Caligari. This historic wizard similarly used a somnambulist named Cesare to commit murders. They also find a diary detailing how the director is pleased that a somnambulist was finally brought in, so that he might "become" Caligari. When they bring Cesare's body into the director's office, the director goes berserk and is placed in a straitjacket and thrown into a crazily painted cell with a huge, triangular door. The film returns us to the beginning with Francis telling the old man that the director, a "madman," never again left his cell. But then we discover the twist. Francis and the old man are *themselves* patients in the asylum. Jane is really another patient, as is Cesare. Jane believes she is a queen and so cannot wed Francis. Cesare leans against a wall picking at a clutch of flowers. Francis raves, "You all think that I'm insane! It isn't true—It's the director who's insane!!" Thus, the story inverts our expectations of the evil superintendent. Francis is here justifiably and only imagines that he is in a standard asylum plot. Finally, Caligari enters, the true director, no longer portrayed in ghoulish face paint. A group of attendants put Francis in the straitjacket and toss him into the cell. Caligari happily thinks that he can "cure" Francis now, since he realizes that Francis believes he is "that mystic Caligari." Here the film ends.[28]

The asylum in *The Cabinet of Dr. Caligari* suits the style of the film. It is exaggerated and geometrically distinctive. The courtyard where the inmates wander about has a floor painted like the sun's rays, with three large archways in the background and stairs leading into the building behind it, smaller arched windows spaced above. The patients include a woman with her doll "baby," a raving old man with a shock of white hair and matching beard, and a semi-catatonic

Woman in White, Jane. Though we learn that Francis is mad, Caligari would become the cinematic model for the evil, demented asylum master. Everything communicates his dark powers: his black suit, white gloves, tall hat, circular spectacles, ghastly makeup, and the streaks splintering his white hair. His servant, the living-dead Cesare, would also be archetypal, having numerous celluloid descendants, most famously Michael Myers in *Halloween*.

The Cabinet of Dr. Caligari offers itself to multiple interpretations. It can be decoded as a metaphor for Weimar Germany, as famously hypothesized by Siegfried Kracauer. The co-writer of the film, Hans Janowitz, had indeed been an officer in the German army in WWI and, explains David Skal, was "persecuted by a military psychiatrist, and forced to undergo various mental tests against his will." In America, the film shocked and impressed early reviewers. A *New York Times* writer said it is "sufficiently unlike anything ever done on screen before." A *Tribune* writer called it a "Psychopathic Film." For the *Los Angeles Times*, it was "Weirdly New." Warned Mae Tinee in the *Chicago Daily Tribune*, "Keep the children away from the thing!" The film's American impact can be witnessed in the shadowy and twisted imagery of the Universal horror cycle of the 1930s and noir shockers like Hitchcock's *Spellbound*. Caligari's descendants surely include Tod Browning's *Dracula* (1931) and Hannibal Lecter in *The Silence of the Lambs* (1991). But Caligari himself was prefigured. One can see his antecedents Count Fosco, Svengali, Stoker's Dracula, and even the villain of D. W. Griffith's 1909 short *The Criminal Hypnotist*. In that film, an evil hypnotist wonders if he can't make a woman do bad things under hypnosis that she wouldn't otherwise think about doing.[29]

The mad asylum ruler came into his own in American cinema in 1925 with *The Monster*, starring Lon Chaney. This movie, based on a successful Broadway play set in a sanitarium, owes much to Poe. In the story, a novice detective goes searching for a missing local and stumbles, literally, into a decrepit madhouse. The patients have taken over, led by the brilliant and insane Dr. Ziska (Chaney), who is conducting experiments in mind transference. The institution is pure gothic—the heroes find hidden rooms and doors, dark hallways, a skeleton, smoke, poison, and monstrous henchmen. In the basement, Dr. Ziska fiendishly works on his ultimate invention: a "death chair" that can transfer one person's "soul" into another's body.[30]

The Monster visualizes classic asylum themes. Dr. Ziska is brilliant but insane, wearing alternately an aristocratic garb or a white lab coat. His face is painted a deathly white, his name is foreign-sounding. His asylum inverts order with its confusing, diabolical interior juxtaposing a stately exterior. The mad are in charge; the good are imprisoned. Monstrous, racialized henchmen reinforce Ziska. One, a hulk named Caliban and played shirtless in blackface by Walter James, is a "servant" who is a "dumb," "poor creature." He seems to derive his look from popular Frankenstein imagery: big, mindless, and dangerous. Ziska's other crony foreshadows future film Igors. His name is literally Rigo, but this is not wordplay; there was no movie "Igor" yet (the first "Ygor" is in 1942's *The Ghost of Frankenstein*). James Whale's 1931 *Frankenstein* has a more "Igor"-like character in the servile, crazed hunchback Fritz. Regardless, Rigo is the prototypical, mad assistant. He also recalls Cesare, in that he is kept in a hypnotic state by the evil asylum master, to be awakened at will. Warns Dr. Ziska, "sometimes he gets out . . . does terrible things." Other asylum devices are formalized in this film. The hero must rescue a maiden in white. The monstrous superintendent works on his evil experiments in the subbasement. The place is topsy-turvy; not only does the architecture boggle the mind but Ziska's ultimate goal is to bend gender. He wants to put a man's mind into a woman's body. Poe recognized the farce of a world turned upside-down in "Dr. Tarr and Prof. Fether," and this movie certainly taps into this. Ziska flips from genteel man to lab-coated maniac, his "guests" are treated insanely, his henchmen are cartoonish, and his "death chair" spells death only for him, as it turns out.[31]

The Monster was a brick in the growing celluloid architecture of the movie madhouse. When the economy collapsed in 1929, new monsters arrived. These beasts were at once familiar and novel, and their relationship to the asylum addressed concerns about hubris, the proletarian masses, and social disintegration. Universal Pictures provided a kind of documentary of nightmares in its celebrated Depression horror cycle. Dracula, Frankenstein, the Mummy, and the Invisible Man all received iconic treatment, and all were dirty outsiders who vented their wrath on a society not living up to its promises. And the asylum informed all of them. Tod Browning's *Dracula* lorded over the asylum and controlled the deranged. Most of the final third of the movie takes place in Seward's madhouse. *The Mummy*, a beast awakened by Anglo-Saxon hubris, takes revenge upon the living by driving them insane. Speaking of the man who chanted the life-giving Scroll of Thoth, a character says, "He was laughing when your father found him. He died laughing. In a strait jacket." The potion that makes Claude Rains invisible in 1933's *The Invisible Man* also makes him into a homicidal maniac. Complained H. G. Wells of the cinematic adaptation of his book, "Instead of an Invisible Man, we have an Invisible Lunatic!"[32] The most famous Depression monster of all, however, is Frankenstein.

Mary Shelley's creation had made itself familiar in American culture long before 1931. In James Whale's famous 1931 film, the creature is depicted as a mad beast with a massive brow suggestive of evolutionary backwardness. He is monstrous by virtue of his degeneracy, but he is also a sad, pathetic beast. Like the incarcerated insane, he cannot lead a normal life, and he cannot help but cause others pain.[33]

Reflecting the science of the times, *Frankenstein* makes much hay of the brain. It begins when Dr. Victor Frankenstein's assistant Fritz tries to steal a brain for his boss. Fritz is clumsy and accidentally knocks over the jar containing the healthy brain and so instead takes the "abnormal brain of a typical criminal." Prior to this, Fritz watches as a doctor describes the abnormal brain to his medical class, describing its "scarcity of convolutions on the frontal lobe" and the "distinct degeneration of the middle frontal lobe." This corrupt organ will be the one that drives the monster. Following the logic of containment, Frankenstein's monster is kept in a dungeon chained to the wall, recalling abuses made public by Dorothea Dix. The chained beast, however, will escape.[34]

In the 1942 film *The Ghost of Frankenstein* (the fourth movie in the franchise), the monster is released from his tomb, goes on a rampage, and is captured by the police. The townsfolk don't know what to do with him, so they chain him up and call him a "madman." The creature's only chance of release is through the actions of Victor Frankenstein's second son, Ludwig. Ludwig's mad science credentials stem from the fact that he's an asylum doctor who specializes in taking out the brains of the insane, fixing them, and then putting them back inside the skull. This follows the logic of the first film, which tells us that brain deformities cause criminality. But logic has little to do with

The Ghost of Frankenstein. Ludwig tries to put his deceased doctor-friend's brain in the monster's head, while Ygor (Bela Lugosi) wants to put his own brain in the creature, giving him a new lease on life. The monster himself, played zombie-like by Lon Chaney, Jr., desires the brain of a little girl he has befriended. Ygor ends up winning this lunatic lottery with Ludwig's duplicitous assistant doing his brain transfer. Sadly, the Ygor-brained Frankenstein loses his sight, as his blood type differs from the monster's. He is eventually killed, though, like in every other Frankenstein picture, he'll rise again. Capitalizing on fears of the congenitally mad getting loose and then having to be pursued by unhinged mind doctors, *The Ghost of Frankenstein* offers an early model of a formula that would be replayed many times.[35]

As the Universal cycle ground on, ridiculousness increased, reaching its pinnacle with *House of Frankenstein* (1944). This film includes plots to transfer brains into and out of: the Wolf Man, Frankenstein, the Hunchback, and some assistants.[36]

A more sophisticated humorous take on the monstrous asylum, *Arsenic and Old Lace* (shot in 1941 but released in 1944) features an escapee named Jonathan Brewster who looks a lot like Boris Karloff's Frankenstein. In the stage play, Karloff actually played Brewster. In the movie, Karloff was unable to appear (he was busy doing the play on Broadway) so a look-alike played the look-alike. The plot is that an old, genteel American family has devolved into a pair of homicidal maniac aunts and a nephew who thinks he's Teddy Roosevelt. The aunts "mercifully" murder old men who board at their house and the nephew buries the bodies, believing they are victims of yellow fever as he digs the Panama Canal in the basement. When Teddy's "normal" brother Mortimer discovers this, he tries to get Teddy sent to Happydale Sanitarium, where he can take the fall for the murders without getting the death penalty. The hijinks build when another brother, the aforementioned Jonathan Brewster, appears. He is a psychopath, having recently escaped from a prison for the "criminally insane." His unstable plastic surgeon, who accompanies him, has unfortunately given him the appearance of Frankenstein in a disguise effort. The juxtaposition of Happydale, the "good" asylum for the innocuous Teddy, and the prison asylum where the Frankenstein character resides, tells us something about the process of monsterization. The dream of asylum safety and shelter was not entirely dead; it was important that the degenerate be quarantined in oubliettes suitable to their monstrosity. In the end, the aunts and Teddy wind up in Happydale and Jonathan is carted back to the bad asylum. The family's devolution is terminated when we discover that Mortimer is, in fact, really the cook's son. His blood is not tainted.[37]

Arsenic and Old Lace makes fun of the madhouse monster, a creature born at the start of asylum fiction and given new life in Progressive America. Unchained and loosed upon the world, the hereditarily insane beast reiterated deep fears of democratic failure and social upheaval. In early twentieth-century America, a WASP middle class beset by "alien" immigrants, "degenerate" criminals, and growing numbers of institutionalized insane invited the formulation of new scientific explanations and technologies of control. Virtues of mental hygiene and genetic purity permeated a discourse of madness and captivity. Control over self and others married in the machinery of reform. Incarceration proved as attractive as it was elusive.

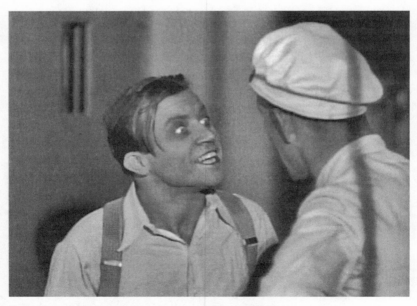

Renfield speaks with an asylum attendant in *Dracula* (1931)

CHAPTER 4

FREUDIAN RESCUES

> Dr. Riggs wasted no time searching for the cause of my slipping
> into such a slough but offered me tools to help pull myself out . . .
> I followed the schedule prescribed, studied the lessons assigned,
> worked in the shop, walked, exercised, rested, played, mixed. His
> methods worked. No cure could have been more permanent. There
> has been no similar illness since.
>
> —Olive Higgins Prouty, *Pencil Shavings* (1961)

Sigmund Freud has all the makings of a classic American villain. He's foreign, aristocratic, domineering, mesmeric, surveilling, and he hates our country. An image that comes to mind is him looking sternly at us, cigar wielded as if to emphasize a judgment he is about to make.[1]

Yet Freud is also heroic. He articulates certain American ideals. He is bold and ambitious, a searcher of new frontiers, and a striving professional. One might call him a psychological entrepreneur, having invented a brand-new therapeutic technique. Psychoanalysis promised to unlock the shackles holding us back from our true potential. This fit with America's long-standing, self-help culture. Though his writing could be impenetrable, his ideas were accessible. For the pop culture asylum, Freud meant something specific. He would help break patients, and doctors, out.[2]

Freud initiated a new-model asylum superintendent. The stereotypical psychoanalyst did not impose his Svengalian will but rather held up a mirror for us to see our flaws. His authority mimicked that of the expanding consumer market, silently interpreting subconscious desires in order to produce real-world satisfactions.

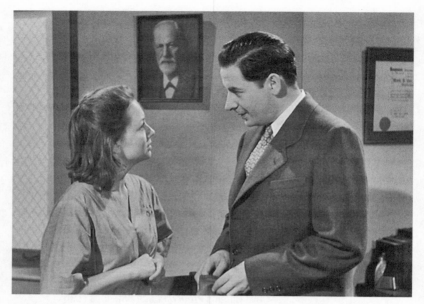

Dr. Kik speaks with Virginia in his office under a watchful portrait of Freud in *The Snake Pit* (1948)

Freudians believed that they could cure a wide variety of illnesses, even schizophrenia. They hoped to empty the asylums without resorting to drastic treatments, pushing back against hopeless, hereditarian diagnoses. Recalled one asylum doctor, in the mid-century, there existed an "almost blind faith in psychoanalysis . . . Those of us who were true believers 'knew' that a sufficiently deep analysis would cure any mental illness." But there was a price. Freudian observation became self-observation. The nightmare asylum, and the superintendent, became internalized.[3]

SHADOWS AND LIGHT DURING THE GREAT DEPRESSION

In the final chapter of his 1957 memoir *Days of the Phoenix*, influential literary critic and Freudian Van Wyck Brooks connected his mental breakdown and commitment with the economic cataclysm that nearly wrecked America. Titled "A Season in Hell," he tells us that the Great Depression was a time of "disillusion and despair" gated with the words "Abandon hope, all ye who enter here." Brooks experienced his own season in hell, becoming a resident in several "houses of the dead," where friends and family treated you as though "you had actually arrived in the land of shades." Similarly, in the 1950 memoir *Snake Pit Attendant*, the anonymous attendant reflects that "the events of 1929 made America insanity-conscious. Normal and healthy men suddenly took to leaping out of high office buildings, gulping gas, and weeping like children. Others, with less brains—or more perhaps—repaired to private sanitariums or state institutions, depending upon the value of their stocks or the size of their bank accounts. It was a rare family indeed that did not have at least one member in Bedlam."[4]

The Great Depression is an apt place to situate Freud's takeover of the asylum. While sitting down with an analyst for hours on end, week in and week out, was not very practical for most inmates, Freudians did enter the high walls. The massive Manhattan State Hospital, for instance, had a "dedicated psychoanalytic clinic" by 1927. Influential doctors like Harry Stack Sullivan and Frieda Fromm-Reichmann advocated analysis as a means of resolving serious psychoses, and most psychiatrists contended with his theories on some level. One driving factor in the takeover was the fact that mental hospitals were getting worse.[5]

Overcrowding had become a serious issue. On average, institutions operated at 10 percent overcapacity, but, as Gerald N. Grob notes, this does not capture the brutal reality of regional variation. Three states in 1938 were above 40 percent overcapacity, ten others over 22 percent. As the Depression set in, public investments declined, affecting new construction, facility upkeep, and hiring. In other words, institutions got less effective and scarier looking.[6]

The asylum was changing in other ways as well. The old idea of shocking patients back to reality was making a comeback, thanks to new biological rationales. One technique involved injecting "horse serum" into the veins. This fever-inducing method began in the 1910s, and it was tried on Zelda Fitzgerald in the 1930s, but it did not produce lasting, positive results. More common was insulin coma therapy, in which doctors pumped patients with insulin to induce a series of blackouts. A sugar solution then pulled them back into consciousness. Occasionally, patients died. Another shock therapy involved the injection of the drug Metrazol, which produced massive, convulsive seizures. The theory behind this was that schizophrenia could not coexist with epilepsy. In 1938, electroconvulsive therapy was introduced, it being portrayed as a gentler way of inducing convulsion. Before sedatives came into the picture, patients would experience extreme, physical reactions to ECT, often incurring compression fractures of the spine and dislocated jaws. But shock treatments were neither malicious nor haphazard. They were carefully planned and vigorously discussed. Contemporary evidence indicated that they improved the lives of many patients. But many Freudians, in public at least, opposed shock therapies on the account that they did not deal with the "real" underlying issues that arose from traumatic, childhood experiences.[7]

Life inside the mental hospital changed too, in ways congruent with the evolution of industrial labor. There was increased regimentation and routine, if the asylum memoirs are at all indicative. Schedules were closely monitored, including toilet access; medications were handed out with regularity and precision. Modern psychology and psychoanalysis techniques often combined with interventions such as the "cold pack" and hydrotherapy. The cold pack (also known as "wet pack," "the sheet," or simply "pack") involved wrapping patients tightly in cold, wet sheets and blankets, sometimes with alternating hot and cold bags placed at the head and feet. This technique could have an insidious disciplinary quality. Most likely the first film representation came in the bizarre 1922 Harry Houdini picture, *The Man From Beyond*. Here, the great escape artist plays a man frozen in a block of ice for a century and then thawed out in modern times. When he goes wild after finding a reincarnation of the girl he loves, he's thrown into a padded cell, wrapped in sheets, and doused with water from a shower above. An intertitle describes it as "a little treatment they had back in the dark ages" that the medical establishment "wouldn't stand" for today. Houdini escapes, of course.[8]

Houdini aside, a new dream of escape emerged as Freudianism ascended. This was the escape effected after "solving" one's illness through talk therapy. Pop culture offered plenty of examples. In the 1932 detective procedural *One Drop of Blood* by Anne Austin, special investigator James "Bonnie" Dundee is trying to solve a murder at the upscale Mayfield Sanitarium. The murder weapon is a small statue of a discus thrower, and the victim is the esteemed psychiatrist Dr.

Koenig. Early on, Dundee figures out that the murderer is no lunatic, but rather a cool, rational killer, based on the orderliness of the
crime scene. The trail eventually leads to a nefarious plot by the business manager, Baldwin, who is trying to move in on the profits with
the help of an evil psychiatrist from California. Baldwin has already
sent one rich wife to a madhouse (using a rigged Ouija board) and, at
Mayfield, takes advantage of the opportunity for "fraud in a private
institution for the treatment of mental diseases." In other words, an
evil capitalist is at fault, one who is trying to subvert a hospital from
place of healing to machine for graft. This Depression-friendly narrative shifts the classic burden of evil from the institution to greedy
managers.[9]

Mayfield Sanitarium is more Freudian paradise than monster factory. Explains a District Attorney,

> Only a small minority of the patients have been "committed"—
> that is, adjudged insane in court. Those are in a locked ward, of
> course. Then there's quite a large group of more or less mild psy-
> chopathic cases, voluntary patients—cases of senility, incipient
> paresis, epilepsy, manic depression, chronic alcoholism, amne-
> sia, aphasia, and victims of all sorts of complexes, psychoses and
> neuroses, harmful, usually, to no one but themselves. In addition,
> the place has become the most fashionable "rest cure" and con-
> valescent home in the state. Society women go there to indulge in
> "nervous prostration" or the luxury of being psychoanalyzed, and
> rich men to be "boiled out" after a prolonged spree.

Here is a place of recovery not imprisonment, which makes use of
the latest scientific principles and subtly references the benefits of
analysis for those who can pay. Note that "society women" get the expensive, time consuming process of psychoanalysis. At one point, a
female patient remarks that "complex" is "a very popular word here."
In this regard, a "girl doctor" who works here takes on significance.
As Eli Zaretsky and others point out, women were overrepresented
as analysands and followers of Freud, and female psychoanalysts ac-
counted for much of the growth of the profession. Analysts like Helene
Deutsch and Karen Horney became famous, fighting back against
simplistic Freudian arguments such as the "castration complex."

Reflecting the times, in *One Drop of Blood*, an attractive female doctor plays both the object of Dundee's adoration and establishes herself as an intelligent, observant physician.[10]

Another genre, the alcoholic's memoir, also illuminates the nascent Freudian asylum. Only a small portion of the institutionalized were in for "dipsomania," as chronic alcoholism was called, so these perspectives do not qualify as "typical." However, once inside and dried out, alcoholics offered a unique perspective apparently unmediated by derangement or investigative agenda. Notably, they were often sympathetic, understanding that in getting them off the bottle, institutions had saved their lives.

In a classic of this genre, *Behind the Door of Delusion* (1932), newspaper editor Marion Marle Woodson writes as "Inmate Ward 8." The premise is that we have gotten the asylum all wrong. They are not dungeons for the railroaded but are residences for troubled souls who *need* to be there. Though, once inside, their lives are still horrible, not because of the torture meted by bad attendants and mad doctors, but rather by the loneliness of the long stays. Woodson goes to great lengths to dispel the illusions accrued in a century of gothic writing. The straitjacket is not like the "the Spanish Inquisition" but rather "only a device to protect the patient from himself." Women attendants are not "of the brawny, 'fishwife' type" but are of normal size. The attendants don't use physical violence so much as "mental superiority, and a manner and tone of voice which I believe are acquired only through experience in handling the insane." Though there is some force, it is humanely applied to control the out-of-control with Woodson writing, "necessary physical restraint of patients must not be confused with brutality."[11]

Evidence of popular misconception is ghoulishly manifested in the visitors who come just "to be shocked, and are disappointed if they are not." He sarcastically reports, "taxpayers, sir, are entitled to free admission to any of the entertainments paid for out of 'our money.' And chief among the legitimate amusements provided by the state through the medium of 'our money' is a trip through the insane asylum, with the creepy thrills incident hereto." The author also critiques standard psychiatric pretensions to understand mental illness. Doctors do not "have some mysterious knowledge of how to treat the brain to overcome insanity." All they can do is to try to "remove the physical cause" of the illness and then let nature's "recuperative forces" do their work.[12]

This is hardly the damning reportage of a Bly or Beers. The difference seems to be connected to the Freudian revolution. For instance, the Viennese master apparently informs Woodson's reaction to his incarceration. He worries about "what sort of complex I am acquiring. I find myself snappish with the other patients quite often. I associate with them less and less . . . Psychoanalysts call that state of mind a dread complex or dread neurosis, and hint, encouragingly, that the fellow who gives way to it is teeter-tottering at the top of a steep hill down which a greased slide leads straight to paranoia." In other words, Freud helps him to diagnose a potential pitfall on the road to wellness. He speaks of "obsessionary recurrent periods of craving" for alcohol, psychoanalytically explaining what later doctors would attribute to physical addiction. Yet like many of his contemporaries, he tempers his Freudianism with humor and skepticism. When an old patient yells out in the middle of the night, a physician says it is "a fear complex. He can't help it." But he notes that the attendants "have a different opinion. 'Just pure cussedness,' is their verdict."[13]

Perhaps the most telling influence of Freud in this asylum relates to the changing notion of heredity. Woodson notes that, presently, doctors are "sharply divided on the question of what forms of insanity are the result of heredity." This represents a change from when "practically all physicians were agreed that the vast majority of insanity cases were the result of heredity." He does not state explicitly the cause of the change, but he indicates that physicians believe now that most mental illness is triggered by "organic physical ailments, social or other germ diseases, injuries, and a variety of other causes, including nervous shock or tension" as well as "so-called shell shock or . . . worry." This commingling of psychological and physical causes reflects the sea of changes underway.

Three years after *Behind the Door of Delusion*, popular writer William Seabrook published his memoir of his time at Bloomingdale Hospital. The book is titled *Asylum*, but, like Woodson, Seabrook quickly disabuses us of its gothic signifiers.

They now call it a "mental hospital," as all such places do—but asylum is still what everybody knows it is, and it proved so truly an "asylum" for me that I have a friendly feeling for the good old word. Asylum from the storm; sanctuary; refuge. That's what the dictionary says the word still means, primarily. That's what it meant to me. That's why I don't mind using it. That's why I call this book *Asylum*.

Even more so than Woodson, Seabrook makes the case that this is a place of healing not horror. Attendants are not brutal but work hard to restrain the deranged without the aid of muffs or cuffs. The superintendent "turned out when you got to know him to be human." There are no "hidden padded cells, dungeons or torture chambers." Nobody is here because they've been framed. There is no "Count of Monte Cristo, no heirs or heiresses in chains, no skeletons in closets." The patients are here because they need to be here. Because they have lost control.[14]

A gentle conception of warranted control is at the heart of Seabrook's lively and well-written narrative. Once in Bloomingdale, he is reduced to a child's state, sent to a room with no lock and with the light always on, given warm milk to drink and crackers to eat. He's escorted about to various activities, spoken to softly, and bathed regularly. As he sums up, "So here I was, an inmate of this extraordinary locked-and-barred kindergarten, for the same good reason as the rest. We were a bunch of grown men, most of us mature, who had lost control of ourselves in one way or another and who had to be controlled by others . . . that is, treated like a bunch of children . . . that is, put back in the nursery."

This reduction of liberty is not insidious but necessary. Everything we think is mistaken, not because the inmates are *not* unfree, but rather because they have forfeited their *right* to be free. This harkens back to Benjamin Rush's paradoxical argument for the asylum to be a place of total control for the recovery of liberty. He updates Rush's dream by demonstrating that the old nightmares are gone. Solitary confinement, physical abuse, and padded cells are now safely in the past. Today's doctors provide picnics, walks, dances, and baths. They use psychoanalysis too, though he notes that it is "just one useful instrument among many."[15]

Seabrook's asylum experience is a decisively *modern* one. Modern novels played with perspective and upended literary conventions such as linearity and realism. They reflected the disorientation of modern life and undermined the conceit of certainty. In Seabrook's narrative, an ironic, playful style jars loose the old gothic madhouse tone and projects a less certain, though optimistic future. Seabrook winds up cured, as do many other patients. And he's as surprised as anyone. Freudianism has helped him see that madness is not a hereditary taint but rather a temporary accident that can be fixed. His description of the notorious "pack" tells it all. While horrifying in its capacity to incapacitate, Seabrook settles into his cold pack and is "soon as peaceful as a four-month fetus." His doctor actually has to stop this treatment for fear it will become "another habit, like dope, veronal or whiskey." Infantile regression threatens to create a new neurotic fixation. This is framed as a humorous anecdote and it fits since "a good deal of the stuff that goes on in such an institution *is* funny, de facto, whether it ought to be or not, and that any picture which leaves it out would be sentimental buncombe." His publisher fights him on this angle. Can all his reports be true? *Yes.* To the point where fact meets fiction: "This sounds like cheap vaudeville, but the Napoleon hallucination is one of the commonest. We had three Napoleons."[16]

Only at one point in the book does Seabrook give us a villain. But Dr. Quigley's crime is merely that he is a "floorwalker-managerial type, equipped with petty but sufficient delegated authority over patients and attendants alike. So that he was more manager, more supervising boss than doctor, and the nature of his job was such that he would perhaps inevitably have been unpopular." Dr. Quigley exerts his power by refusing Seabrook prunes and by treating him inconsiderately. But in the end, Seabrook admits that even Quigley isn't so bad. His mild nemesis serves only to highlight Seabrook's message of safe, Freudian passage back to health.[17]

SMALL TOWNS AND SEA VOYAGES

While the Freudian asylum did not vanquish the gothic dungeon or the factory of monsters, it marked a transition toward a much different place. As Foucault notes, though Freud would "deliver the patient from the existence of the asylum," he "regrouped [the asylum's] powers, [and] extended them to the maximum by uniting them in the doctor's hands." By removing the hereditary, biological explanations for mental illness, the Freudian turn helped to undermine the institutional focus of psychiatry and facilitated the rise of psychopharmacology and self-diagnosis. Yet Freud was no mere liberator. Even in positive portrayals, the great man's suspect foreignness and mind control powers reared up. For example, the heroic Freudian in *The Snake Pit* is called "Dr. Kik," his real name being unpronounceable and "foreign." In the 1940s, a number of films and books gave us paradoxical shrinks who were at once intimidating and sympathetic, brilliant and inaccessible, distant and welcoming.[18]

Henry Bellamann's bestseller *Kings Row* (1940) offers a snapshot of the contradictions. The setting is Kings Row, a "good, clean town. A good town to live in, and a good place to raise your children." Just east of town is "the State Asylum for the Insane" with its "many wings" and "ample grounds." This asylum is not frightening. "At night, with its hundreds of windows gleaming through the high trees, it had a palatial and festive air." But all is not as it seems. The opening portrait practically begs us to peel away the surface to uncover what lurks beneath.[19]

The two protagonists in *Kings Row* are Parris Mitchell and Drake McHugh. Parris is an introverted intellectual raised by his German aunt, and he travels to Europe to become a psychiatrist. Drake is an all-American kid who wants to enjoy his life and find economic success. Both will face shattering setbacks at the hands of older men, who happen to be doctors. Dr. Tower is a brilliant recluse who lives with his daughter and a mad wife whom he confines. He's something of a phantom, a man who "gave the contradictory impression of being dead to the world about him but keenly—even painfully—aware of some other world inside." Tower becomes a mentor to Parris and teaches him about the science of the mind. His cynical, worldly philosophy reinforces the Freudian message that we delude ourselves in imagining we are on the course of civilized progress. Says Tower,

> Everybody is busy trying to spot the shining goal toward which we must be tending. If we are evolving, it must be toward something. Just there, my guess is, they are mistaken. We aren't going anywhere at all. It's hard for us to believe that we are simply adjusting. Heaven knows that's a noble enough end, and a perfectly

ample excuse and reason for everything. But the whole structure of the human mind is so damned flimsy and weak that it has to have a framework. Since there isn't any, the mind invents one—something to hold on to, to lean on, something to keep itself from spilling all over like milk poured out of a glass. Usually, it invents a cage for itself.

Rather than making a grand future for the boy, Tower poisons his daughter (and earlier, his insane wife), and then shoots himself. Reading Tower's journal, Parris discovers that his mentor had gone completely mad and had committed incest.[20]

Drake's nemesis is Dr. Gordon, the town physician. When Drake is injured in a railyard accident, Gordon amputates both of his legs. The operation is unnecessary, but Gordon is a sadist and he doesn't approve of his daughter's love for Drake. When Louise threatens to "out" her dad as a monster, he threatens a one-way trip to the asylum. He intones, "I have only to call Dr. Nolan on the telephone there in the hall, and have you in a cell—behind bars—in one hour."[21]

In the end, both Parris and Drake wind up picking up the pieces of their lives. Drake recovers with the help of the love of a working-class girl, and Parris becomes a mind doctor working at the town asylum. The message, it seems, is that the old Victorian world and the small-town life it extolls is not all it's cracked up to be. The town is full of malicious gossips, and the respected doctors endanger the young generation. In the face of the old resistances, youth must forge its own path.

The state hospital in *Kings Row* is a place where the irrational and inconvenient are sent away for the good of social harmony. For instance, it is repeatedly suggested that Benny Singer, a developmentally disabled Jewish boy, should be committed. He's called the "town idiot" and teased remorselessly until he finally shoots into a gang of toughs and kills two. For this, he is hanged. Parris, being unable to convince his colleagues that Benny is not mentally responsible, helplessly has to stand aside. Another person, the eccentric Lucy Carr, lost her mind when her husband went broke, and she was sent away to an asylum a few times. Now, she lives at home under the care of her husband. She outfits herself in garish dresses with "innumerable strings of beads" around her neck and "many cheap rings" on her "deformed-looking, helpless little hands." Folks think she should be locked away for good. Queries the sage Colonel Skeffington, "Did you ever notice . . . how everybody's always ready to send somebody else to the asylum? It's a fact. First thing occurs to them." He goes on, "It's a bad thing to have a lunatic asylum in town. Keeps it in everybody's mind. I think a lot of people go crazy just because the building stands out there at the end of Federal Street. It's too confounded convenient." For Benny and Lucy, the asylum provides no sanctuary. This is unfortunate, because, as Parris learns on returning from his psychiatric schooling in Europe, "the 'asylum,' as Kings Row continued to call the State Hospital," is a true place of healing. He is astonished "how superior all American equipment was. The scrupulous hygiene, the smooth efficiency in all mechanical and material phases of administration." The only problem is the inferior staff, who are here for political rather than meritocratic reasons. The issue boils down not to the institution but to fixable issues of personnel and budgets.[22]

Both in the asylum and out of it, Parris uses Freudian treatments. He is a searcher of hidden truths beneath "neurotic" behaviors, and he patterns his inquiry, and indeed his whole mien, after Freud. He's distant and authoritative; he grows up speaking with a European accent; he learns his craft in Vienna; he privileges talk over drugs; and his opinions are irreverent, brilliant, and clearly designed to cut through superstitious views of madness. At one point, he references Freud's famous arguments about civilization as a repressive reaction to sexual aggressions and the death drive. He tells a local minister that the State Hospital is a "monument of the failure of man to withstand the pressures of the civilization he has himself created." Not only does Freudian discourse influence Bellamann's characters, it also influenced the reader's expectations. For many, Freud meant sex, sex, sex. Noted one reviewer, Kings Row featured a "whole horde of half-witted, sensual creatures preoccupied with sex."[23]

Kings Row was a success and quickly found its way onto the screen, making a star of the young actor named Ronald Reagan who played Drake McHugh. Reagan's heart-wrenching recognition of his double amputation—"Where's the rest of me?!"—would remain a cultural touchstone and serve as the title of one of his memoirs. The scandalous issues in the book—most prominently incest—had to be dealt with by the screenwriters in the face of the Production Code.

In the movie, Dr. Tower kills his daughter because he knows she has "dementia praecox." The murder then is not about incest but about saving Parris from a life with a madwoman, as Tower himself has endured. Thus does the film keep Freud in mind even when it changes the plot, implicitly making a point Freud himself might have made. Schizophrenia cannot be treated by the talking cure.[24]

As Bellamann's book became a hit, it became clear that he was writing about a real place, his hometown of Fulton, Missouri. This happened to be the home of the Fulton State Hospital. Like in the fictitious Kings Row, the asylum at Fulton provided a major source of town revenue while simultaneously generating local concern and even embarrassment. One of the subplots of the book has Parris and Drake making money by selling off asylum land to the state. They are innocent of insider dealings, but this mirrored popular Fulton rumors about asylum doctors profiteering in this manner. The wider reading public would have been unaware of this connection. Its importance is that it shows that Bellamann wrote what he knew. The asylum represented a politically ensconced source of revenue, taxation, and local legend.[25]

In *Kings Row,* the asylum plays an ambivalent role. It is a place where heroic Freudians heal the minds of the troubled, but it's also a source of fear ("I was always afraid of that asylum—of being locked away forever," ruminates one resident; "it must be a terrible place to live," says another) and subject to unsavory political pressures. In another novel that also became a hit film, *Now, Voyager,* a private asylum serves a more positive Freudian function.[26]

Olive Higgins Prouty was an established writer with a major hit, *Stella Dallas,* under her belt when she published *Now, Voyager* in 1941. The third in a trilogy about the Vale family, the book sold relatively well, though it moved only half the number of units as her previous book, *Lisa Vale.* When Warner Brothers adapted *Now, Voyager* for the screen, however, it struck gold. The studio's fourth-highest grosser of 1942, *Now, Voyager* earned Bette Davis her fourth Best Actress nomination in four years (she lost to Greer Garson), as well as a Best Supporting Actress nomination for Gladys Cooper who portrayed her tyrannical mom.[27]

Now, Voyager is a melodramatic love story about a woman named Charlotte Vale. She lives under the thumb of her domineering mom, "one of the last of the old Victorian matriarchs in existence, still ruling her family with a rod of iron." Driven to an emotional collapse, Charlotte goes to the Cascade Sanatorium, a gentle institution run by the wise Dr. Jaquith. Here, Jaquith helps Charlotte discover her inner strength, encouraging her to voyage across the Atlantic. Onboard the ship, she finds love with a married man, Jerry Durrance, and after her return to Boston, she finally breaks free of her mother's control. Mom does not handle the loss well. She has a fit and soon drops dead. Vale goes on to become a surrogate mother to Jerry's daughter, whom she discovers on a friendly visit to Cascade. The story begins aboard the ship and uses the technique of flashback to fill out the background.[28]

Prouty described the novel as one about a "spinster who finally finds escape from the domination of her mother through doors opened by a nervous breakdown." The novel and film rely on cultural traditions of the hysterical woman saved by the strong and masterly male, the power of love, and, in deference to Freud, the capacity of analysis to liberate. Dr. Jaquith first comes across a bit off-putting, "with that brusque manner of his, but kindly, in spite of the frequent interpolations of blunt humor." He tells Charlotte that she has "free-will" and is the captain of her own life. Charlotte, thus, becomes self-assured and independent, discovering that she does not need a man to be complete. Her breakdown is not a mere product of her gender either. (Her love interest Jerry has also had one.) Rather, it is the consequence of the hurtful burdens of the old world of domestic tyranny. Mother tells Charlotte to be submissive and peevish, ideals that make little sense to the modern age. By finding her freewill, Charlotte masters herself and breaks Mother's hold over her. Dr. Jaquith (who gets more lines in the film version at the request of actor Claude Rains) is more of a guru than a physician. He helps Charlotte free herself and find her own voice.[29]

Now, Voyager offers a positive mental institution in Cascade Sanatorium. The film makes a point of having the cruel mother voice popular concerns about institutions so as to let the wise psychiatrist knock them down. When Charlotte's sister Lisa recommends that she visit Cascade, Mother scoffs, "Probably one of those places with a high wire fence and yowling inmates." Dr. Jaquith placidly corrects her, "Well, I wouldn't want anyone to have that mistaken notion. Cascade is just a place in the country. People come there when they're tired.

You go to the seashore—they come here." Mom then attacks "psychiatry," asking her daughter if the "very word" does not "fill you with shame." Jaquith, patiently again, corrects, "There's nothing shameful in my work—or frightening, or anything else. It's very simple, really, what I try to do. [directs the script: '(A quiet, direct appeal to Charlotte.)'] People walk along a road. They come to a fork in the road. They are confused, they don't know which way to take. I just put up a signpost: not that way, this way."[30]

Trussed in a stiff nineteenth-century dress with lace at her throat and played with demonic coldness by Gladys Cooper, Mother represents the dead hand of Victorian America. Her aristocratic tone (Cooper, appropriately, is British) condescends and belittles. In the novel, Prouty paints Mother as opposing the "independence" that Charlotte craves. She criticizes her daughter's clothing, makeup, and post-voyage inclination to do what she likes. When Charlotte tries to tell her that Jaquith says independence merely means "reliance upon one's own will and judgement," Mother goes after that "snake-in-the-grass." She asserts she has no use for "those new-fangled alienists and psychoanalysts." Charlotte corrects her. Jaquith is a "psychiatrist." She emphasizes his medical bona fides, contrasting him not only with the old gothic nightmare of institutional quackery but also with the simplistic pop-Freudianism that so many enlightened doctors sought to distance themselves from. Her internal dialogue reinforces his power: *"I see what Doctor Jaquith means now! She cannot hurt me. She's just a little shrunken old lady who loves authority with only her money to wield it. She has no power over my integrity and my decisions. I see now! I see!"* The good doctor and his asylum have given Charlotte the strength to break free from her neurotic mother. He empowers her, guiding her gently to the endgame of Freudian analysis—the freeing moment of catharsis.[31]

Like Bellamann, Prouty based her asylum on a real place. Cascade is a version of the Austen Riggs Center in Massachusetts. Prouty had once suffered an emotional collapse and had stayed here. As she explains in her memoir *Pencil Shavings*, "The theme of *Now, Voyager* is a woman's nervous breakdown and her recovery. Much of the action takes place in a sanitarium similar to the Riggs Foundation in Stockbridge and one of the important roles is that of the doctor in charge." In the book, Cascade is described as a bucolic place, nestled

amid apple orchards, woods, pastures, and three brooks that join
to create a waterfall. The film plays a pleasant orchestral score over
sunlit establishing shots, a decided break from most previous asylum
movies. Austen Riggs was similarly stately and pleasant. Like Charlotte, Prouty's own upbringing was very strict and "Victorian," and her
mother controlled her with guilt, stopping her from heading to New
York after college. The Austen Riggs sanitarium, with its kindly superintendent, freed Prouty to see her writing as a vocation apart from her
family duties. Dr. Jaquith similarly empowers Charlotte by showing
her it is okay to do what you want and to develop as a person.[32]

Olive Higgins Prouty did not push psychoanalysis *per se* in her
book. However, Prouty's Jaquith clearly uses the psychoanalytic talk
therapy and is versed in Freud and not afraid to show it.[33] In reality,
few psychiatrists were trained psychoanalysts, despite the fact that
Freudian theory percolated through the profession quite thoroughly
by 1941. And while Prouty wrote that she had never been psychoanalyzed, her memoirs include lots of references to Freud and Freudian
interpretations, even if given with a grain of salt. This fits with the
broader culture. Americans did not trip over themselves to genuflect
at Freud's feet, though his ideas had, by the forties, become common
sense.[34]

THE FIRST AUTHENTIC FILM STUDY
OF A MENTAL HOSPITAL

As Freudianism rose in public esteem, films and popular books cre-
atively combined the new science with older tropes of asylum imprisonment. In Alfred Hitchcock's *Spellbound* (1945), for example, a
gothic asylum is the setting for a battle between a "good" psychiatrist,
played by Ingrid Bergman, and a "bad" one who is trying to cover up
a murder. Thanks to Bergman's command of Freudian dream therapy,
she uncovers the plot, saves her beau, and ultimately inspires the bad
man to kill himself. The message is that psychoanalysis works, but it
also gives power that can be wielded for evil.[35]

Similarly, in *Strange Illusion* (1945), a good doctor named Dr. Vin-
cent (who happens to teach psychology) helps a young man named
Paul battle a schemer and his psychiatrist associate. The evil shrink,
Professor Muhlbach, has slicked hair, circular glasses, a trimmed

mustache, and a white blazer. He and his partner in crime, Bret Curtis, aim get their hands on Paul's father's estate by killing the dad (which they do) and marrying his widow. But Paul is on to them. Searching for evidence to link the bad doctor and the murderous paramour, Paul checks himself in to Restview Manor, Professor Muhlbach's sanitarium. He finds himself controlled and surveilled, thrust into a room with a two-way mirror, listening devices in the ventilators, and a tapped phone. The plot, with suitably *noir*-ish twists and coincidences, culminates when the cops capture the professor and shoot the paramour.[36]

Both *Spellbound* and *Strange Illusion* speak to mid-century ambivalence in regards to the asylum. Was it still a gothic dungeon, or was it a healing place where analysis could be conducted? *Spellbound* wants it both ways, giving us a mansion where a beautiful analyst saves the mind of the hero through dream interpretation while uncovering an insidious plot by an evil doctor. *Strange Illusion* is more straightforward with Restview Manor, though this bad place gets a modern update with surveillance technologies. The evil superintendent is the Freudian, though a magical variant of dream interpretation helps the hero save the day. Three years after these films, Twentieth Century Fox charged into this tangle of perceptions and added a new phrase to the language. It was called *The Snake Pit*.[37]

Mary Jane Ward's novel almost never saw the light of day. Her literary agent, along with several publishers, rejected it. It might have sat silently alongside her three other unpublished manuscripts had she not chosen to send it on to Random House herself. The editor liked it and had it printed as a small batch, "prestige" title. It would become a massive success, selling over a million copies, becoming a Book-of-the-Month Club selection, getting excerpted by *Harper's Bazaar*, condensed by *Reader's Digest*, and ultimately translated into many languages.[38]

Ward tells the tale of a woman on the edge of sanity. Virginia Stuart Cunningham is an author who winds up committed in an asylum. (Ward herself had suffered a nervous breakdown and had spent eight months at Rockland State Hospital in New York.) She lands in "Juniper Hill," a place that has issues. She must wait in excruciating lines to use the toilet, she's fed strange tasting medicines, and is subjected to shock treatments and wet packs. She encounters unhinged patients,

uncaring attendants, domineering nurses, and mysterious mind doctors. But this is no exposé. The narrator is unbalanced, her perspective often wobbling between first and third person within the same
paragraph. The reader is left wondering what is real and what is not.
One senses that lost minds do not even realize the reality of their
physical incarceration. Early on, Virginia is convinced that she's an
investigative reporter in a prison. We know this is not the case, but
there is nothing funny about her observations. In another instance,
she believes that she is being forced to drink "formaldehyde." We also
know that this cannot be true, but is paraldehyde really helping her
get better? We read how it makes the patients "smell like badly tended
lions" and causes them to drift off into "paraldehyde emptiness."[39]

The title of the book suggests torture. The inscription states, "Long
ago they lowered insane persons into snake pits; they thought that
an experience that might drive a sane person out of his wits might
send an insane person back into sanity." Later, this quote appears in
reference to shock treatments of "insulin, metrazol [and] electricity"
as well as to the shock of being placed in the chaos of crowded Ward
Thirty-Three.

Mostly, the narrator is tortured by her own mind. Virginia's brain
is also a snake pit, punishing her with doubts and hideous illusions.
At one point, she almost exits the narrative completely. Thinking
about how people used to tell her "what an imagination you have,"
she ponders what they would say if she were to put Juniper Hill into a
book. "Don't you know that modern mental hospitals aren't at all like
your trumped-up Juniper Hill," she imagines them saying.

> Why, patients are all so happy and, my dear, they do the darned-
> est things. Of course it's pathetic in a way but it really is a scream,
> what they say and do, thinking themselves Napoleon and all. They
> have a good roof over their heads and they don't have to worry
> about where the next meal is coming from or who's going to pay
> the gas bill. I'd say it's an ideal existence and you've gone and
> made it sound perfectly icky. Why, I've always said if anything ever
> happened to one of my family (it is interesting that they always
> have it happening to one of the family or to a friend, never to
> themselves) I would put them into an institution right off the
> bat and my heavens if I believed your book I'd hesitate. Everyone

knows we don't treat our insane like cattle. They are so much happier with their own kind and they just play around like happy little children all day long.

As should be clear, American pop culture virtually never portrayed asylums as "happy" places. Ward's struggle with reality suggests this imagined criticism is a component of her own insecurities. She knows she is sick, but she doesn't know why or how to find a cure. She doesn't know if the asylum is working, or if the staff are even who they say they are. Everything is up for grabs.[40]

The most frightening scene in the book involves electroconvulsive therapy.[41] Virginia is taken by a "guard" (as she calls the attendant) through corridors and locked rooms, up a cement stairwell, and into a small room. "[T]he moment she saw that room she knew she had been shocked previously and that she did not care for another helping. The room smelled like her old electric egg beater and there was a dull red glass eye in the wall." There is an "operating table," and she remembers suddenly that she is going to have an "operation" and regrets not having fasted in preparation. Dr. Kik comes in, "The Indefatigable Examiner," wearing a "white coat" instead of his usual suit. He is cheerful but unintelligible "with his heavy accent that you had never been able to place. It wasn't German, French, Italian or Scandinavian. Polish, perhaps. He began to talk at a great rate but you could tell he didn't care if you translated or replied." Virginia receives an anesthetic and has a wedge placed uncomfortably under her back. Now, she recognizes there will be no operation. They "were going to electrocute her." She wants her lawyer. She's tied down, and when she opens her mouth to demand her attorney, a gag is thrust in. The doctor becomes "the foreign devil with the angelic smile" and thanks her and then gives a "conspiratorial nod." The actual shock is not described, fitting with the experience of ECT, in which the patient is unconscious and has no memory of it.[42]

Electroconvulsive therapy was still novel in the 1940s, though it was spreading rapidly in mental hospitals. By 1947, nine in ten psychiatric hospitals used ECT. Importantly, given that the Freudian revolution privileged psychological over biological models, there was some public concern about its somatic presuppositions. However, in Ward's book and in many others, ECT is Freud-friendly, demonstrably making intransigent patients more amenable to talk therapy. It was an opening wedge that analysts might use to enter the psyche.[43]

In the movie version of Virginia's experiences, Hollywood conventions replace literary ambiguities. She is the helpless waif, imprisoned by her mental illness and trapped in a scary asylum. Dr. Kik is a Freudian hero, battling institutional inertia, insensitive fellow physicians, rough nurses, and, finally, the place itself. He will free Virginia both literally, from the institution, and, figuratively, from her neuroses. Unlike past asylum films, the studio went to great lengths to portray a "realistic" mental hospital. The movie came out amidst a sharp rise in attention to the condition of state hospitals and director Anatole Litvak felt it imperative to "awaken public interest in this vital matter." The filmmakers even hired three, well-known psychiatrists to gloss the treatments portrayed in the script, and they all ensured a clear, Freudian diagnosis of Virginia's illness.[44]

The film opens with Virginia sitting on a park bench, hearing voices. We get no prefatory hospital "establishing shot." Yet we know something is wrong. Olivia de Havilland, a Hollywood beauty, is wearing almost no makeup, her hair is disheveled, and she dons a torn sweater. As she had told a reporter, she'd done intensive, personal observations of Californian hospitals and of patients who "were in the same state as the girl whose character I would portray." In director Litvak's capable hands, the asylum has become a true *institution*. The nurse tells the patients to "fall in," and a bedraggled line of women enter a massive, brick building, with a high, chain link fence, a massive smokestack, trucks driving out, and groups of uniformed nurses milling about. We watch as the regimented deranged are herded inside. Looking upward, Virginia sees groups of women looking out from a caged-in balcony. Nurses pull out their heavy industrial keys and guide the throng into the interior.[45]

The movie follows the book in establishing the institution as a place both disorienting and scary. But Litvak's camera erases the dreamlike uncertainties of Virginia's experience. We get a straightforward, Freudian explanation that links childhood events and the traumatic death of her first fiancé to her current disorders. In other words, not a somatic but *romantic* explanation, of the sort that, ironically, Virginia fears is being imposed on her in the book. Film flashbacks reveal oedipal issues, complete with scenes of the young

Virginia fawning over her father and battling her mother. Dr. Kik, played with authoritative bearing by yet another Brit (Leo Genn), is dapper, kind, and attractive. In the book, Dr. Kik is many things—"executioner," "Young Jailer," and also "elegant man" and savior. In the film, he is whittled down to elegant savior.[46]

In the novel, Virginia learns only after the fact that she has been psychoanalyzed, and that Dr. Kik has theorized the root of her illness to be guilt over marrying Robert after the death of her earlier beau Gordon. Robert dismisses the idea, and Virginia agrees it sounds more like fiction than science. She muses, "I always think of [Dr. Kik] in connection with that little room with electricity, always a man of science. This changes the picture. I'll have to think of him as a man of romance as well." Later on, a different doctor undermines Kik's theories saying, "We don't know the cause." He speculates a mysterious, physical pathology yet to be unearthed. He even wonders if the shock therapy might have been useless. The reader is ultimately left in the dark, just as Virginia is. The movie, on the other hand, is quite clear about the cause.[47]

As for the ECT, the film's depiction is telling. The caged windows cast frightful shadows behind her as she waits in the hall. When her time is near, she confides, "I'm afraid, I'm terribly afraid." Once she's brought into the ECT suite, an exhausted doctor asks a nurse "How many more are left?" and is answered, "Twenty-three, doctor." The whole process resembles a factory line rather than the scary descent of the book. When Virginia receives a shock, the camera focuses only on the ECT machine, while the jarring soundtrack mimics the throwing of the switch. The fact that Dr. Kik is operating the scary device, but is also heroic, is resolved by way of explanation. As he tells Virginia's husband, ECT is meant to "establish contact" with her. When the husband asks, "Isn't there any other way?" Dr. Kik tellingly replies, "Yes, if we had time, lots of time. There are many things we're short of in State Hospitals, but time most of all." In other words, Virginia must be subjected to electricity because overcrowded hospitals don't have the resources for the lengthy psychoanalysis that would cure them. This neatly demolishes the ambivalence of the book toward Freud. The film does not so much "sell" ECT as it excuses it as a sad necessity. Later, when it appears that Virginia will be released too early, Dr. Kik injects her with Sodium Pentothal to pry free repressed memories.

These drastic depictions of contemporary treatments serve to high-light the narrative of institutional desperation.[48]

Other scenes replace the book's murkiness in concrete and even shocking ways. In the book, Ward Thirty-Three is a "great bore" filled with "eccentricity." In the film, it is a literal hellhole. We see Virginia caught in a crowded pit filled with other tormented souls. As the pro-tagonist voices over and references the "snake pit," we get a dizzying crane shot with the patients writhing about and surrounding her.[49]

The Snake Pit was touted by the studio as the "first authentic film study of a mental case and a mental hospital." Unlike the mansions, dungeons, and laboratories of prior films, here we have the asylum as a factory. Like Dr. Jaquith, Dr. Kik is a Freudian healer, but he's also the servant of an overcrowded institution and beholden to its limits. He tells Virginia's husband that he's taking "shortcuts" due to pressure to let her out early. Trapped within the bureaucratic confines of an unnerving environment, beset by hordes of incoming patients, and without the budget to accommodate them with analysis, his struggle oddly parallels Virginia's in its immensity.

The Snake Pit was a watershed for the pop culture asylum. The book garnered a mass audience, capitalizing on the horror element in its title and working the reader through a nightmare space where reality remained elusive and treatments insidious. The film (one of the top-five grossers of 1949) provides memorable scenes of chaotic wards, barred-windows, shadows, and confinement. It also carries the redeeming message that, with Freudian interventions, even those trapped in the most dysfunctional asylums could be healed.[50]

Mid-twentieth-century pop culture supplied many other Freud-ians. In novels like *The Cobweb* (1954) and *The Horizontal Hour* (1957), fatherly psychiatrists proved capable of effecting great change. In the former book, which takes place in a pleasant home-like institution, the patients are nervous but curable, and most of the drama involves whether or not the idealistic and manly Dr. McIver can promote his patient-community ideal in the face of an intransigent, female man-ager. (He does.) In 1968, the co-writer of *The Snake Pit*, Millen Brand, crafted perhaps the most fantastical pro-Freud effort. In *Savage Sleep*, a young analyst gets a job at the New State Hospital and cures a deeply psychotic patient by delving into his oedipal hang-ups. He takes the role of the boy's father and actually tells him, "Your prick's safe, son." The boy is miraculously cured.[51]

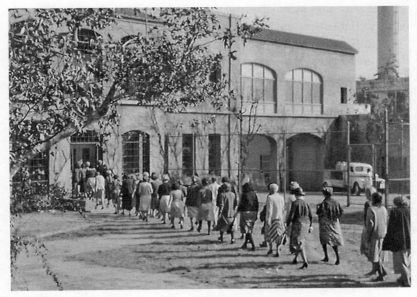

Patients file into a state institution, *The Snake Pit* (1948)

Freud's revolution slowly undid the links between psychiatry and institutions. Unlike past treatments, psychoanalysis did not require asylums (or, in Freud's view, even MDs). The analyst only needed proper training in order to clear away repressions and damaging childhood traumas. As Foucault ominously described it,

> Focused upon this single presence—concealed behind the patient and above him, in an absence that is also a total presence—all the powers that had been distributed in the collective existence of the asylum; he transformed this into an absolute Observation, a pure and circumspect Silence, a Judge who punishes and rewards in a judgement that does not even condescend to language; he made it the Mirror in which madness, in an almost motionless move-ment, clings to and casts itself off.

Freud personified the asylum, becoming both a divine inspiration for mental health and a mystic who could lead individuals to self-cure by becoming their own superintendent. The transformation would help set the stage for a dramatic expansion of the therapeutic impulse that accompanied the collapse of the state hospital system. Even when Freud was later dismissed, his argument that mental health was reachable through self-investigation remained.[52]

Significantly, in mid-century popular culture, all of the major Freudian asylum stories were middle-class, white person stories. The new vision recapitulated old race, gender, and class hierarchies. Freud-influenced plots revealed psychiatric prisons for Anglos, with accented foreigners playing enchanter roles and African American and "ethnic" immigrants as intimidating extras. The reality of institutionalization was never further from the popular depiction than in the case of African Americans and Native Americans. Theirs was a story of neglect. For example, take the case of Junius Wilson. As described in the book *Unspeakable: The Story of Junius Wilson*, this deaf African American was born into Jim Crow poverty, sent to a school for "the Colored Blind and Deaf," and drummed out like most of the rest of his classmates without having been taught American Sign Language. When later accused of attempted rape, Junius was sent to the State Hospital for the Colored Insane (later renamed Cherry Hill) in Goldsboro, North Carolina in 1925. Here, he was castrated. Junius remained at the hospital for the rest of his long life. Though the doctors later recognized that he was not mentally ill, they did not release him. As the hospital director explained in the 1990s, "You didn't have to be insane to be committed back then."[53]

Junius Wilson's story, like many others, went unrecognized by the public, undignified in fiction, unreported in the scientific literature, and unscreened by Hollywood. The State Hospital for the Colored Insane, like others designated for non-whites, was far worse than the snake pits the public was used to hearing about. A 1949 article in *Ebony* magazine noted that, "If for white patients, the result has been institutions that are more jails than hospitals, then for Negroes the situation approaches Nazi concentration-camp standards— especially in the South where three out of every five colored insane are confined."[54]

The concentration camp reference was becoming a common asylum description after World War II. To that story, I turn next.

CHAPTER 5

THE DAWNING AGE OF PARANOIA

> Life was identical with this institution . . . it was simply a larger
> insane asylum, with an atom bomb for shock treatment.
> —Fritz Peters, *The World Next Door* (1949)

Cold War paranoia kicked off on August 6, 1945, when a flash over Hiroshima signaled the end of a seven-year orgy of industrialized death and birthed a new, disturbing age. As poet Allen Ginsberg noted, "the splitting of the atom" brought about a "splitting of the old structures in society and also a sense of the inner world splitting up and coming apart." Inspired by his own stay at a mental institution, Ginsberg would compose a legendary indictment of a world gone crazy with his poem, "Howl." Here, he suggested that we lived in an "armed madhouse."[1]

The madhouse was an apropos Cold War era organizer. In the landmark 1951 novel *The Catcher in the Rye* by J. D. Salinger, young Holden Caulfield goes on a brief, bizarre trip to New York City after being expelled from yet another prep school. He encounters "phonies," battles a pimp, agonizes over girls, and generally tries to get a hold of himself. Significantly, Caulfield narrates his adventures from the confines of a mental institution. He tells us, "If you really want to hear about it, the first thing you'll probably want to know is where I was born, and what my lousy childhood was like, and how my parents were occupied and all before they had me, and all that David Copperfield kind of crap." But he will skip the Freudian childhood ordeals and "just tell you about this madman stuff that happened to me around last Christmas before I got pretty run-down and had to come out here and take it easy." Later, however, it's clear that a childhood

trauma, his brother's death, has much to do with his disturbances.
Salinger uses words like "crazy," "mad," "screwy," and "complexes" to
convey Holden's state of mind, but, as one influential contemporary
reviewer saw it, "It is not Holden who should be examined for a sickness of the mind, but the world in which he has sojourned and found
himself an alien."[2]

The idea that we all belong in the booby hatch is, of course, no
Cold War invention. But Holden's saga spoke to a novel praxis of existential fears and Freudian expressions that saturated his America.
In *The Sane Society* (1955), pop analyst Erich Fromm noted that civilization now faced "schizoid self-alienation." Fromm was not alone in
the opinion that society was ill. Misogynists like Philip Wylie pinned
the etiology on "castrating" mothers. Martinet psychiatrists such as
Fredric Wertham blamed the comic books. Sociologists like David
Riesman and William H. Whyte argued Americans were more concerned with fitting in than with being independent. Hipper theorists
like Paul Goodman posited that America warped youngsters by creating a "neurosis of chronic boredom" and "sexual paranoia." It goes
without saying that by showing us the walls of our new prison, these
intellectuals could offer us the tools of escape.[3]

During the Cold War, this dark vision made sense. Never had we
been so affluent; never did the Apocalypse seem so imminent. Never
had the asylum seemed such a suitable metaphor.

THE MEAT FACTORY: WORLD WAR II LEGACIES

J. D. Salinger stormed Utah Beach on D-Day with the U.S. Army's
Fourth Division, carrying with him the first six chapters of his manuscript *Catcher in the Rye*. He then survived the gruesome battle of
Hurtgen Forest, a place nicknamed "the meat factory," where a yard
of ground equaled a man's life. Later, after entering the desolate remains of Kaufering IV (a part of the Dachau concentration camp
complex), Salinger checked himself into a hospital in Nuremburg for
"battle fatigue." He would eventually admit, "You never really get the
smell of burning flesh out of your nose entirely, no matter how long
you live." His popular 1948 short story, "A Perfect Day for Bananafish,"
struck the postwar pitch. A veteran named Seymour is vacationing
with his wife Muriel. Muriel's parents are worried that Seymour is

dangerous and unhinged. The Army, her father thinks, got away with a "perfect *crime*" by releasing him so early from the "hospital." Muriel chastises her mom over the phone, saying, "Mother . . . you talk of him as though he were a raving *maniac*." Seymour is nothing of the sort. He spends his days at the bar or on the beach, playing with a little girl. One afternoon, after searching the seas with the girl for the elusive and fantastical "bananafish," he goes back to his room, sits on the twin bed opposite his sleeping wife, and blows his brains out with a German pistol.[4]

Salinger knew that the war did not stay on the battlefields. While Americans were justly proud of their role in defeating fascism, the exuberance was shot through with tensions and fears. The dehumanization of military experience undermined the promoted narrative of democratic victory. Though most fiction and film celebrated the heroism and sacrifice of the soldiers, some illuminated the insanity and senselessness of modern combat. For example, James Jones's *The Thin Red Line* (1962) paints a picture of the infantry soldier as woefully unprepared for, and disillusioned by, mechanized death and hierarchical command. The combat scenes are gruesome, and the episodes of heroism are demeaned by selfishness and brutality. One character comes to the conclusion that the whole war is "pointless" and wishes that he might just "go crazy" and leave it all behind. The tedious camp days and the nightmarish night raids create a "schizophrenic" existence. One battle is described by a soldier as a "crazyhouse." Similarly, vet Joseph Heller's *Catch-22* teaches us that irrationality is an irreducible aspect of military experience. As Heller writes, "Orr [a combat pilot] would be crazy to fly more missions and sane if he didn't, but if he was sane he had to fly them. If he flew them he was crazy and didn't have to; but if he didn't want to he was sane and had to. Yossarian was moved very deeply by the absolute simplicity of the cause of Catch-22, and let out a respectful whistle." This "Catch-22" is the "best [catch] there is." It contains all dissent and denudes all criticism.[5]

Sloan Wilson confronted the postwar dilemma in *The Man in the Gray Flannel Suit* (1955). How does one go to the office with the stench of burning flesh still in one's nose? For Tom Rath, the "trick is to learn to believe that it's a disconnected world, a lunatic world, where what is true now was not true then; where Thou Shalt Not Kill and the fact that one has killed a great many men mean nothing, absolutely nothing, for now is the time to raise legitimate children, and make money, and dress properly, and be kind to one's wife, and admire one's boss, and learn not to worry." Tom Rath's quandary captured a paranoid dynamic of Cold War prosperity. The bright new age could not excise the war. "Ever since the war," Rath concludes, "it's been as though I were trying to figure something out . . . I keep having the feeling that the world is nuts, that the whole world is absolutely insane."[6]

American culture worked hard to assimilate this nagging feeling. Some films, like *The Best Years of Our Lives*, presented audiences with sensitive portraits of vets struggling to make a go of civilian life. The most illuminating depiction of battle fatigue came in the form of a documentary by filmmaker John Huston. Commissioned by the U.S. Army in 1945, *Let There Be Light* tells the story of a cohort of vets at the Mason General Hospital, a massive psychiatric facility in Long Island. The camera focuses tightly on the faces, as veterans lose their speech, wobble on unsteady legs, and stare off into the void. The narrator tells us that these are the "human salvage." Huston offered a new look at an asylum as a place of healing and understanding. Even "scary" treatments such as Sodium Amytal are presented as gentle cures. Freudian group analysis is conducted alongside somatic treatments. The men talk about their childhoods and get hypnotized into recalling moments of horror. Unfortunately, Huston's film was out of step with the Army's agenda. It was confiscated by MPs and hidden from the public until 1980. According to Huston, "They wanted to maintain the 'warrior' myth, which said that our American soldiers went to war and came back all the stronger for the experience, standing tall and proud for having served their country well."[7]

Let There Be Light was not the asylum that the public got after the war. The first picture to depict insulin treatment, for example, was a horror feature. Starring newcomer Vincent Price, *Shock* (1946) tells the story of a woman who, while waiting for her soldier husband to return after two long years in a POW camp, witnesses a murder in her hotel room. The killer is Dr. Cross (Price), a psychiatrist who owns a sanatorium outside of town. Once Cross figures out that the woman witnessed his act, he plots to make her forget what she saw, first by means of hypnotic suggestion and later by simply trying to kill her with insulin therapy. Her husband knows about insulin shock. Talking to Dr. Cross, who he does not yet realize is evil, he says, "They use that in the Army on guys who blow their tops." He agrees to go along because, "I *have* seen it work in the Army." Several things are happening here. A vet is speaking well of a drastic treatment that the public, had it viewed Huston's film, might have believed to be effective. Instead, what we learn about insulin therapy is that, while it might have helped some soldiers, it is very dangerous, bringing patients to the brink of doom even under normal circumstances. Foreboding music plays while the white-jacketed Cross and his evil lover peer down on the writhing young wife undergoing the treatment. *New York Times* critic Bosley Crowther condemned the film in wartime terms. "Treatment of nervous disorders is being practiced today upon thousands of men who suffered shock of one sort or another in the war. A film which provokes fear of treatment, as this film plainly aims to do, is a cruel thing to put in the way of these patients or their anxious relations." The film was nothing less than a "social disservice."[8]

The first asylum book by a vet to address the cost of the war is *The World Next Door* by Arthur A. Peters, writing under the pseudonym Fritz Peters. Peters had served with the Twenty-Ninth Infantry Division in the Battle of the Bulge, suffering a postwar mental breakdown and hospitalization. He prefaces his book by explaining that it "is based on actual experience," and he dedicates it, in part, to "the veterans, of war and society, in all psychiatric institutions." Composed along the lines of *The Snake Pit*, Peters paints a picture of life in the strange land of the mental institution. As in Ward's narrative, we are thrust into the mind of a confused person. After strolling outside nude and delirious, David Mitchell is cuffed and taken to a massive building fronted incongruously by beautiful landscaping. He is not sure just where he is. He speculates that he's in a Nazi prison camp. The man tied in the next bed must be a "German spy," the attendants Nazis, and the doctor some sort of Nazi leader. Or he might be in an American military prison. The coffee tastes like Army coffee and the place resembles an Army hospital he'd known.[9]

Eventually, David receives ECT. He likens it to anti-aircraft fire. "Lightning in my head in the ack-ack-pack room. Ack-ack-ack . . . in my battery in the Army they called me ack-ack mitchell, did they not, *n'est-ce-pas*." He's also put in a cold pack, provided occupational therapy in the form of typing, and spends time talking to a doctor about religion and the nature of society. When it is revealed that David once had a homosexual experience, the vocational-rehabilitation specialist takes special interest. At mid-century, homosexuality was considered a mental illness, and, early in the war, some five thousand recruits were dismissed for having "homosexual proclivities." As the carnage progressed, the restrictions became more lax. The vocational specialist wants to know if David is gay, and he responds, "It is true that at that time, in the beginning, I was willing to be a fairy, or whatever you want to call it," but now he had decided it was not for him. The matter is dropped.[10]

Ultimately, David emerges from his psychotic state and leaves the asylum, admitting that the experience had "increased my sense of my own wholeness." But the war is something he can never get past. He senses his delusions might even be a *rational* response to a "corrupt and seemingly insane society . . . a society in which wars, insane asylums, prisons, electric chairs, concentration camps, courts of law, were accepted as logically and humanly inevitable?" "Certainly," David thinks, he is not "wrong to object to it, fight against it." Most alarmingly, he posits that the asylum is no haven in a heartless world but rather a metaphor for it. For what is the world but "simply a larger insane asylum, with an atom bomb for shock treatment."[11]

The war was something of a mixed blessing for the asylum. On the plus side, the Freudian emphasis on "environmental stress over predisposition" offered hope for the battle fatigue epidemic that amounted to one in five American casualties. Even treatments like Sodium Pentothal and ECT could fit the Freudian model, as doctors used them to "break through" and prime patients for analysis. In the novel *Captain Newman, M.D.* (1961), a fictionalized account of the experiences of an Army Air Corps doctor, Sodium Pentothal ("flak-juice") helps soldiers "access" what they otherwise would repress. In the film version, we see a caring Gregory Peck penetrate the defenses of Bobby Darin, who writhes his way through a Pentothal-induced breakthrough to score an Oscar nomination.[12]

But there were negatives as well. The war tightened the labor market considerably, and the staffs of the low-paying mental hospitals found better wages elsewhere. The government stepped in to fill the gap. Of the nation's conscientious objectors (COs), some three thousand served in state institutions.[13]

The COs were horrified by what they witnessed. After the war, a group of them established the National Mental Health Foundation and sponsored the publication *Out of Sight, Out of Mind.* Written by a CO named Frank L. Wright, Jr., in this book we read about patients who bleed to death through their anuses, squish about in human excrement, freeze in overcrowded wards, get beaten by laughing attendants, eat directly off the floor, suffer from bedbugs while tied to mattresses, pull out damp wads of tobacco from urinals to chew on, and sometimes receive lethal doses of sedatives from vindictive staff members. Eleanor Roosevelt asked "everyone" to read the book in her popular newspaper column.[14]

A gathering pack of reports reinforced the critique, capped by Albert Deutsch's 1948 exposé *Shame of the States.* Deutsch was a crusading journalist, writer, and self-taught historian, and his book provided perhaps the most-quoted resource for the mid-century asylum reformer. Deutsch takes us into the abyss. Chronic overcrowding, atrocious food, and general neglect has created hellholes, like the incontinent ward at the Philadelphia State Hospital for Mental Diseases, a "Dante's Inferno" in which hundreds of nude men, covered in their own excrement, rot away amid "shrieks, groans, and unearthly laughter." The book provided photos of patients eating with their hands, wearing cloth for shoes, and squatting naked while eating off the floor. Images of exposed bricks peeking through water-mutilated plaster and toilets sitting opposite dishes in makeshift pantries added mute witness to human neglect.[15]

Deutsch wants us to know that this horror has no relationship to the clichés we've been raised on. He is well versed in the pop cultural asylum.

> I knew that the history of the institutional care and treatment of the mentally sick was strewn with "asylum horror" tales revolving around individual scapegoats and that, through the decades, the customary way to resolve the problem was to oust a superintendent, a staff physician, a nurse or attendant who served as a convenient scapegoat for the public's guilt.

I knew that, to find the real causes of the conditions I witnessed, I would have to seek beyond the scapegoat, beyond the lurid incident, back to the deep-seated sources of chronic evils and abuses, back to the real culprit—the *state hospital system*.

The *system* is at fault. Hospitals are underfunded, overcrowded, and inefficient. Isolated from the rest of society, asylums have become backwaters loaded with bureaucrats who hide their mediocrity behind a seniority system that neither recruits nor recognizes talent. Medical treatments have nothing to do with the real horrors. Deutsch applauds the use of Metrazol, insulin, and electroconvulsive therapy (though he recognizes there is a "violent controversy" over ECT). The problem is not shock but rather the lack of it. Like Upton Sinclair, Deutsch looked to inspire federal help, and like Sinclair, what the reader mainly takes away is queasiness.[16]

Perhaps no single investigation was more read than Albert Q. Maisel's *Life* magazine photo essay, "Bedlam 1946." In this piece, Maisel effectively connected the old gothic fears of tyranny and control to the new postwar climate. In the first paragraph, he describes a basement ward (the "Dungeon") beneath images of a towering, brick edifice. In the second, he likens state hospitals to concentration camps. In these "man-made hells," the "patient-prisoners" are fed a "starvation diet," receive "little and shoddy clothing at best," sleep on bare floors, undergo "forced labor," contract disease, and are sometimes beaten to death. Photos of nude, crouched inmates in various states of despair accompany the article, along with images of hands clenching prison-like bars and shots of overcrowded wards. By way of reference, *Life* had already printed images of the dead and living-dead liberated from Nazi camps in late 1945.[17]

Summoning the Nazis brought immediacy to the problem of the asylum. Others added their own Nazifications. In *Out of Sight, Out of Mind*, a psychiatrist is described as a "paunchy potentate" who "you sort of expect to see [everybody] salute, click their heels, and say, 'Heil, Bancroft!'" Another attendant is reminded of his stay in a "Nazi prisoners' camp" when he looks out at the yard. In Ellen Philtine's *They Walked in Darkness* (1945), an autobiographical novel about the wife of a psychiatrist living in an overburdened state institution, a cruel doctor greets a helpful German analyst with a "Heil, Hitler!" In *Shame of the States*, Deutsch argues that, just as the Nazis believed that the insane did not deserve to live, in America we have our own "euthanasia" policy. Commenting on the neglect that leads to raging asylum epidemics, he bitterly reflects, "No, indeed, we are not like the Nazis. We do not kill off 'insane' people coldly as a matter of official state policy. We do not kill them deliberately. We do it by neglect."[18]

Buttressed by Nazi metaphors, the Cold War asylum added a new kind of horror that would be called "Orwellian." This related to the fascism that drenched the twentieth century in blood. "Totalitarianism," the form of tyranny associated with the Nazi and Soviet systems, referenced a world in which the state claimed complete dominion over a person's life, engendering slave-like subservience and fear. George Orwell's *1984* (1949) proved a publishing sensation in America and spoke to this dread. In the book, Winston Smith lives an abject life under the watchful eye of Big Brother, a Stalin-esque monstrosity that inspires total acquiescence with the help of the Thought Police. In the bleak future state of Oceana, Big Brother combines gestapo and KGB into a totalitarian world of discipline and control. In Orwell's nightmare vision, the citizen is pressured into a self-loathing self-discipline. This was a compelling and potent brew of contemporary fears, and it, in turn, reenergized older concerns about the lurking dangers to liberty. The Cold War madhouse could become a bleak place of surveillance and abuse, cloaked in the doublespeak of "healing."[19]

FILM NOIR

Perhaps no genre better reflected the new totalitarian encroachment than film noir. Roughly spanning between 1940 to 1960,[20] this cinematic field reflected a culture living with new uncertainties and fears. Dark shadows, devious characters, femmes fatales, tormented heroes, and a subtext of violent sexuality all spoke to Fromm's "schizoid self-alienation." The audience was encouraged to empathize with transgressors and underworld denizens. The Freudian jargon that often pops up in these films is targeted to help the audience analyze and uncover evil plots.[21]

Noir suited the asylum and vice versa. In *The Snake Pit*, caged windows cast long, dark shadows on the walls, metaphorically confining Virginia Cunningham as she knits her brows and awaits her shock treatment. In *Spellbound, Shock,* and *Strange Illusion,* private sanitariums are settings for malign plots and twisted psychiatrists. In these movies, the old "dungeon" asylum is replaced by a more formal space in which analysts lounge in book-lined offices and monitor patients with the help of uniformed attendants and nurses. The gothic style is still here; secrecy, torture, and control lurk not far beneath the surface. Yet innovations complicate things. In *Strange Illusion,* for instance, technological surveillance is evident in its one-way mirror room, embodying Foucault's notion of the "internalized gaze" of the panopticon. In *Spellbound,* a heroic female analyst helps Gregory Peck recover lost memories and free himself, even as a bad shrink tries to destroy him. Mingling good and bad, dark and light, is a noir specialty. I'll examine two films, *High Wall* (1947) and *Screaming Mimi* (1958), to illustrate this.

In *High Wall,* a World War II veteran named Steven Kenet, suffering from a combat-related head injury, returns home to find himself accused of murdering his wife. He confesses but, when the police doctor recognizes he is mentally deranged, he is sent to the Hamelin County Psychiatric Hospital. Suitably introduced at night and surrounded by the eponymous high wall, we learn that Kenet has a "subdural hematoma of the left frontal lobe" that has caused "both physical and emotional changes." He's put in a small cell with a lone mattress on the floor, grated windows, and a small, barred door portal. Like some other Freudian asylums, this place has a saving grace in the form of a gentle and assuring doctor. The beautiful Dr. Anne Lorrison helps him, through narco-synthesis, discover that he has been framed. Kenet breaks out and, with the help of Dr. Lorrison (who falls for him), finds out that the real murderer is his wife's boss with whom she'd been having an affair. With more narco-synthesis, Kenet gets the man to confess. The film's asylum locale and strained Sodium Pentothal-based plot did not pass muster with the *New York Times,* whose critic called it "morbid and socially cynical" before concluding it was "Just the thing for your holiday entertainment—unless, of course, you are sane."[22]

War experience informs *High Wall.* Kenet served and married a woman while on leave; their child is an almost entirely unknown creature to him. His wife covets his high rank and commensurate pay, and, after the war, she doesn't want him to take a pay cut at the university, even though that's where he wants to work. So he must continue flying in Burma, which still results in a salary loss. This forces his wife to get a secretarial job, exiling her from the domestic ideal, and here she has an affair with her boss. Although Kenet is a war hero (he has a Distinguished Service Cross and a Silver Star), he cannot navigate postwar life, his wife and his brain trauma conspiring to send him to the asylum. Director Robert Taylor would later say that with this film, "I suddenly saw a chance to bring directly to the American people the experience of the war. In the American pictures, this experience is treated as a kind of ballyhoo concept. *The Best Years of Our Lives* came after *High Wall*."[23]

Just as with *Spellbound* and *The Snake Pit*, a kindly analyst using the latest techniques serves as redeemer in *High Wall*. With Sodium Pentothal, at the time commonly depicted as a wonder drug, Kenet discovers that he did not really murder his wife. The administration of the drug and the sleep-like state induced is realistically shown, though the plot-resolving flashbacks are smirk inducing. Dr. Lorrison also helps him by diagnosing his desperate need to "escape from reality," and her kindness effectively neutralizes the depressing situation of hospital life. Lorrison provides a proper postwar model of feminine, domestic support, juxtaposing Kenet's own viperous one, and literally becoming a mother to his otherwise orphanage-bound son. She supports Kenet and helps solve the crime.

High Wall uses film noir language to modernize the asylum. Wrapped in shadows and rainy nights, the narrative takes us along with a troubled war hero to unmask a duplicitous plot that emasculates and quarantines him. We wind up rooting for an asylum escapee, committed on false pretenses but who nonetheless receives treatment from a doctor who is both professional and domestic. In sum, this film contains plenty of paradoxes. The asylum is frightening but redeeming, it's understaffed but has caring staff, and the asylum doctor turns out to be the polar opposite of the hero's scheming wife. In *High Wall*, a noir sensibility captures the fears of postwar assimilation and provides a happy ending to a veteran's nightmare.

A more bizarre example of the noir asylum is Fredric Brown's pulp, *The Screaming Mimi*. Published in abbreviated form in *Mystery Book Magazine* in October 1949 and then by E. P. Dutton as a novel, the story relates the adventures of a boozy, down-and-out reporter named William Sweeney. We begin on a summer night with Sweeney chugging his way through a bender on a park bench in Bughouse Square, a place "bright with lights, but dark with the shadows of the defeated men who sit on the benches." On Sweeney's way home, he encounters a beautiful woman in a white gown sprawled in the doorway of an apartment building, guarded by a large dog. As she slowly rises, it's apparent that she has been seriously injured, a large red slash on her abdomen. The police arrive but are kept at bay by the fearsome dog. Then "the incredible thing happened." The dog gets up on his hind legs and, with his teeth, unzips the gown. The dress drops, and the woman now stands completely naked. A cop shoots the dog and the woman is taken off in an ambulance. The dog, who turns out to be both the woman's protector and stage-prop for her stripping act, survives.[24]

We learn that there have been a series of murders in the city, and this waif, Yolanda, appears to be the only surviving victim of the killer. But nothing is as it seems. Yolanda not only sets the story in motion, but she also turns out to be the killer herself. Through a series of discoveries that rely on Freudian interpretations of past traumas, we see that as a youth she was attacked by a knife-wielding, asylum escapee. She had a breakdown and was institutionalized. Her psychiatrist fell in love with her and helped get her out, quitting his job to become her manager. Yolanda, née Bessie Wilson a quiet girl from Wisconsin, became a vivacious Chicago stripper. Her new personality "splits" again when she turns into The Ripper, who performs a ritual of "transference" using a horrible, little statue called "The Screaming Mimi."

The madhouse motif carries through the novel. We open at Bughouse Square. The femme fatale works at a strip club named El Madhouse. She is an unwell, asylum patient, sent there in the first place by an escapee. Her ex-asylum doctor runs her degraded life. The Woman in White here is both victim *and* killer, an appropriate example of noir's wiggling of moral expectations.[25]

The book inspired two films, the first being 1958's *Screaming Mimi* starring Swedish bombshell Anita Ekberg. The film differs a bit from the book, lingering on Ekberg's sultry S&M-style stage act and the unique screen presence of famed burlesque queen Gypsy Rose Lee (playing a predatory lesbian dominatrix). The film also plays up the bad shrink role of Dr. Greenwood (as the movie calls him), who is shown closely monitoring Virginia (as Bessie is renamed) in a cell-like room in the Highland Sanitarium. He is a classic Svengali, his power gleaned from controlling an unattainable beauty, he, at one point, actually says to her, "You must do as I say!" The film ends with Virginia, draped in a white overcoat, getting taken to the asylum in a wagon by uniformed attendants. The movie was too much, or just too odd, for the late-fifties audience (and for Brown himself). It was yanked after a short run as part of a Columbia double feature.[26]

Other film noirs similarly used asylums to plunge audiences into paranoid environments. *Shock* (1946) matches scenes of madness with a stormy night, lightning illuminating the asylum. *Shock* also combines a femme fatale with a Woman in White in Elaine, coldly captivating in her starch white nurse's dress. Vincent Price's Dr. Cross winds up a kind of murderous Tom Rath, until, at the very end, he refuses to kill his patient and strangles Elaine instead. *Kiss Me Deadly* (1955), based on Mickey Spillane's book of almost the same title (he has a comma after *Me*), starts at night on a desolate road with a blond in a pale trench coat fleeing an asylum. Mike Hammer takes her in, his sense of honor overpowering his jaded, narcissistic personality. We eventually discover that this Woman in White was sent to the "funny farm" as a means of extracting information about a key to a locker containing (in the film but not the book) a suitcase of nuclear materials. In *The Enforcer* (1951), Humphrey Bogart talks to a patient in a wet pack in the "State Hospital for the Insane," musing, "The lunatic's the only one who makes sense." In *Possessed* (1947), Joan Crawford goes to a "Psychopathic Dept" in a hospital and is thrust into a room that resembles a cell. A doctor laments, "This civilization of ours is a worse disease than heart trouble or tuberculosis and we can't escape it." Luckily for Crawford, a good Freudian doctor brings her back to sanity. Then there are bad, femme fatale shrinks in films like *Nightmare Alley* (1947), *Ring of Fear* (1954), and *Shock Treatment* (1964). These temptresses wield analysis like a knife.[27]

MENTAL ADJUSTMENT

Acclimatizing to the new landscape of fear and abundance strained the jangled nerves of the nation. Mental health became politicized, securitized, and federally underwritten. The National Mental Health Act of 1946 and the subsequent National Institute of Mental Health represented millions in tax dollars. Mental hospital admissions almost doubled between 1940 and 1956, with mental patients occupying the largest share of hospital beds in the country. For those not inside, tranquilizers like Miltown and self-help books kept keels steady. In darker expressions, federal resources poured into CIA "psychological warfare."[28]

Erich Fromm felt there was a connection between the craze for "adjustment" and the Cold War. As he observes in *The Sane Society*, "In recent years there is an increasing emphasis on the concept of security as the paramount aim in life, and as the essence of mental health." Fromm worried about psychiatry telling us that a bunkered war footing was normal, that we must battle Communism with shopping sprees and bowling alleys. He saw in Aldous Huxley's dystopian *Brave New World* our final destination if we continue down the soothing path. What Fromm hoped for was a psychology that could help break through the walls of fear and conformity. But such was not the reality of the field. Rather, psychology had become "the apologist for the status quo." Fromm concluded that "the crowning achievement of manipulation is modern psychology . . . these professions are in the process of becoming a serious danger to the development of man, that their practitioners are evolving into the priests of a new religion of fun, consumption and self-lessness, into specialists of manipulation, into the spokesmen for the alienated personality." Fromm's own formula for mental health is vague. Regardless, his worries cut to the root of adjustment.[29]

Adjustment was the sine qua non of mental health for postwar psychoanalysis, and Ego Psychology was its cheerleader. Practiced by luminaries in the mental health field, Ego Psychology focused on accommodating oneself to a tough world. As William Menninger explained in *Psychiatry in a Troubled World*, the role of the ego was to "help the personality adjust to the demands placed upon it by the environment." Unless "equilibrium and harmony" are established, "the individual develops a neurotic symptom." Ego Psychology became a tool to help mitigate the id's impulsive demand for gratification and substituting "the reality principle for the pleasure principle" (to quote Freud). It was an important moment in the "psychiatrization" of America. No longer should psychiatrists be associated with the "insane." As Menninger explains, "minor personality disturbances" must become the meat of analytical treatment. The psychiatrist could help us all. This would be, uncoincidentally, the "golden age" of the screen analyst.[30]

Perhaps the most sensational adjustment tale of this era is *The Three Faces of Eve* (1957). Here, one woman's maladjustment takes the form of multiple personalities. Thanks to a pair of wise analysts, she recovers and adjusts. Just as Ward put "snake pit" into America's pop vernacular, *The Three Faces of Eve* (along with Shirley Jackson's *The Bird's Nest*) put multiple personality disorder (MPD) into the national conversation.

The Three Faces of Eve tells the story of Eve White, a "neat, color-less" twenty-five-year-old housewife. Interestingness is on the way. Like the femme fatales who stepped outside the bounds of propriety in the film noirs, within her there lurks a second, darker personality, Eve Black. In an age that disciplined women via accusations ranging from "momism" to over-seductiveness, Eve Black was dangerous, a creature who denies sex to her husband as well as responsibility for mothering her child. Black's escape from the confinements that Betty Friedan would later define as "the feminine mystique" manifests in her activities, dress, shopping habits, language, and bearing. Her eyes are "bright" with a "look of childish deviltry." A clinical psychologist finds her to be "far healthier" than her domesticated host in a Ror-schach test. But as the book makes clear, Eve Black is *mal*adjusted. According to a report the psychiatrists receive from another set of doctors, "*Eve Black has a achieved a violent kind of adjustment in which she perceives herself as literally perfect, but, to accomplish this break, her way of perceiving 'the world' becomes completely disoriented from the norm.*" Notably, Kevin Young finds that this personality tellingly manifests a racialized blackness along with her name.[31]

The authors, who are the psychiatrists who treat Eve, are care-ful not to offer too pat an explanation for her problems. Her expe-rience as a child being forced to touch her dead grandmother's face is presented as having something to do with them, as is the "mon-ster" living beneath the waters of a stagnant ditch where a man once drowned. But they resist the lure of tidy Freudian justifications, saying "no single incident of fright or stress, such as our patient's experience as a child at her grandmother's funeral can plausibly be assumed to account in full for the disorder she developed." Their strategy is to hedge somewhere between the power of trauma and other, less understood processes. They even go so far as to say, "A better definition and understanding of consciousness and of personality must be found before any reliable explanation can be offered of such a patient as the one presented here." However, they do offer a remarkable Cold War analogy. They ask us to imagine "an organized conspiracy by a vast secret party" that "suddenly rises and overthrows the existing government" of Eve's mind. Eve Black, a shadow self to a demure feminine ideal, is akin to the Communist forces the paranoid culture obsessed over. They even use "the recent political history of France" (where Communist-supported Pierre Mendès France became Prime Minister) as a referent.[32]

Ultimately, a third personality named "Jane" emerges to save the day. Jane "accepts the usual evaluations of concepts by her society yet still maintains a satisfactory evaluation of herself." Her dominance ultimately leads to a "coalescence." The book thus becomes a glorious event of "adjustment therapy," the ultimate ambition of postwar psychiatry. The asylum serves as a place to stop the advance of Eve's illness, while true healing comes from talk.[33]

One of the most fascinating aspects of *The Three Faces of Eve* is how the authors explicitly mock Freudian schemas. They even go so far as to provide a detailed summary of Freud's famous "Wolf Man" dream (formally, *From the History of an Infantile Neurosis*) in order to smash it. The two psychiatrists dismissively conclude, "No objective evidence is offered anywhere in the paper to support [Freud's] interpretations." This skeptical stance reflects the air of scientific detachment that runs throughout the Eve account. Drs. Thigpen and Cleckley want it known that Eve's condition is real, complex, and understandable only through the most rigorous analysis. Their elbows were sharp enough to earn a review by Dr. Joost A. M. Meerloo in the *New York Times* that scolded their unfair "diatribe against Freudian concepts." Yet the doctors did not really dismiss the Freudian revolution. Their approach involved a heavy dose of psychoanalysis, from their focus on Eve's childhood and sexuality to their reliance on the "psychoanalytic hour." Their concern is that psychoanalysis by itself cannot offer the reproducible, evidentiary base required for grasping the mysteries of the brain.[34]

The Hollywood version of Eve's experience is not so complicated. Dr. Luther (Lee J. Cobb sitting in for both Thigpen and Cleckley) is heroic, Freudian, and businesslike. The film follows the plot, but with a smoothness and certainty that the book lacks. For example, when Eve Black emerges, we hear a sultry, jazz clarinet riff, announcing that the femme fatale has arrived. Eve's husband is clueless; Dr. Luther is brilliant; and the basis of her condition is entirely childhood-trauma based. The recollection of a traumatic experience cathartically helps Jane to emerge and save the day. The film closes with Jane finding happiness with her new husband, Earl, and their infant daughter. In the book, Eve marries Earl Lancaster as "Evelyn Lancaster," and, though the authors wish her well, they concede they are "unable to predict" whether or not the "beautiful integration" of her personalities will hold.[35]

The movie's portrayal of the asylum is instructive. This "psychiatric section of the university hospital" could be any university building, busy and functional. The nurses are quiet and professional, and nobody is raving about in the dayroom. When Eve complains to Dr. Luther that she is in a "nuthouse," he corrects her, "it's a hospital. You don't see any bars or anything like that, do you?" The asylum doctor here turns out to be ineffective, a man utterly mortified when Eve Black hits on him. This serves the narrative too. Modern asylums might not be horrible, but without Freudian interventions, they are useless. When Dr. Luther arrives, things shape up. Eve Black tries to seduce him, to earn his retort, "Do you want to be shut up in one of these places for life? One *with* bars?" This is the slide into the abyss, a recognition of the snake pits awaiting if she does not obey.

The Three Faces of Eve struck box office gold. The real-life Eve, however, ultimately had to sue Twentieth Century Fox for the rights to her own story. MPD became fitted into a genre writers were more comfortable with—horror. The cementing of this trope came in 1959 with the publication of Robert Bloch's *Psycho*. In this book, an unassuming, young motel manager listens as his dead mom, whom he has previously murdered, berates him as he carries out ghastly acts. Like Eve, Norman Bates has three faces. There is Norman the little boy, Norma the dress-wearing psychopath, and Normal the well-adjusted adult. The book closes with him locked up in a "small, barred room" in the State Hospital. Here, in a bizarre twist on the "convergence" of personalities that ends *The Three Faces of Eve*, a "fusion" takes place. He becomes Mother.[36]

BREAKING DOWN

In a culture that placed a premium on adjustment, the nervous break-down held a privileged place. Like the bomb, nervous breakdowns could strike at any time. As Judith Kruger's doctor-husband explains to her in her 1957 memoir *My Fight for Sanity*, "We all have our break-ing points. I'm not immune to a breakdown. No one is. Now it's hap-pened to you." A few examples of this signature psychological debacle shed light on the Cold War asylum. In memoirs by Judith Kruger and Robert Dahl, breakdowns lead to asylum trips and Freudian interven-tions. In Vladimir Nabokov's *Lolita*, something much more cynical is suggested: Adjustment is a worthless dream and the asylum a point-less locale in a landscape of mindless pleasures.[37]

In *My Fight for Sanity*, Judith Kruger has everything going for her: an attentive, medical student husband, a devoted mother, and a new-born baby. Unfortunately, she discovers she cannot fulfill her feminine role. "I wanted to smile for him," she writes of her husband, "to be fresh and crisp when he walked in the door, to lie in bed with him at night. But it was impossible." She develops suicidal thoughts. Eventu-ally, her husband commits her to the "State Hospital." On her way, she remembers that shock treatments cause memory loss, so she writes down her name and other pertinent information on a note card.[38]

The asylum is so crowded that she's forced to sleep in a converted utility closet. Her terror intensifies when she receives her first electro-convulsive treatment. In this episode, a nurse rolls a "large white ma-chine" up to her bed, telling her, "We're going to make you feel better," and then asks if she has any dental work that can be removed. Tied to her bed, she thinks, "I'm going to throw up. Can I run someplace? Hide from them? These things on my feet. Scared. Scared stiff." She hears the doctor say "Shock!" and then blacks out, waking up in the shower attended to by a nurse.[39]

Kruger's account of the State Hospital provides a kind of elabora-tion of Ward's Juniper Hill. It is overcrowded and filled with bizarre in-mates and imperial, distant doctors. Seemingly normal conversations about recipes and jobs get infected by "strange words" like "'shock' and 'solitary' and 'O.T.' and 'secondarys,' 'spinals,' 'coma,' 'Staff,' and 'parole.'" The portable ECT machine serves as a particularly morbid example of how institutions process inmates with indifference. To relieve the stress, one jokes, "Well, here we go again, girls! Another day, another shock. Nothing like a good shock to start off the day." But this is not funny. "Some of the women giggled, but their eyes weren't laughing."[40]

Kruger realizes her only means of adjustment is to submit to the power of the doctors, mimicking the submissive, domestic role she had aspired to at the start. "Their weapon is authority. I have nothing to match that. I must be docile, bending, meek, and willing." Once released, she recognizes that she is still unwell and so seeks analysis. A good Freudian is able to break through and help her escape the nightmare. He unearths her oedipal attraction to her father and her competitive resentment to her mother. He tells her, "Most of us make an adjustment as we grow older. It's not something we're aware of. We just come to accept the fact that we can't have the parent we favored." Judith finally concludes that she envies her husband's penis, that she lusted for her father, and that she failed to identify with her mother. The breakthrough is like an asylum treatment: "A shock. A jolt. Shock of knowing. Learning. Forced learning. Painful. Shameful." As in *The Snake Pit*, the analyst, not the institution, saves her.[41]

Robert Dahl offers up a similar cure in his memoir *Breakdown* (1959). Dahl was a family man with a promising career at a national charitable foundation when the crisis struck. He felt "pulled to pieces," and when his wife has a miscarriage and becomes suicidal. His doctor advises that he commit himself, and he eventually winds up in a dismal and crowded state hospital called River's Edge. River's Edge is a "prison" where they "control your body and your mind." Worse, "If they choose, if they decide for your good or the good of society, they can change you into another person through drug, electricity or surgeon's knife." A young doctor even jokes, "You wouldn't want us to make a turnip out of you? We could, you know, with a little surgery." Eventually, Dr. Agoston (with appropriate "heavy accent" and "big cigar") saves the day. Dahl learns that he had never cut his "infantile" ties to his mother. He escapes by talking his way out.[42]

At this point, it might appear that Freud reigned unchallenged. Recalls psychiatrist Yale Kramer,

In the late forties and fifties, college campuses were saturated with the new science. You read Freud in Soc Sci I; your professors talked about it, taught it, and lent you books on it. Your friends were in it, going to be in it, or had been in it. Your sophisticated friends' parents talked knowingly about it, hinting personal experience; your own parents looked nonplused and slightly dazed when you mentioned it. When you took your girlfriend to the movies, you went to see Hitchcock's *Spellbound*. Later that night, you joked with her in bed about the Id and the Super-Ego.

Yet a current of distrust swept alongside, always, even in the mid-century, Freudian heyday. Perhaps nothing reveals this as much as *Lolita*.[43]

Vladimir Nabokov's tale follows Humbert Humbert, a tortured pedophile who marries a woman in order to get close to her twelve-year-old daughter. Like *The Catcher in the Rye*, this is a story narrated after the fact from the confines of an institution. As Humbert notes, he began writing, "fifty-six days ago . . . first in the psychopathic ward for observation, and then in this well-heated, albeit tombal seclusion [jail cell]." The book opens with a fictitious "Forward" by a doctor who tells us we are about to get "a case history" that "will become, no doubt, a classic in psychiatric circles." But the book is nothing of the sort. At multiple points, Nabokov ridicules Freud, psychiatry, institutionalization, and all manner of pop-psychologizing. His success is in his tapping into the ongoing critique of conformity that runs beneath many Cold War–era writings. Humbert Humbert's sick urges are explained in psychological terminology, indicting the reader for wrapping immoral compulsions in neat, analytical packages. "While my body knew what it craved for, my mind rejected my body's every plea. One moment I was ashamed and frightened, another recklessly optimistic. Taboos strangulated me. Psychoanalysts wooed me with pseudoliberations of pseudolibidoes." In an effort at self-cure, Humbert spends time in a number of sanatoria. At one, he recovers by way of mockery.

> I owe my complete restoration to a discovery I made while being treated at that particular very expensive sanatorium. I discovered there was an endless source of robust enjoyment in trifling with

psychiatrists . . . By bribing a nurse I won access to some files and discovered, with glee, cards calling me "potentially homosexual" and "totally impotent." . . . I added another week just for the pleasure of taking on a powerful newcomer, a displaced (and, surely, deranged) celebrity, known for his knack of making patients believe they had witnessed their own conception.

The Freudian asylum only works because Humbert Humbert sees through its folly and empowers himself via scorn. He's never "healed." Nabokov seems to be telling us that madness is an artificial label placed on those who tread outside of the bounds of morality. Even worse, America seems to be engendering it. This is a land overstuffed with fakery and hypocrisy. Like in Poe, we are forced to identify with an unappealing character, sympathizing with a self-aware madman whose urges at once titillate and alienate us. Nabokov happily references Poe throughout, offering up disquieting references to Poe's famous ode to his pubescent wife, "Annabel Lee." The asylum is nothing more than false refuge in a culture that cannot "adjust" to its own contradictions. Nabokov's book, one might predict, both attracted and repelled Americans, just as Humbert Humbert was designed to do.[44]

"POLITE TOTAL POLICE CONTROL"

Many addressed worries of adjustment and social breakdown. Perhaps the Beats offered the best critique. In "About the Beat Generation," Jack Kerouac argued that the earliest Beats were crushed during the Korean War (1950–1953), when a "sinister new kind of efficiency appeared in America." He speculates that perhaps it was because of TV, and the rise of "the Polite Total Police Control of Dragnet's 'peace' officers." Though this first generation "vanished into jails and madhouses, or were shamed into silent conformity," a new group of Beats emerged with Rock n' Roll, James Dean, and other hip phenomena.[45]

The best-known Beat work, Kerouac's *On the Road*, shows how freedom is made by taking to the highways and living among the demimonde. This is madness, he acknowledges. In the most-quoted line in the book, Sal Paradise (a thinly disguised Kerouac) proclaims, "The only people for me are the mad ones, the ones who are mad to live, mad to talk, mad to be saved, desirous of everything at the same time, the ones who never yawn or say a commonplace thing, but burn, burn, burn like fabulous yellow roman candles exploding like spiders across the stars and in the middle you see the blue centerlight pop and everybody goes 'Awww!' "[46]

Madness as escape from conformity is a theme that runs throughout Beat works. As Nora Sayre explains in her memoir/analysis of the 1950s, the Beats "talked about 'going bananas' and 'flipping,' 'laughing academies' and 'bug-houses' and 'funny farms'; the words freed them from feeling stigmatized for having lost control. Nothing, they were saying, was abnormal, nothing should be forbidden; it was rewarding to be deviant." The Beats reveled in their madness, using it as a hammer to break through the walls of conformity and censorship. In a well-known Beat hangout, Slim Brundage's College of Complexes, clients were called "schizoids."[47]

Madness for many Beats was more than a metaphor. Jack Kerouac, Allen Ginsberg, Carl Solomon, Gregory Corso, and William Burroughs all spent time in mental institutions. Both Ginsberg and Burroughs were homosexual, and, at this time, the psychiatric community classified this as a mental illness. After he was sent to the New York State Psychiatric Institute as part of a plea deal for getting caught with stolen goods, Ginsberg tried to find catharsis. Instead, he found himself ignored and bored, hard evidence of a mental health system more interested in quarantine than in cure. In his journals, he notes that it was here that he came up with the notion of America as "a nation of madhouses." Ginsberg's observation of the effect of ECT on another patient, Carl Solomon, would play out in his nightmarish visions. He'd write to Kerouac how Carl "speaks in a sinister tone to me about how the doctors are driving him sane by shock therapy." Carl even demanded (but didn't receive) a lobotomy, seeing it as a heroic form of suicide. Allen knew about this treatment firsthand: he'd OK'd psychosurgery for his own mother.[48]

"Howl" is Allen Ginsberg's primal scream against the monstrosities of postwar capitalism, militarism, and conformity. He first recited it at San Francisco's Six Gallery on October 13, 1955, and published it in 1956 in the iconic *Howl and Other Poems*. Following a very public, obscenity trial in 1957, "Howl" gained national celebrity. The poem speaks to the paranoia of the times. He despairs, "I saw the best minds of my generation destroyed by madness, starving hysterical naked."

THE DAWNING AGE OF PARANOIA

The poet's vision is of a split America, both repressive and loose, an "armed madhouse."[49]

The asylum figures prominently in "Howl." In Part I, Ginsberg ties institutionalization with war, riffing "yacketayakking screaming vomiting whispering facts / and memories and anecdotes and eyeball kicks / and shocks of hospitals and jails and wars." He references Carl Solomon's treatments, including insulin, hydrotherapy, OT, ECT, and Metrozol, and makes full use of asylum horror. At "Pilgrim State's Rockland's and Greystone's foetid / halls," the "dream of life" becomes a "nightmare." In Part II, Ginsberg summons forth the demon Moloch, the monster that symbolizes both capitalism and soulless technology. Again, the asylum enters, with "Invincible / madhouses!" listed among suburbs, factories, and bombs. Moloch is our own creation, a monster we know.[50]

Part III recalls Ginsberg's hospitalization to sum up the dilemmas of his generation, repeating the refrain "I'm with you in Rockland" nineteen times. Though Carl Solomon had never been in Rockland, the name conjures a stony formation against which things break, and ties to the "Moloch" section with its "sphinx of cement and aluminum" that "bashed open their skulls and ate up their brains and imagination." (Also Rockland was known to be the locational basis for *The Snake Pit*.) This section evokes the irrationality of those incarcerated, with bizarre phrases and accusations taking us to the "abyss" before ending with a peaceful vision of Solomon visiting him in a cottage in the West. Ginsberg makes one final connection, linking the "hospital" with the ultimate Cold War horror—nuclear war.[51]

"Howl" is a freewheeling, devastating critique, circuiting the madness of the asylum to a mad society and finally to the insane logic of nuclear war. The madhouse served as the perfect culmination of the Cold War disease. He'd write to Kerouac that his mental hospital was both "Orwellian" and "Kafkesque," as if run by "machine men from the NKVD." Just as the asylum is totalitarian ("doctors are in control and have the means to persuade even the most recalcitrant"), so too is America.[52]

Kerouac would describe American "Civilization" as an infernal conjunction of "relativity, jets and superbombs and supercolossal bureaucratic totalitarian benevolent Big Brother structures." Similarly, he lamented the plight of the hobo amid "increased police surveillance of highways, railroad yards, sea shores, river bottom, embankments and the thousand-and-one hiding holes of industrial night." Looked at this way, the whole of American society was becoming an institution. Standardized housing, standardized testing, the military industrial complex, the freeway system, homogenized entertainment, "motivational research," psychological testing, mental health, and surveillance, all this pointed in just one direction—control. Explains the narrator in Kerouac's *The Dharma Bums*, "The only alternative to sleeping out, hopping freights, and doing what I wanted, I saw in a vision would be to just sit with a hundred other patients in front of a nice television set in a madhouse, where we could be 'supervised.'" And the Beat rebellion was just the beginning.[53]

CHAPTER 6

THEY'RE COMING TO TAKE YOU AWAY

The installations they do nowadays are generally successful. The technicians got more skill and experience. No more of the button holes in the forehead, no cutting at all—they go in through the eye sockets. Sometimes a guy goes over for an installation, leaves the ward mean and mad and snapping at the whole world and comes back a few weeks later with black-and-blue eyes like he'd been in a fist fight, and he's the sweetest, nicest, best-behaved thing you ever saw . . . A success, they say, but I say he's just another robot for the Combine.

—Chief Bromden in Ken Kesey's
One Flew Over the Cuckoo's Nest (1962)

Crazy as it sounds, the most influential of all asylum fictions was composed in a mental institution. In the summer of 1960, a young Stanford graduate student named Ken Kesey worked as a night attendant at the Menlo Park VA hospital, clacking away at the big typewriter in the nurse's office when he could. Sometimes he directly quoted the patients who stumbled by. He called his book *One Flew Over the Cuckoo's Nest.*[1]

In this chapter, I'll look at Kesey's book[2] and explore some of the dark corners of the 1950s and 1960s pop culture asylum. I'll examine psychosurgery, warehousing, and drugs, and show how, despite the Freudian rescue, the asylum remained a brutal metaphor for social control. As the first generation of Cold War kids came of age, their eyes opened to a whole catalogue of resentments. Perhaps unsurprisingly, they often used humor to express their discontent. Kesey's book, like Poe's "Tarr and Fether," is funny. So, I end this chapter with a cartoon frog singing to a patient in the windowsill of a psychiatric hospital.

ONE FLEW OVER THE CUCKOO'S NEST

One Flew Over the Cuckoo's Nest is a fable about independence and
liberty, configuring the asylum as an Orwellian metaphor for classic
enemies of the republic. Kesey draws liberally from multiple sources:
the agrarian legend of the white frontiersman resisting civilized ef-
feteness (with a noble Vanishing Indian at his side), Christian symbolism, the myth of the vampire female, and slavery. Yet his is a modern
project. McMurphy's rebellion is above all a guerilla action.[3]

The plot is straightforward and told from the perspective of a
giant, schizophrenic half-Indian named Chief Bromden. We learn
how the arrival of a bold delinquent named Randle P. McMurphy
turns the ward of an Oregon mental hospital upside-down. Under
McMurphy's leadership, the patients challenge tyrannical Big Nurse
by gaining control of their own therapies, playing basketball, gambling, going fishing, and eventually sneaking booze and prostitutes
in for a midnight party. They become "sick *men* . . . No more rabbits."
McMurphy duly receives punitive ECT and an eventual lobotomy.
The novel ends when Chief Bromden mercy kills the zombified hero
before busting out of the institution. Scholars have glossed Kesey's
use of myth, religion, metaphor, and poetics. They have also critiqued
his crude racial and gender stereotypes. I will focus on his transformation of dark asylum themes and how *Cuckoo's Nest* intervened in
the larger culture.[4]

Kesey's asylum is a closed-off, isolated, tightly monitored space,
like a prison or factory. The inmates wear green uniforms and serve
at the whim of a martinet and her subhuman drones. Gothic elements
are here. There are torture rooms (i.e., the "Shock Shop"), the windows
have mesh wire and cannot be easily broken, the doors are impossible to transgress, and everything is creepily suffused in "fog." But the
primary characteristic is modern control. The staff doses the patients
to keep them quiet and tracks them from a glass office. There are
modern amenities such as swimming pools, TV, and "chicken twice a
month." But modernity is anything but benign.[5]

The control apparatus here is totalizing. The touted patient democracy is a sham; the votes simply reflect the will of Big Nurse. An
infernal managerial system begins with group therapy in which the
patients report on each other and continues with the brutal African

American attendants who enforce Big Nurse's rule. Kesey describes these attendants in a nasty, racist way. "The blacker they are, [Big Nurse] learned from that long dark row that came before them, the more time they are likely to devote to cleaning and scrubbing and keeping the ward in order." One attendant is even described as "a twisted sinewy dwarf the color of cold asphalt."[6]

In this undemocratic, bureaucratic, racialized matriarchy, Kesey taps into the longstanding trope of imperiled whiteness. Anglos tremble under the grip of militarized tyranny and its (Black) slave legions. What this erases, of course, is the fact that control and surveillance are deeply embedded aspects of the non-white, and particularly African American, historical experience. As Frederick Douglass reflected, "At every gate through which we pass, we saw a watchman—at every ferry ground a guard—on every bridge a sentinel—and in every wood a patrol. We were hemmed in upon every side." Notes Simone Browne, "Surveillance is nothing new to black folks." The nightmare of enslavement, control, and surveillance here is the white nightmare of racialized degradation. In Kesey's hands, this sets the stage for his critique: the modern world is a great, emasculating reducer of independence.[7]

Nurse Ratched is the pivot upon which Kesey's narrative turns. She embodies the mechanical characteristics of the evil Combine. "Her face is smooth, calculated, and precision-made, like an expensive baby doll, skin like flesh-colored enamel, blend of white and cream and baby-blue eyes, small nose, pink little nostrils." She carries "no compact or lipstick or woman stuff, she's got that bag full of a thousand parts she aims to use in her duties today—wheels and gears, cogs polished to a hard glitter, tiny pills that gleam like porcelain, needles, forceps, watchmakers' pliers, rolls of copper wire." Inside her glass booth she watches and records, a kind of central processor in a ghastly computer network.[8]

To contextualize Big Nurse, we must begin by noting how the asylum has long been depicted as a repository for fearsome, desexed females. Nearly every major asylum account offers examples of brutal, female matrons, nurses, and attendants. Elizabeth Stone's 1841 narrative includes "a tall, black eyed, masculine looking female" who pushes everyone around. In Fanny Fern's *Ruth Hall* (1853), we meet Mrs. Bunce, who is "gaunt, sallow and bony, with restless, yellowish, glaring black eyes, very much resembling those of a cat in the dark;

her motions were quick, brisk, and angular; her voice loud, harsh, and wiry." In Elizabeth Packard's *Modern Persecution* (1875), there is Elizabeth Bonner, a "large, coarse, stout Irish woman, stronger than most men; of quick temper, very easily thrown off its balance, when, for the time being, she would be a perfect demon, lost to all traces of humanity. Her manners were very coarse and masculine, a loud and boisterous talker, and a great liar, with no education, and could neither read nor write." Nellie Bly relates the "coarse, massive" female attendants who curse and spit tobacco in the wards of Blackwell's Island. Similarly, the female attendants in Florence Seyler Thompson's *A Thousand Faces* (1920) are "large of stature, well-built, very strong, and coarse." Margaret Starr's *Sane or Insane? Or How I Regained Liberty* (1904) gives us Madam Pike, a "short, muscular woman . . . with hands, arms, and limbs indicating unusual strength." Pike has a voice "deep in tone" and the unsettling ability to stare at a patient for minutes on end without blinking. She is a "vindictive, cruel, heartless shrew." Olive Higgins Prouty cannot resist giving us the brusque nurse Miss Trask, a foil upon which to juxtapose Charlotte's kindness toward young Tina. *The Snake Pit* (1946) has the aptly named "Miss Wildebeest Hart" who orders the patients around, treating them like naughty children. And the nerve clinic in Sylvia Plath's 1958 short story, "Johnny Panic and the Bible of Dreams," has secretary Miss Milleravage, "a large woman, not fat, but all sturdy muscle and tall on top of it." She hauls the narrator into the ECT room. "Against her great bulk I beat my fists, and against her whopping milkless breasts, until her hands on my wrists are iron hoops and her breath hushabyes me with a love-stink fouler than Undertaker's Basement."[9]

Kesey's innovation is to elevate Nurse Ratched to *uber-commandant* of an entire asylum and to emphasize her control over men not women. Her rule is mediated by neither doctors nor superintendents. The "supervisor," we learn, is another woman, who also serves Ratched. Explains patient Harding, "The doctor doesn't hold the power of hiring and firing. That power goes to the supervisor, and the supervisor is a woman, a dear old friend of Miss Ratched's; they were Army nurses together in the thirties. We are victims of a matriarchy here, my friend, and the doctor is just as helpless against it as we are." Ratched is desexed and rough, "big as a damn barn and tough as knife metal." What ultimately breaks her is McMurphy's act of tearing open her dress and exposing her breasts, re-sexualizing her and thus reducing her power.[10]

Like Ratched, the inmates evoke older themes while simultaneously transforming them. Many have illnesses not somatic in origin. Billy Bibbit is afflicted by a low self-esteem-based stutter resulting from his domineering mother. The Age of Freud elevated emasculating motherhood to existential villainy. Take away mom and all references to her and Bibbit becomes independent. Harding has the "illness" of homosexuality. Notably, he is the patient most at odds with the manly McMurphy. His condition is exacerbated by Ratched, who belittles him in group therapy, reinforcing the then-current canard that gays were "made" by their moms. But unlike earlier tales of the railroaded sane, in *Cuckoo's Nest* the inmates are clearly incapable of dealing with the modern world. The subtext is that the modern world is to blame. These patients are "rabbits" beaten down by the system.[11]

Keeping with tradition, Kesey's asylum is a monster factory, though again, he offers striking innovations. The monstrous patients are merely "mistakes." Ruckly's botched lobotomy makes him a "robot." Ellis has been "overloaded" by ECT and is now "nailed against the wall in the same condition they lifted him off the table for the last time, in the same shape, arms out, palms cupped, with the same horror on his face. He's nailed like that on the wall, like a stuffed trophy." These monsters are unintended. They are now sad "machines with flaws inside that can't be repaired."[12]

But there are no Freudian rescues. Kesey personally believed that "Freud was full of shit." In *Cuckoo's Nest,* he ridicules the idea that neuroses are located in early childhood traumas. We get plenty of laughable Freudian aphorisms in the monologues of Harding, the effete intellectual who McMurphy replaces in the leadership role. Yet Freud is still here; he informs in the novel's subtext. As Ruth Sullivan shows, a crafted, oedipal situation is evident. Consistent with many contemporary Freudians, the mother-figures in the book are terrifying. Chief Bromden's mom belittled his dad. Harding's wife is sexually aggressive and domineering. Billy Bibbit's mother practically seduces him ("She wrinkled her nose and opened her lips at him and made a kind of wet kissing sound in the air with her tongue, and I had to admit she didn't look like a mother of any kind").[13]

Another innovation is Kesey's making the Women in White into males. The inmates are thoroughly unmanned. Big Nurse is a "ball-cutter," lobotomy is "frontal-lobe castration," and Group Discussion is "a pecking party" (where Big Nurse pecks "at your everlovin' *balls*"). When the men finally stand up for themselves, they do so in an act of masculine regeneration, with a party that includes prostitutes. Asserting themselves sexually over hookers and then Big Nurse herself, they recapture their agency. Breakouts, both metaphoric and real, follow.[14]

Situating *Cuckoo's Nest* within its militarized, historical moment is vital to understanding Kesey's project. He had avoided military service, but his generation served in percentages far higher than any ever had. The book uses martial references to establish its tone. Asylum escapees are "AWOLs." Big Nurse, an Army veteran, runs her ward with military discipline, down to using a mirror to spot-check the latrines. She plans "her next maneuver" after she is foiled by McMurphy. When she busts the patients after they have their party, Harding muses, "We shall be all of us shot at dawn. One hundred cc's apiece. Miss Ratched shall line us all against the wall, where we'll face the terrible maw of a muzzle-loading shotgun which she has loaded with Miltowns! Thorazines! Libriums! Stelazines! And with a wave of her sword, *blooie*! Tranquilize all of us completely out of existence." McMurphy is a Korean War vet who received a Distinguished Service Cross "for leading an escape from a Communist prison camp." Though he was dishonorably discharged (foreshadowing his inability to be tamed by Big Nurse's discipline), he is war-heroic, a John Wayne–type who might run up to the machine gun nest and toss in the decisive grenade. He defies the ordeal of punitive ECT, telling Big Nurse, "Hooee, those Chinese Commies could have learned a few things from you, lady." Bromden is also a veteran who "was hurt by seeing things in the Army, in the war." When the inmates go on a fishing trip, the boat is captained by an inmate who was a PT boat captain in World War II (just like John F. Kennedy). In sum, the asylum breaks men just as the military breaks men; yet their heroism depends upon a violent ethos of resistance.[15]

The book also reflects contemporary concerns about corporate bureaucracy. Metaphors of business, machinery, labor, and factories abound. A few examples: Nurse Ratched's name sounds like "ratchet," a toothed mechanism that only moves in one direction (it is also a verb, meaning "to cause to move by steps or degrees," suggestive of the process of factory motion). She manages from her "glass Station" like "a watchful robot," and becomes upset when "something keeps her outfit from running like a smooth, accurate, precision-made machine." She takes notes all day and enters the data into a machine. She "accumulates her ideal staff" and "dreams of . . . a world of precision efficiency and tidiness like a pocket watch with a glass back." The men carrying out the medical procedures are "technicians." The ward itself is reminiscent of a "cotton mill" and also "a factory for the Combine." The name "Combine" evokes both the mechanical farming implement that levels fields and the big, corporate "combinations" dominating the economy; it is "a huge organization that aims to adjust the Outside as well as [Big Nurse] has the Inside." The Combine is manifested in "things like five thousand houses punched out identical by a machine and strung across the hills outside of town, so fresh from the factory that they're still linked together like sausages."[16]

The Combine captures Kesey's ultimate innovation—the infernal continuity between asylum and society. From the group therapy that Dr. Spivey wants to be "a little world Inside that is a made-to-scale prototype of the big world Outside" to the belittling observations to the mollifying drugs, this place *is* America. Writes Foucault, "Our society is not one of spectacle, but of surveillance . . . the circuits are the supports of an accumulation and a centralization of knowledge . . . We are neither in the amphitheatre, nor the stage, but in the panopticon machine, invested by its effects of power, which we bring to ourselves since we are part of its mechanism." The inmates of Kesey's asylum police themselves. As McMurphy learns to his horror, the ward inhabitants are largely self-committed. They spend their days monitoring each other and recording the results in a logbook. And though Big Nurse is evil, she is essentially just a component of something larger. She is a part of a machine, and parts are, after all, replaceable. In the culminating event of the book, when McMurphy finally attacks her, he must first smash "through that glass door" to get at her.[17]

Kesey's argument was prefigured a year earlier. In Erving Goffman's *Asylums*, based on his experiences at St. Elizabeth's Hospital, we are introduced to the "total institution." Total institutions, he explains, are places where inmates are sequestered and subjected to rigid control. Once inside these "forcing houses for changing persons," patients are modified to suit the system. Goffman's intake description sounds like a primer for McMurphy's confrontation with the Combine. And Goffman is not concerned with the evolution of institutional practice. For him, the asylum is transhistorical, an island in a timeless archipelago of total institutions. As Michael E. Staub notes, in Goffman's institution, personnel don't matter; the institution *itself* is the oppressor. Staub argues that the two works are "complementary rather than comparable." One might add that Kesey's book fictionalizes Goffman's total institution and makes characters count for narrative purposes. To fantasize our way out of total control, we need protagonists and antagonists. Kesey also goes further than Goffman in one major respect. For Goffman, the asylum is a discrete place, if however symbolic of "free society." For Kesey, the asylum *is* society. Through the Combine, we learn that America is nothing but a single, vast, total institution.[18]

MAKING ROBOTS

Big Nurse finally ends McMurphy with the operation of "last resort," the lobotomy. The medical history of the lobotomy properly starts with Egas Moniz, a Portuguese neurologist. He performed the first leucotomy (which would become "lobotomy" in the United States) in the mid-1930s. In this decade of new "shock" treatments, the idea of attacking the brain directly was not unreasonable. Moniz received a Nobel Prize for his efforts in 1949. Walter Freeman and his associate James Watts brought the procedure to America in 1936, and it slowly made its way into the asylum repertoire in the 1940s. The process involved boring through the skull, and Freeman dreamed of a quicker operation that would empty the crowded back wards and free patients from their hellish existences. It mattered less whether the person who left was the same one who entered. As Freeman explained in his co-authored book *Psychosurgery*, for a patient's relatives, "a cheerful drone . . . is more bearable than a complaining one." Freeman began by following Moniz's procedure, but he really desired a better, faster, less complex cerebral adjustment. Working on cadavers, he happened upon an idea inspired by something in his own kitchen—the icepick. He inserted the pick into a tear duct and whacked it with a hammer, driving the point through the orbital plate and into the frontal lobe. Then he moved the pick laterally. He had to admit that his new transorbital lobotomy looked "medieval," especially since, in lieu of an anesthetic, he would stun patients first with a blast or two of ECT. But, within hours, the patient would be up and on their feet, wearing sunglasses to hide the splotchy bruises inking their eyes. Notably, many more women were lobotomized than men, and they were lobotomized far more often for sexual transgressions.[19]

Fictional lobotomies started soon after factual ones. E. B. White, author of *Charlotte's Web* and other beloved books, wrote a piece for *The New Yorker* in 1939 titled "The Door," in which a disturbed and confused patient appears to escape the procedure by leaving a room. The public got a full serving of lobotomy in Robert Penn Warren's Pulitzer Prize–winning, 1946 novel, *All the King's Men*. This fictionalized treatment of Southern demagogue Huey Long traces the rise and fall of "Willie Stark." Like Long, Stark meets his demise at the hands of a disgruntled doctor. In Long's case, the assassin was Carl Weiss, a physician aggrieved over the senator's attempt to remove his judge father-in-law via redistricting. For Stark, the assassin is Adam Stanton, a refined asylum doctor who has previously taken the narrator to his hospital to watch a prefrontal lobotomy on a "catatonic schizophrenic." The narrator is surprised to learn that there exists a surgery for "being nutty." He surmises, "I thought you just humored and gave them cold baths and let them make raffia baskets and got them to tell you their dreams." He is mixing classic warehouse treatments with newer Freudian interventions. "No," counters Dr. Stanton, "you can cut on them." Stanton explains that he is going to give his patient a "different personality." Currently, the man only "sits on a chair or lies on his back on a bed and stares into space," but soon he will be back among the living. Burden convinces the doctor to let him watch.[20]

The lobotomy in *All the King's Men* is not the procedure pioneered by Walter Freeman. Dr. Stanton slices his scalpel across the patient's head and peels back the skin. After sopping up a "considerable" amount of blood, he drills "five or six holes" and then uses a saw to open up the skull like a "high-grade carpenter." Stanton then wields an "electric gadget" that cuts out chunks of brain, leaving a burning odor reminiscent of Burden's childhood memories of horses burning in a barn. Eventually the patient gets sewn back up, "the little pieces of brain which had been cut out ... put away to think their little thoughts quietly somewhere among the garbage."²¹

Dr. Stanton is a progressive man of science. His solution reflects the new trend that saw mental illness as rooted in biology. As a science writer summarized in 1955, "There is a revolution in psychiatry: a change in emphasis from psychology to biology." Stanton's gory procedure is shocking to read, but most lobotomy coverage was actually quite positive. In 1937, the *New York Times* boasted that the new "psycho-surgery" can turn "wild animals into gentle creatures." The article did, however, include the disclaimer that some "leading neurologists" were "very skeptical." A few years later, an AP report told of "More than fifty 'hopelessly' insane persons" who were now "living and back at work" thanks to the "new wizardry of surgery." In 1946, *Time* magazine reported that "lobotomy centers" were "swamped" with requests. By 1949, the *New York Times* editorialized that the technique had "justified itself."²²

Lobotomies hit their height between 1949 and 1952, with some five thousand procedures carried out each year in America. But this golden age was short-lived, and critics grew louder. In a powerful 1951 essay, "The Operation of Last Resort," Irving Wallace told how the operation "is the center of a heated, world-wide controversy." The debate was between neuropsychiatrists, who argued that lobotomy "prevents insanity and suicide" and "usually makes men happier," and their opponents, who thought it "converts patients into docile, inert, often useless drones." The bulk of Wallace's account follows a patient called "Larry," who is lobotomized to keep him out of "an asylum." Larry winds up "happier" but also a far different person from his former self. Though Wallace leaves his opinion as to the operation's necessity unsaid, the story is horrifyingly told and includes a photo of a doctor injecting an anesthetic into the shaved head of a patient strapped to an operating table. It is hard not to be shocked when Wallace writes, "The thin knife had removed his worries. It had also removed his old personality."²³

Lobotomy tapped into historical fears of slavery and control. In the bizarre 1952 novel *Limbo* by Bernard Wolfe, psychosurgery proves a false answer to modern problems. The book features a neurosurgeon named Dr. Martine who flees the H-bombs of World War III to find solace on an uncharted isle off the coast of Africa. He lives here eighteen years, assuming a leadership position in the indigenous society and raising a son named Rambo. His most important task is lobotomizing the violently agitated among the populace. He does this because the natives formerly used a very crude method to "chase the devils from the head" via a rock and a chisel. After the real world intrudes on his island paradise, Martine must leave and find his way in a post-apocalyptic America. He discovers that tensions between a reconstituted Russia and reconstructed America are leading to a new war. One thing Martine knows, however, is that lobotomies are not the answer. As he tells the mad-doctor/dictator Helder, who wants to lobotomize everyone, "I can slice up the worst homicidal maniac's prefrontal lobes and give you a real lamb of a pacifist, sure, the best little basket case you ever saw—but he's not a human being any more, just a lump!" Most horribly, Dr. Martine must blast his own mortally wounded son's brains out: "First successful lobotomy he had ever performed. As he had to. Last he would ever perform. As he had to." *Limbo* preaches that lobotomies are no good because they destroy our virile, if flawed essence. The answer to war lies in Freud's theories, particularly the recognition that aggression is disguised "masochism" that can be addressed if appropriately analyzed. Wolfe's argument boils down to a Freudian critique that lobotomies only address the symptoms without getting down to the sickness itself. *Psychiatric Quarterly* praised his book.[24]

Famed playwright Tennessee Williams also found literary use for the lobotomy. In *Suddenly Last Summer* (1958), a monstrous old Southern belle named Mrs. Venable tries to get a handsome, young doctor to lobotomize her niece. The reason: she doesn't want the girl to tell the world that her dead son was a gay dilettante cannibalized by the young boys he was soliciting. Mrs. Venable is not concerned with the doctor's reasonable advice regarding the surgery. He tries to explain that it is "new and radical" and that "there is a good deal of risk." She does not care. She only wants her niece to stop "smashing my son's reputation." In the end, with the help of truth serum, Venable's niece escapes with her brain intact. The play concludes with Mrs. Venable being led off stage by the doctor after she tries to smash her niece with her cane, perhaps in hopes of short-circuiting the need for psychosurgery. Her final words: "Lion's View! State asylum, cut this hideous story out of her brain!"[25]

Suddenly Last Summer references Williams's life, including his own tortured sexuality and his sister Rose's stays in mental hospitals and lobotomy. Although the lobotomy is a punishment as far as Mrs. Venable is concerned, it is also held up as something of value to those who might really need it. As the good doctor explains, lobotomies offer hope to the dangerously deranged. He tells of the pride and relief he experienced after performing one on a wild, obscene woman. The issue then is the misuse of a potentially dangerous procedure.[26]

Starring Elizabeth Taylor as the niece, Montgomery Clift as the doctor, and Katherine Hepburn as Mrs. Venable, the 1959 movie *Suddenly, Last Summer* owes as much to the film *The Snake Pit* as it does to Williams's play. Like *The Snake Pit*, we begin in a state hospital. In fact, most of the action takes place in the asylum, rather than in Venable's house as in the play. The opening credits roll over a brick wall that fully occupies the screen. The camera pans to a small metal plaque, "Lion's View State Asylum," establishing the story as one of imprisonment. Next, we go inside a dreary dayroom, where lost women stare at walls, play with dolls, and hunch over chairs and tables. The camera focuses on one woman lifting her doll up to catch the rays of a setting sun. Later, we see her prepped for a lobotomy, the first one in the state (it is explained this is 1937; the same year, coincidentally, that Williams erroneously dated as his sister's real-life lobotomy). The procedure is filmed up until the first incision, including the tracing of a line across a shaved skull as a group of doctors look down from a decrepit balcony.

Keeping with the times, Clift plays the doctor as a brave Freudian, the savior of the damned in a warehouse state hospital. He doesn't like doing lobotomies, and the superintendent even scolds him for it. Unlike the character who in the play has an "icy charm," Clift is sensitive and gallant. In other words, he's more like the movie version of Dr. Kik than he is of Tennessee's creation. In another nod to *The Snake Pit*, Catherine flees her room and stumbles into the chaotic men's dayroom, where a spiral staircase and aerial shots summon the famous crane shot of that film. *Suddenly, Last Summer* deviates from the play in other ways as well. In the play, the truth serum helps convince a lobotomist that he need not operate. In the movie, Clift races against time, battling with a superintendent who wants to operate immediately, him pushing for just "one more day" to "break through that block to the truth." The film also has a love story tacked on. When Clift injects Taylor with the truth serum, she swoons, "Hold me! I've been so lonely," and they passionately kiss. Clift tells the rest of the family, "Catherine's going to be alright," hence neatly sewing up the story with Taylor at his side.

In *Suddenly, Last Summer* lobotomies are sad and occasionally necessary. Avoiding them is best. Analysis seems to be the best alternative, but there was also another option. As Frank G. Slaughter makes clear in his 1958 novel *Daybreak*, a pill can also do the trick.

Daybreak concerns Dr. James "Jim" Corwin, a man of integrity and intelligence who experiences a crisis and finds new purpose at an institution. As the book opens, we find Corwin at the prestigious Lakewood Hospital prepping a prefrontal lobotomy. The patient is "another charity case, from a locked ward at Rocky Point, a state hospital for the insane." Corwin is assisting the famous and pompous Dr. Anton Ziegler, a "squat, china-bald Viennese with drill-sergeant eyes, whose voice was a perpetual bark." As he preps the patient, Corwin wonders at the ultimate purpose of it all. Performing lobotomies feels like working on an assembly line. At the same time, he recognizes that this man and others like him are suffering a living death, "buried in their cells as irrevocably as though they were already underground." Yet he cannot quiet the voice asking him if he might be destroying "the bridge linking [the patient], however remotely, to the angels?"[27]

Tragedy strikes when Corwin's cheating wife dies in an automobile crash with her paramour. Distraught, Corwin flees south, serving as ship's surgeon aboard the *Creole Belle* as it winds its way down the Mississippi. Onboard, he encounters the beautiful and mysterious Lynn Thorndyke, on whom he must operate to repair a ruptured ovarian follicle. It turns out that Lynn is depressed and wants to die, and so after saving her, Corwin refers her to an analyst friend at a mental hospital in Baltimore. Lynn is diagnosed as a catatonic schizophrenic and gets shipped to a southern state hospital called Leyden. Jim decides to get a job at Leyden so that he might help the girl.

Like other madhouses of literature, Leyden first appears quaint and pastoral, but looks are deceiving. Corwin quickly notices the bars, the screens in the windows, the guards, and the "nameless odor" of "sweat, formaldehyde, and despair." Once inside, he learns that the "real reason" he was hired has to do with his lobotomist credentials. As the vast, pompous superintendent Thaddeus Meeker explains, turning "lunatics" into "lambs" on a "large enough scale" will provide both a docile workforce and save him money on attendants. In other words, the superintendent wants to create robots.[28]

Corwin at first goes along, performing Freeman-style transorbital procedures. The first man he operates on, Enoch Williams, is already basically dead, "The body, sprawled in corpselike abandon, scarcely seemed to breathe." The operation brings Enoch back to life. Many more operations follow, but similar miracles are hard to come by. Some patients turn into "perambulating zombies," others into "literal robots." The lobotomy, Jim finally concludes, offers no dependable cure. True healing can only happen with intensive psychoanalysis.[29]

Daybreak asserts that the tragedy of mental health care is that there are too many patients and not enough analysts. Thus, the appeal of dramatic treatments like lobotomy. As one doctor explains, the problem is that most psychiatrists operate in private practice, dealing with rich "neurotics," while the state hospitals are "deluged with people in desperate need of such treatment—and we can do little more than lock them up. When someone of Dr. Ziegler's stature introduces a program of lobotomy you can hardly blame Dr. Meeker for trumpeting its virtues to the skies." Superintendent Meeker's slave labor operation is an outcome of the logic of cheap legislatures and corrupt bureaucracies.[30]

Fortunately, Frank G. Slaughter offers a spectacularly optimistic message of hope: drugs. Specifically, reserpine (a.k.a. Serpasil) and phenidylate (a.k.a. Ritalin). These medications work by providing a "bridge" to lost minds, helping analysts access underlying casual traumas. Corwin saves Lynn from an imminent lobotomy by dosing her with drugs, and then he marries her. The fatherly Freudian thus enters the asylum and saves a Woman in White from an evil superintendent who would convert her into a robotic slave. Meeker gets his comeuppance when Corwin exposes him for the fraud he is, and he subsequently gets replaced by a Viennese Freudian named Dr. Frankel. The author's afterward touts the new miracle drugs and even thanks "the medical service division of Ciba Pharmaceutical Products" (makers of Serpasil and Ritalin) and Smith, Kline and French Laboratories (who make Thorazine).[31]

Published three years before *Cuckoo's Nest*, *Daybreak* offers escape from lobotomy while still leaving room for meaningful asylum psychiatry. After Kesey's work hit the stands, psychiatric solutions became more suspect. In Elliot Baker's novel *A Fine Madness*, another big, virile man is locked up and lobotomized. An even more outrageous rebel than McMurphy, Samson Shilltoe is not to be beaten by the icepick.

In *A Fine Madness*, a brilliant poet-rebel hurtles through life drinking, womanizing, and being an all-around bad boy, pursued by cops, psychiatrists, and various, amorous females. Samson Shilltoe is anything but an ivory tower intellectual. He looks like a "prizefighter" or a "prairie scout," with a "high forehead and big chin" that "placed him on the prow of a ship with the ocean spray hitting his eyes." He's the quintessential Natural Man, a primitive brawler whose rugged lust for life makes him irresistible to the female sex. His physical abuse of girlfriend Rhoda is explained as being a part of his nonconformist character and is "hilariously" depicted without evidence of remonstrance from Rhoda. For example: "He threw a roundhouse right, but she stepped inside it."[32]

Samson is in constant battle with the forces that try and tame him. Once a woman had tricked him into marriage, and when she became pregnant, he suggested, "one little left jab in the stomach." She fled to her parents' house. Samson now gets accosted by her lawyer demanding delinquent childcare payments. Others similarly want something from him. His agent wants him to keep writing and reading his poetry. Cops chase him after he tries to frame a man who is having an affair on a woman friend. A neighbor accosts him for his mistreatment of her husband. Finally, he's pursued by Dr. Oliver Wren, the psychiatrist Rhoda pays to help remove his writer's block.[33]

The pursuits end when Samson returns to Dr. Wren's asylum (he's already fled once) to retrieve the unfinished epic poem he left there. He's caught by two "gorilla" attendants and receives a lobotomy. Described in agonizing detail, we read how the white room and strange men remind him of the concentration camp he'd entered in World War II, when "the skeletons in tight, bleached skins had clapped their hands." But unlike that camp, these occupants are "well fed." During the procedure, the doctor offers droll commentary while a conscious Samson thinks random thoughts. Despite their penetrations, the doctors cannot still his mind. The lobotomy fails. Afterwards, he completes his epic poem, undefeated.[34]

The movie based on the novel is much campier. Sean Connery plays Samson in an apparent effort to escape being typecast as a debonair spy, but he cannot escape his James Bond-ness. He's altogether more charming and handsome than the character in Baker's novel. Playing up the humor and playing down the violence, his domestic abuse is explained to be pure theater. He doesn't punch Rhoda until the very end of the film, and she literally *asks* him for it. The director, Irvin Kershner, who would go on to direct *The Empire Strikes Back*, seems swept into the misogyny of the times.[35]

A Fine Madness provides cinema's first description of Walter Freeman's procedure, with a bespectacled "Dr. Menken" standing in for the lobotomist. Menken's black-rimmed glasses echo Freeman's, while spooky sci-fi music marks him as a mad scientist. Menken begins with a violent chimpanzee named "Jo Jo" (in seeming reference to historical chimps Becky and Lucy, who had their frontal lobes removed in the earliest lobotomy) and then switches to a plastic skull model with ghastly eyeballs. Menken demonstrates inserting the pick into the orbital plate, orgasmically thrusting it in and sliding it about until the eyeball pops out and flies across the room. Chided by Freudian observers, he rebuts them, saying his technique is the only salvation for violent patients. In the novel, the lobotomist is not ludicrous, and he tellingly says that his main concern is one of demand. Angry schizophrenic men are simply becoming harder to find, thanks to the fact that "in a matriarchal society, increasing in conformity daily, catatonic excitement in the male was becoming almost as extinct as the dodo." Samson is a perfect candidate because the matriarchy hasn't crushed his spirit.[36]

Though lobotomies lost their luster in the medical community by the late 1950s, cinema and fiction took quite a shine to them. The idea of an extant procedure that could turn you into a robot was simply irresistible. For instance, ape-people in the distant future use them to crush human willfulness. In *The Planet of the Apes* (1968), co-scripted by *The Twilight Zone*'s Rod Serling, simians lobotomize an astronaut. Steeped in heavy-handed social critique, this movie gives us much to ponder. The apes are racially stratified (the orangutans being the masters, gorillas the soldiers, and chimpanzees the discriminated-against underdogs), and they dominate the humans. Though the apes are primitively stuck with horses, carriages, adobe huts, and simple firearms, they have no problem hammering through skulls to great effect. (In the source novel by Pierre Boulle, the apes are far more advanced, so brain surgery seems less out of place there.) When a visiting astronaut (Charlton Heston) locates a missing crewman among the apes, he wonders why his friend does not recognize him. We soon see why—a long scar on his head signifies lobotomy. Rants Heston, "You did it. You cut up his brain, you bloody baboon!" He tells the apes, "You took his identity." Dr. Zaius, the leading ape scientist, agrees, calling brain surgery "a kind of living death."[37]

This film is doing more than simply using a lobotomy as shorthand for robot-making. It is offering up a warning. As the ape "anti-vivisectionist society" struggles to save Heston from his own lobotomy, we ponder lone voices in the wilderness of modern injustice. Serling, whose social conscience broadcasts loudly in the script (as does that of his co-author, Red-baited Michael Wilson), is telling us to watch out lest we lose all that we hold dear in the name of Cold War security. Serling and Wilson depict a racially oppressive state, twinning discriminatory and totalitarian threats. The lobotomy becomes a metaphor for a panoply of contemporary liberal nightmares. Awaiting brain surgery, Heston rages that he is in "a madhouse." Hardly could a stronger, or stranger, use of the lobotomy be mustered.[38]

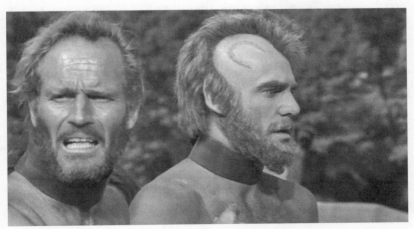

Charlton Heston and an astronaut lobotomized by an ape in *Planet of the Apes* (1968)

GOD FORSAKEN

The Cold War asylum was not only a metaphor. These were places of much concern. Americans slid down the social ladder and into the nightmare space that João Biehl calls the "zone of social abandonment." One finds artistic expression of this in the plays of Tennessee Williams. In *A Streetcar Named Desire* and *Suddenly Last Summer*, asylums are off-stage graveyards for unmentionable, family problems. In *Streetcar*, Blanche DuBois, a deteriorating "neurasthenic personality," gets carted off to the state hospital on the arm of a doctor, parting with the famous line, "I have always depended on the kindness of strangers." She arrives at this point after being raped by her sister's brutal husband amid the poverty and squalor of their turbulent existence. Living with it is just too much for her. The asylum doctor arrives with a standard-issue "Matron" who, "divested of all the softer properties of womanhood," is "a particularly sinister figure in her severe dress." Williams had walked through a ward at a state hospital with his sister in 1937, and he was affected by this space "full of narrow beds and wooden benches, with a catatonic young girl crouching under one of them."[39]

A realistic depiction of social abandonment can be seen in Dariel Telfer's 1959 debut novel *The Caretakers*. In this book, Canterbury state hospital destroys all who enter, staff and patients alike. The tale centers on a pair of young nurse affiliates named Kathy and Althea. Both experience life-changing traumas. Althea, raped by a lecherous doctor, goes into the "living death" of catatonia and is taken away by him, he proclaiming his love for her. Kathy is nearly murdered by a patient and survives to find peace in the arms of a journalist.[40]

The asylum in *The Caretakers* is bleak. Treatments are scarce, doctors are either emotionally out-of-touch or downright dangerous, and the staff is terrorized by patients and physicians alike. Other characters include Lucretia Terry, who "was not a woman; she was authority personified and she wanted the world to know it . . . She was a dictator;" Dr. Donovan Macleod, competent but cold; and Dr. Andreatta, a Portuguese Don Juan who sneaks around raping nymphomaniac patients. *The Caretakers* sold well, reviews praising its "nauseating realism."[41]

In 1963, United Artists released a film adaptation of Telfer's book. But Hollywood had its own agenda. The movie is more homage to

The Snake Pit than a blast at systemic mistreatment. And like with *The Snake Pit*, male Freudian screenwriters substantially changed a woman's original work. The focus shifts from the two female protagonists to a male analyst, who enters a dismal institution in order to save a damsel in distress. The film begins by following Lorna, a woman who has a breakdown in a movie theater and gets carried off to Canterbury in an ambulance. While the movie drops in on her slow progress from time to time, her purpose is to take us inside so we can meet Dr. MacLeod (spelled slightly differently from the novel) and witness his efforts to bring humanity and light to an institution ruled by the ruthless nurse supervisor Lucretia Terry (Joan Crawford). MacLeod (Robert Stack) is a dreamer and pioneer, his goal to replace such asylums with innovative outpatient facilities. He initiates a group therapy program while being challenged at every step by Lucretia, who is essentially a pre-Forman Nurse Ratched. The two battle over the soul of the hospital.[42]

The movie keeps with *The Snake Pit*'s depiction of scary treatments, such as an ECT scene in which Lorna is blasted by Dr. MacLeod while being pinned down by nurses and attendants and watched by a crowd of young affiliate nurses. The scene alternates between Lorna's arching back and twisting legs and a close-up of the ECT dial. As in *The Snake Pit*, electroconvulsive therapy is explained by a Freudian doctor as a means of breaking through a patient's defenses so analysis can take place. When a cruel nurse tells Lorna many more shocks are coming, the infuriated Dr. MacLeod sends her off. The final scene shows MacLeod's triumph. Freshly liberated patients file in to the new day hospital, where they get group therapy and get to go home to their families at night. In this Freudian fantasy, Hollywood demonstrated it was not ready to deliver Telfer's story. Criticism had limits.

INSTITUTIONALIZATION IS FUNNY

In 1966, Napoleon XIV (Jerry Samuels) released a novelty song, "They're Coming to Take Me Away, Ha Ha." The number is not so much sung as it is spoken over a rhythmic tambourine and drum, with Napoleon telling us how his lover rejected him and drove him insane. The chorus, sung with a voice rising in pitch (thanks to a new device called the Variable Frequency Oscillator) and sirens playing in the background, makes committal funny:

> And they're coming to take me away Ha Ha
> They're coming to take me away ho ho he he ha ha
> To the happy home with trees and flowers and chirping birds
>   and basket
> weavers who sit and smile and twiddle their thumbs and toes
> They're coming to take me away ha ha

The B-Side of the album is even crazier. It's just the song in reverse. The bizarre ditty became a massive success, selling five hundred thousand copies and hitting number three on the charts. But the triumph was ephemeral. Radio stations began getting a lot of complaints, "mostly from nurses," according to one program director. The track was pulled from major markets, even as it sat high in the charts. There was at least one protest, with youths in New York carrying signs saying, "We're coming to take WMCA [a New York station] Away! Unfair to Napoleon in Everyway."[43]

Humor, Freud tells us in *Jokes and their Relation to the Unconscious*, reveals the desires of the unconscious, as well as offering a means of circumventing repressive social structures. The Cold War may not seem funny, but, in dark times, humor buds like mushrooms. Director Stanley Kubrick, for instance, tried at first to make a tense and dramatic screenplay out of the 1958 nuclear war thriller *Red Alert*. But the parts that seemed most ludicrous also seemed most true. So, he made it into a comedy. *Dr. Strangelove, or How I Stopped Worrying and Learned to Love the Bomb*, unlike in the source novel, annihilates the planet in mushroom clouds to the accompanying voice of Vera Lynn singing "We'll Meet Again." This happens because a deranged general named Jack D. Ripper triggers Russia's Doomsday Device in an effort to strike first and "win" the Cold War. There is perhaps no better imagery of MAD-ness than Major "King" Kong gleefully riding a nuke to Earth like a bucking bronco, waving his cowboy hat and hollering. Likewise, Joseph Heller's *Catch-22* pivots on the absurd premise that since war is insane, the military must operate along insane lines. Like *Strangelove*, *Catch-22* patently shows the contradiction of free and rational thought in a system structured around total militarization. Such humor is rife in anti-authoritarian, Cold War–era products like *The Dirty Dozen* (1967), where an army psychiatrist says that, since the Dozen are "the most twisted, most antisocial bunch of psychopaths I have ever run into," he "can't think of a better way to fight a war."[44]

The inverted world of the asylum is a perfect place for humor. In *Cuckoo's Nest*, there is a scene in which McMurphy pretends he is watching a banned baseball game on a TV. As Big Nurse is "hollering and screaming," McMurphy avidly scrutinizes the dark screen, inspiring the other patients to stop working and conspiratorially join him. Nurse Ratched rants, "You're committed, you realize. You are . . . under the *jurisdiction* of me . . . the staff . . . Under jurisdiction and *control.*" Acting silly frustrates a system dependent upon rigid, agreed upon rules.[45]

Madhouse follies are in evidence in numerous Cold War cultural artifacts. In Ralph Ellison's 1952 novel *Invisible Man*, the nameless African American protagonist takes a white trustee into a bar and sparks a *Maison de Santé*–style revolt among the black asylum patients who are there on a field trip. In *Snake Pit Attendant*, written by a man who spent many years in the "bughouse racket," a "war" erupts when "several Negroes started a rebellion one day in my ward." In Poe's story, recall, the asylum battle is a Revolutionary farce. In *Attendant*, the Founding Fathers figuratively look on. "There were several pictures of noted Americans on the wall, including one of Patrick Henry whom I believe is responsible indirectly." Poe tells us that the tar-covered attendants looked like "a perfect army of what I took to be Chimpanzees, Ourang-Outangs, or big black baboons of the Cape of Good Hope." In *Attendant*, a particularly frightful attacker "was large and overgrown, with long arms like a gorilla." He is taken down with a blow to the head. Although the struggle ends with the arrival of state troopers, "Casualties on both sides were heavy."[46]

The French film *The King of Hearts* earned large, art house crowds in the late sixties with a story about mental patients taking over a town in World War I France. The gist of the tale is that the townsfolk and the asylum keepers run off when the fighting got near, and so, when a British soldier arrives looking for a bomb, he finds a people oblivious to the horrors of war. This is a great Cold War parable; it takes madness to find bliss in a world of conflict. It also correlates with an argument made by radical professor Herbert Marcuse. In *One-Dimensional Man* (1964), Marcuse found our society so totalizing and oppressive that all dissent had become impossible. Unless, that is, we participate in a Great Refusal, "the protest against that which is." The idea sounds mad. To refuse to accept reality is a hallmark of insanity; yet it is also, in this formulation, rational.[47]

Madhouse humor need not be confined to comedic works. Mary Jane Ward's *The Snake Pit* has her protagonist sneakily thinking that she is an undercover journalist. *Invisible Man*, which is comedic in only the darkest sense, also wields asylum humor to great effect. In one episode, the protagonist awakens after an explosion to find himself in a factory hospital. He hears a machine begin to hum, and his bed rises to the point where he is face-to-face with a doctor. "A whirring began that snapped and cracked with static, and suddenly I seemed to be crushed between the floor and ceiling. Two forces tore savagely at my stomach and back. A flash of cold-edged heat enclosed me. I was pounded between crushing electrical pressures." His head is "encircled by a piece of cold metal like the iron cap worn by the occupant of an electric chair," and he listens to a calm discussion among the medical men. One says that surgery is the best option for him. The other demurs, "The machine will produce the results of a prefrontal lobotomy without the negative effects of the knife." Using the lingo of psychology and the machinery of mad science, the hero's humanity is eliminated via an infernal ECT device. One of the doctors, noticing him "dancing," says, "They really do have rhythm, don't they? Get hot, boy! Get hot!" The scene is utterly ridiculous, the humor pitch black, and the critique excruciating.[48]

Director Sam Fuller fully grasped the asylum's humor potential. In *Shock Corridor* (1963), reporter Johnny Barrett goes undercover as a mental patient to solve a murder. As he prepares, he assures his girlfriend that even if he doesn't solve the crime, "my experiences alone will make a book, a play, or even a movie sale." (This indeed happened with one-time attendant Ken Kesey.) Johnny gets in via a Freudian ruse, claiming he lusts for his sister. The pipe-smoking analyst's diagnosis is that Johnny be institutionalized until he can "resolve the underlying sexual conflict." Shot in film noir style with slanting shadows, tilting angles, and sharp corners, Fuller's hospital subjects patients to an endless corridor. Like Kesey, Fuller makes a metaphor out of the place. Johnny interviews three patients who each represent some aspect of Cold War paranoia. There is the Korean War vet who was brainwashed by the Communists and then discarded as unpatriotic; a Black man who attended an Anglo university and lost his mind due to the abuse he took; and a scientist who built the atom bomb and is now unable to cope with reality. Each of these men is hilariously dysfunctional. The veteran thinks he's Jeb Stuart. The African American is convinced he's a founding member of the Ku Klux Klan. The nuclear scientist acts like a six-year-old child. Johnny ultimately solves the murder (it's an abusive attendant), but he loses his mind in the process. The doctor solemnly tells his girlfriend, "A man can't tamper with the mind and live in a mental hospital and subject himself to all kinds of tests and expect to come out of it sane." John becomes a "catatonic schizophrenic," a permanent resident of the asylum. The theme, which Fuller hits us over the head with, is that America itself is the asylum, a dysfunctional place that cannot deal with its contradictions and thus submerges them, making us mad in the process.[49]

A subgenre that tapped asylum silliness might be called "horror humor." In 1960s Miami, TV host M. T. Graves rose out of his coffin to greet his viewers, "inmates incarcerated in hospitals, prisons and in your own little homes!" In the classic 1963 *Twilight Zone* episode "Nightmare at 20,000 Feet," William Shatner plays a young man fresh out of a mental institution. He'd been sent there after having a "teensy weensy breakdown" on an airplane. Now he's on another plane, returning home, and he sees a monster on the wing. The furry humanoid tears into the aircraft's structure, but only when he's watching it. He grabs a gun and shoots the beast off, sending the cabin into chaos. Once grounded, we see him being carted off. Rod Serling assures us the man is now free from the "fear of recurring mental breakdown."[50]

Finally, there is the purely ridiculous. In *The Disorderly Orderly*, a Jerry Lewis vehicle, a nefarious plot is underway to expand a hospital. Says a doctor, "We should have more nuts in this place! Do you realize that this whole country is cracking up?" Then there is the seven-minute, animated short "One Froggy Evening." In the short, a construction worker discovers a box dated 1892 in the cornerstone of the building he's demolishing. Inside is an apparently immortal frog. The animal begins to sing and the worker dreams of dollar signs. Investing all his savings in a theater, he puts the frog on stage, sadly to discover that the creature only performs for him, croaking for everyone else. Becoming destitute, the man sleeps in a park. When a cop hears singing and approaches, he tries to explain that it is the frog loudly performing "Figaro." Off he goes to the "Psychopathic Hospital," a big brick building situated behind an iron gate. Here the frog sings with abandon, arms wrapped wistfully around a cell window bar. The man stares at the wall in consternation. Upon his release, he deposits the frog in the cornerstone of a new building. Fast-forward to 2056. A new demolition man uncovers the frog in the box. With visions of dollar signs, he scampers off. We can only assume he's destined for personal destruction.[51]

Later dubbed "Michigan J. Frog" after the Michigan Rag he sings, the frog parodies the American Dream. He is the pipe fantasy of the little guy trying to rocket up the class ladder. In this case, dreaming can slide you disastrously into the asylum. Incidentally, "One Froggy Evening" was released in 1955, the year that witnessed the apex of institutionalization in America. There were 559,000 patients in state hospitals.

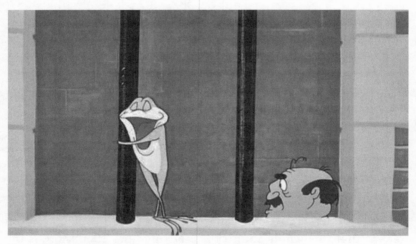

Singing in the asylum, "One Froggy Evening" (1955)

CHAPTER 7

THE ASYLUM NEXT DOOR

I also remembered Buddy Willard saying in a sinister, knowing way that after I had children I would feel differently, I wouldn't want to write poems any more. So I began to think maybe it was true that when you were married and had children it was like being brain-washed, and afterward you went about numb as a slave in some private, totalitarian state.

—Sylvia Plath, *The Bell Jar* (1963)

T he best-selling novel of 1966 was the potboiler *Valley of the Dolls* by Jacqueline Susann. Critics mostly trashed it. With lines like, "No one sticks in show business because it's got good hours or steady dough. Every kid who goes into it thinks she can make it," one does not expect to plumb the depths of pathos. But Susann's book was, in its way, a brilliant, escapist epic. It follows three women as they chase their dreams in the entertainment industry and learn important lessons about the male-dominated world of fame and glory. They discover that love isn't a two-way street, that sex is a fleeting commodity that must be milked for all it's worth, that friends will betray you, and that "dolls"—meaning pills—can help smooth out the jagged bits but can also bury you. One character becomes so addicted to dolls that she lands in a mental hospital. Though not often remarked upon, this element of the story is significant. True to literary forebears, Susann's asylum serves as a warning for women who overstep and lose control.[1]

This chapter explores the asylum's guest-starring role in the early years of the modern Women's Movement. Mental institutions long played the part of prison for inconvenient women, beginning with Mary Wollstonecraft's *Maria* and continuing through the writings of

Elizabeth Stone, Elizabeth Packard, Louisa May Alcott, and others. Not only did these writers portray asylums as prisons, they also analogized the asylum with the home, making superintendents and wards into dark reflections of patriarchal power. After World War II, a Cold War bunkering of domesticity fostered yet darker metaphors. In the works discussed below, the asylum helped add shape to the discourse of female struggle. Explained Betty Friedan in her breakout book *The Feminine Mystique*, the home had become a locked place where women imbibed the draught of subservience and medicated their unhappiness with glossy magazines and drugs. Freud reigned supreme as spectral superintendent, controlling with his message of female inferiority. Friedan hoped to supply the keys of escape. Indeed, Second Wave feminism took *escape* as a motivating theme. The phrase "Women's Liberation" emphasizes it.[2]

Though not usually classified by academics as "feminist," *Valley of the Dolls* utilizes themes of empowerment and liberation. The main character, Anne Welles, flees a stuffy New England village and later refuses to marry a wealthy New Yorker because she's not prepared to surrender her "freedom." Similarly, when co-protagonist Neely O'Hara lands in the asylum, she instantly recognizes Haven Manor as a trap. She gets out, but she cannot overcome the prison of her own vices. The third of the trio of protagonists, Jennifer, kills herself (with pills) once she realizes that her husband misogynistically disapproves of her getting a mastectomy. The adventures of this tragic threesome reflect a culture of boundaries. Even women who ostensibly know the score fail in the face of society's stifling institutions.[3]

Other writers of the period, such as Sylvia Plath, Anne Sexton, and Joanne Greenberg, similarly used the asylum to inform their critique of patriarchy. The home, like the hospital, looked pleasant on the outside, and the occupants even behaved as if everything was fine, but something was definitely amiss. Escape beckoned.

THE FEMININE MYSTIQUE AS ASYLUM BREAKOUT

The Feminine Mystique opens with a creeping sense of horror. Housewives are mysteriously finding themselves filled with foreboding. On the surface, nothing appears to be wrong. They have nice houses equipped with dishwashers and swimming pools, loads of free time to shop and dress the kids in the latest fashions, and affluent husbands to dote on. Yet they are experiencing nervous breakdowns, suffering "bleeding blisters," enduring "new neuroses," and popping tranquilizers "like cough drops." "Sometimes," writes Friedan, "a woman would tell me that the feeling gets so strong she runs out of the house and walks through the streets."[4]

Like a good mystery, Friedan first offers us a tantalizing hint: it is a "problem that has no name." Friedan notes that family life had created not contentment but rather "a strange discrepancy between the reality of our lives as women and the image to which we are trying to conform." She goes on to name the problem. It is "the feminine mystique." The mystique lurks in houses and percolates through magazines, TV shows, and books aimed at women and girls. It "brainwashes" females and slowly destroys their health.[5]

The house, Friedan explains, is a "trap." It insidiously welcomes women only to become their prison.[6] Like the Combine, this trap includes not just the physical home but also the larger society that draws energy from it. In Orwellian fashion, the feminine mystique tells women to love their trap and chides them for feeling unhappy. Friedan uses the analogy of Korean War POWs and concentration camp victims to buttress her argument. Like housewives, inmates in these places are reduced to "passive non-identity." In making this comparison, the familiar language of the asylum emerges. The "prisoners literally became 'walking corpses.' Those who 'adjusted' to the conditions of the [concentration] camps surrendered their human identity and went almost indifferently to their deaths. Strangely enough, the conditions which destroyed the human identity of so many prisoners were not the torture and the brutality, but the conditions similar to those which destroy the American housewife." Though not being led into the gas chamber, the housewife endures a living death, trapped in her "comfortable concentration camp." Friedan continues,

> Have not women who live in the image of the feminine mystique trapped themselves within the narrow walls of their homes? They have learned to "adjust" to their biological role. They have become dependent, passive, childlike . . . American women are not, of course, being readied for mass extermination, but they are suffering a slow death of mind and spirit.

The confinement, the "treatments" (tranquilizers, Freud, childcare books, booze, endless chores), and the sense of "unreality" are literally killing her.[7]

In Friedan's asylumized home, we find the familiar figure of the Woman in White, but the narrative causality is reversed. The housewife is not imprisoned because she is weak; she is weak because she is imprisoned. Escape is imperative, but it will be difficult because her institution is secured within a vast cultural apparatus. Ergo, the breakout must be vast and cultural as well. "The key to the trap," she explains toward the end, "is, of course, education." Perhaps something along the lines of the government's massive GI Bill. The imagery she selects to emphasize her point is apropos. College is "educational shock treatment."[8]

Friedan's book was a watershed, but it also tapped deep currents, which accounts for its rapid fit into American culture. The dream of escape from un-homelike peril (to crib from Freud's notion of the "uncanny") is the same one that motivated the captivity flights, nunnery escapes, and sentimental gothics of earlier times. Just as Elizabeth Packard had found herself trapped in the patriarchal prison of her home even after her release from Jacksonville State Hospital for the Insane, Friedan finds that a woman's independence is structurally imperiled by conditions beyond her making. In postwar America, a new set of historical circumstances added fresh layers. Now there was a concerted effort to drive women back into the house and away from the "male" sphere of work. Coming back to civilian life after a calamitous Depression and World War II, millions of men demanded priority in industry, urging women to retreat to the nuclear household and produce babies. This trend was compounded by Cold War insecurities that configured the home as a bunker of safety. Perhaps nothing underlined this as did a famous stunt in *Life* magazine in which a newlywed couple honeymooned in their backyard bomb shelter. Friedan appropriately historicized the appeal of the mystique: "We were all vulnerable, homesick, lonely, frightened. A pent-up hunger for marriage, home, and children was felt simultaneously by several generations; a hunger which, in the prosperity of postwar America, everyone could suddenly satisfy."[9]

But the price paid was onerous. America had regressed into somnambulism. "The American spirit fell into a strange sleep; men as well as women, scared liberals, disillusioned radicals, conservatives bewildered and frustrated by change—the whole nation stopped growing up. All of us went back into the warm brightness of home, the way it was when we were children and slept peacefully upstairs while our parents read." This infantilization made us forget earlier generations of women's rights crusaders. Just as the asylum curated a bucolic appearance that belied the hell within, so too did the American media cultivate a perfect image of happy homemaking that jarred against the real ennui and despair.[10]

With the home as a modernized asylum, the superintendent was equally recognizable—Sigmund Freud. Or, perhaps more accurately, the Ghost of Freud. In a remarkable chapter titled "The Sexual Solipsism of Sigmund Freud," Friedan places blame squarely on the famous man.

> The feminine mystique derived its power from Freudian thought; for it was an idea born of Freud, which led women, and those who studied them, to misinterpret their mothers' frustrations, and their fathers' and brothers' and husbands' resentments and inadequacies, and their own emotions and possible choices in life. It is the Freudian idea, hardened into apparent fact that has trapped so many American women today.

She concedes that Freud was a "genius" whose ideas helped in the "emancipation" of women by destabilizing the sexual repressions of the Victorian world. Yet Freud was also a product of his world, "a prisoner of his own culture," and his ideas about women simply did not belong in the Atomic Age. Penis envy? Maybe in a Victorian situation where a woman "might wish herself a man." But not today, when women could participate socially and educate themselves. Yet such archaic ideas had become scripture, thanks to archons of analysis like Marynia Farnham and Helene Deutsch.[11]

According to Friedan, Freud's original sin was that he was "not concerned with changing society, but in helping man, and woman, adjust to it." Adjustment to second-class status was Freud's worst bequest to the female sex, and his superintendence of our culture makes us all victims. Adjustment is everywhere; it accounts for all of the ills that corrode our democracy. It "provided a convenient

escape from the atom bomb, McCarthy, all the disconcerting problems that might spoil the taste of steaks, and cars and color television
and backyard swimming pools. It gave us permission to suppress the
troubling questions of the larger world and pursue our own personal
pleasures."[12]

Friedan's escape protocols are couched in the language of psychology, appropriate for an asylum-like imprisonment. She was a
psychology major in college, and *The Feminine Mystique* reflects this
background. She'd even been analyzed and had been told that "deep-
seated hostilities towards my mother" were at the root of all her problems. She had rebelled against this and had found therapeutic release
in her own explorations. As she explained in an interview, her work
had made "the difference between Betty Friedan in a mental institution or out." Some have argued that Friedan's focus on "self-help"
skewed the modern feminist project at birth, reducing deeper political problems to mere psychological hurdles. This may be true, but
to separate the political from the psychological in *The Feminine Mystique* is to dismantle the methodological platform she used to launch
what was a startling and powerful attack on patriarchal structures.
Further, in the Age of Freud, millions of women understood the language of psychology; Friedan's challenge was easily grasped. Concepts like complexes, neuroses, oedipal relationships, and even the
domineering Viper Mothers who smother their sons (and sometimes
inadvertently make them gay) are taken at face value in *The Feminine
Mystique*. Friedan's innovation was to flip the causality of these plights
on their head. Women are not neurotic because of biology but rather
as a result of their incarceration in America's totalizing, culturally reinforced madhouse. Her own psychological blend tapped into "human
potential" arguments by thinkers like Abraham Maslow that she studied as a graduate student in Berkeley. Such psychologists liberated
themselves from mainstream adjustment ideology, forwarding a rhetoric of liberation that coincided with the counterculture.[13]

Friedan's "trap," with its prima facie argument for escape, found
resonance in popular books, songs, and films in the years ahead.
Fashionable novels like *Valley of the Dolls* succeeded by commenting
on the trap and offering sympathetic portrayals of women stifled by
the unreality of middle-class domestic expectations. This is not to
say Susann's book and similar fare should be classified as feminist

challenges to the status quo. Rather, they used a rhetoric of empowered escape to help build forward bases for raids into the male provenance of worldly success and respect. One popular novel that makes use of Friedan's home-as-asylum framework, *Diary of a Mad Housewife*, is worth briefly assessing.[14]

Sue Kaufman tells the story of Bettina Balser, a woman who at first blush seems to have it all: a nice apartment, great clothes, beautiful kids, fancy friends, and a well-paid, ambitious husband. But she is miserable. She can't sleep, she can't function, and she starts popping tranquilizers and sleeping pills. She becomes her own superintendent. Drugs, bath and shower "hydrotherapy," and excruciating self-analysis ensue. Nothing works. Like Friedan, Bettina just cannot play the "Feminine Passive Role." As the story unfolds, we discover that her husband is selfish, that her kids are driving her crazy, and that the social pressure of living a jet-set lifestyle is wearing her down. Her predicament ultimately becomes a warning fable about postwar prosperity. Wealth created impossible expectations; the happy nuclear home is an illusion; and trying to adjust makes you unhinged. Bettina eventually embarks on an affair, but this proves no answer to her malaise. Surprisingly, in the end, she resigns to accept her domestic role, breaking off the affair and exulting privately in the fact that her husband had his own nervous breakdown following his own botched affair. Peace comes with learning that she can't play the role of super-wife to the "Renaissance Man." Happily, her husband can't be that man anyway. The reader is comforted to know that a quiet life of unostentatious normalcy is best.[15]

With shades of Kate Chopin's *The Awakening*, Bettina's attempt to escape her domestic trap leads to suicidal thoughts, though she pulls herself back from launching herself from her high-rise apartment. Like Edna Pontellier, Bettina's luxurious digs become a prison. First, she tries to break away, reconfiguring the control apparatus, and playing the medicating, Freudian superintendent. When this fails, she adulterously forces a crisis, which, in turn, leads to catharsis. Her wistful comments about sitting placidly in a tract home watching the Million Dollar Movie with a TV dinner seems calibrated to tell the reader (undoubtedly titillated by the paperback's promise of the "startling bestseller that ripped the lid off the New York marriage scene") that the glamorous life is not all that it's cracked up to be. In

Bettina's imprisonment and attempted escape, she learns that only a more realistic vision of marriage can save her. This is not the sort of liberation narrative Friedan had in mind, but neither is it an abject capitulation to the mystique. Like *Valley of the Dolls*, Kaufman's book plays with the emergent discourse of domestic discontent, as well as with its asylum aspects, to offer up an ambiguous, yet resonant, message of discontent.

PRIVATE TOTALITARIAN STATES: THE ARGUMENT OF SYLVIA PLATH AND ANNE SEXTON

Sylvia Plath killed herself in February 1963, the same month *The Feminine Mystique* came out. At the time of her death, Plath was a recognized, if lesser known, poet, with a well-received collection under her belt, *The Colossus and Other Poems*. She would leave behind a body of work that dealt with the conundrum of the cosseted, frustrated, yet modern female. Like Friedan, Plath configured the home as an asylum, but she also wrote about real mental institutions. In her most famous work, *The Bell Jar*, a fictionalized version of her younger self is committed several times. Published under the pseudonym "Victoria Lucas" in England, *The Bell Jar* would not see print in America until 1971. It would become a sensation.

The Bell Jar appeared to be a *Catcher in the Rye* for young women. One early British critic called it "the first feminine novel in the Salinger mode." Like Salinger's book, Plath's is a first-person account of a youth undergoing a mental breakdown, and it too is chock full of clever observations, pathos, and humor. But *The Bell Jar* is neither retread nor homage. It is something much darker, and its implications are that, for many women, there is no light at the end of the tunnel. In *Catcher in the Rye*, the troubled narrator tells his story to an asylum doctor, unburdening himself of his worry that the adult world isn't all it's cracked up to be. In the end, he finds a kind of peace for himself. In *The Bell Jar*, the narrator openly contemplates and then attempts suicide, feeling utterly trapped by her situation. She winds up institutionalized, and the results are ambiguous at best. She cannot escape the domestic trap, and what's worse, her cohorts don't even see it. College girls "playing bridge and gossiping and studying . . . sat under bell jars of sorts."[16]

Plath had mental institutions in mind as she developed her book. Between 1954 and 1959, she'd written a series of short stories that dealt with her experiences of mental torment and commitment. In "Tongues of Stone" (1955), she paints a bleak picture of a girl who gets institutionalized and receives insulin treatment. This pitch-black fugue includes a scene where the protagonist hopes that the sun "would stop at the height of its strength and crucify the world, devour it for once and for all." Life is not worth living; she hides a glass and breaks it into shards, presumably to slit her wrists later. The story ends on an ambiguously happy note. She tells the nurse that she feels "quite different" after her treatment and is now ready to leave. Plath knew she needed to expand on these ideas. She wrote in her journal in 1959 that there is an "increasing market for mental hospital stuff. I am a fool if I don't relive, recreate it." In fact, Harper and Row initially rejected *The Bell Jar* because it was yet another madness narrative entering a crowded field.[17]

The Bell Jar concerns a young woman named Esther Greenwood. She's just getting out into the world, heading for New York City, one of a select group of guest editors for a major women's magazine. She experiences the daunting cosmopolitan environment of the metropolis, with its erotic encounters and volatile friendships. Upon her return to the suburbs, Esther finds that she has been rejected for a prestigious writing course at Harvard. She descends into a deep depression, which prompts her mother to send her to a psychiatrist. Suicide attempts and asylums follow.

Plath is clearly referencing her own experiences. In 1953, at age twenty, she had been awarded a guest editorship at *Mademoiselle* in New York and had stayed at a women's hotel there (the Barbizon in real-life, the "Amazon" in the book). Later that summer, after being turned down for a Harvard writing class, she had attempted suicide in the manner described in the book. She'd then gone to McLean Hospital in the fall of 1953 (in the novel, McLean's Belknap and Wyman Halls become "Belsize" and "Wymark"). Though Plath wrote *The Bell Jar* in England nearly a decade later, her book was about coming of age as a precocious 1950s female and the prison that her own adult life had become. She was depressed and confined in a dreary series of homes with two young children in tow, and her husband was a philanderer.

Like Friedan's book, *The Bell Jar* takes on the domestic trap. Esther's boyfriend Buddy Willard (patterned on her old real-life beau Dick Norton) tells her, "In a sinister, knowing way that after I had children I would feel differently, I wouldn't want to write poems any more. So I began to think maybe it was true that when you were married and had children it was like being brainwashed, and afterward you went about numb as a slave in some private, totalitarian state." After Esther learns that she will not be attending Harvard, her hope for a future liberated by academe dims. En route to the suburbs, the car becomes a loony-bin wagon, "The gray, padded car roof closed over my head like the roof of a prison van, and the white, shining, identical clapboard houses with their interstices of well-groomed green proceeded past, one bare after another in a large but escape-proof cage." In this suburban hell, she is left to her own thoughts, ultimately determining that escape can only happen in the form of death.[18]

Reflecting the "mental health stuff" that Plath was thinking about, Esther internalizes her own Freudian superintendent, using the language of neuroses and complexes to describe her struggles. For example, she tells her boyfriend that she can never marry because she is "neurotic." The lack of choice, or rather a set of choices that each seem to lead to a form of imprisonment, makes her miserable. Her mom sends her to see a psychiatrist named Doctor Gordon. Gordon is the epitome of the condescending male, an enlightened and infuriating patriarch who observes and judges. Esther sits "curled in the cavernous leather chair," facing him "across an acre of highly polished teak." Gordon is both "good-looking" and "conceited," wielding his authority with questions like, "Suppose you try and tell me what you think is wrong." Immediately she thinks, "That made it sound as if nothing was *really* wrong, I only *thought* it was wrong." This is the asylumized world of the feminine mystique, the Freudian prison in which one's real problems acquire a sense of unreality. Esther does not want to concede power. Indeed, as she explains elsewhere, her problem is that "I hated the idea of serving men in any way." She does not want to get married. "I wanted change and excitement and to shoot off in all directions myself, like the colored arrows from a Fourth of July rocket." Doctor Gordon recommends ECT. This is how she winds up in the doctor's "private hospital."[19]

Gordon's hospital is beautiful and secluded, with an idyllic veranda and pleasant lawn. But we know there is darkness within.

"What bothered me," Esther thinks, "was that everything about the house seemed normal, although I knew it must be chock-full of crazy people. There were no bars on the windows that I could see, and no wild or disquieting noises." With a poet's eye, Plath peels its ghastly layers one detail at a time. First, Esther sees that nobody is moving. "I made out men and women, and boys and girls who must be as young as I, but there was a uniformity to their faces, as if they had lain for a long time on a shelf, out of sunlight, under siftings of pale, fine dust." Then she finds that some people "were indeed moving, but with small, birdlike gestures." These people have been changed; the institution has gotten to them. Like her suburban home, the sanitarium is a place that constrains personal ambitions, shapes behaviors, and corrals minor rebellions within its architecture of control. At one point, Esther notes that a suicidal woman is laughingly disregarded by a nurse (described as "dumpy and muscular"), who points out that the windows are made to prevent her from jumping to her death.[20]

Next comes the ECT. The burly nurse and Doctor Gordon team up to pin Esther down. The nurse's "fat breast muffled my face like a cloud or pillow," a "vague, medicinal stench" emanating from her body. Gordon buckles metal plates to her head and gives her something to bite. "Then something bent down and took hold of me and shook me like the end of the world. Whee-ee-ee-ee-ee, it shrilled, through an air crackling with blue light, and with each flash a great jolt drubbed me till I thought my bones would break and the sap fly out of me like a split plant." Plath's description certainly fits with the literary horrors of ECT. One thinks of *One Flew Over the Cuckoo's Nest*, in which McMurphy climbs up on the table, has a "crown of silver thorns" put on his temples, and then gets his blast: "light arcs across, stiffens him, bridges him up off the table until nothing is down but his wrists and ankles and out around that crimped black rubber hose a sound like *hooee!* and he's frosted over completely with sparks." Biographers note that Plath's real-life, horrifying, early ECT experience was due to the fact that she received her treatment in the pre-"modified" days, possibly going without the benefit of "muscle relaxant or anesthetic" nor any "professional care or support afterwards."[21]

But there seems to be more going on here than just a bad experience. ECT represents the helplessness felt when one's life is not under one's own control. In Plath's 1958 short story, "Johnny Panic and the Bible of Dreams" (1958), the narrator is pinned down by "five false priests in surgical gowns" who place a "crown of wire" on her head and then blast her with electricity. "I am shaken like a leaf in the teeth of glory. His beard is lightning. Lightning is in his eye . . . The air crackles with his blue-tongued lightning-haloed angels." That ECT device is monstrous and surveilling, a "box [that] seems to be eying me, copper-head ugly." In her poem "The Hanging Man," we read, "By the roots of my hair some god got hold of me. / I sizzled in his blue volts like a desert prophet." ECT, suffused with references to God, angels, cyclopes, and priests, communicates a patriarchal grip on the subjugated female body. *The Bell Jar* layers this with specific Cold War nightmares. The book opens, "It was a queer, sultry summer, the summer they electrocuted the Rosenbergs." This is a reference to the 1953 execution, via electric chair, of Ethel and Julius Rosenberg. Plath opposed the execution, as did many intellectuals. Esther is duly horrified, commenting, "I couldn't help wondering what it would be like, being burned alive all along your nerves." This image, scorched into the reader's brain on page one, is reinvoked with the "great jolt" and "crackling . . . blue light" later.[22]

More ominous is the suicide-ECT connection. After a failed attempt to hang herself, Esther wonders if she should give up on suicide. But then she remembers "Doctor Gordon and his private shock machine. Once I was locked up they could use that on me all the time." Here is an association between torture and institutionalization. Esther does not want to be quarantined, her brain blasted indeterminately. She also understands how commitment speeds a downward spiral for the middle-class person. "They would want me to have the best of care at first, so they would sink all their money in a private hospital like Doctor Gordon's. Finally, when the money was used up, I would be moved to a state hospital, with hundreds of people like me, in a big cage in the basement." This is the living death, a fate well known in asylum literature, and Plath wanted none of it. Most American readers knew about Plath's suicide before they read her book, so connections between electrocution, ECT, incarceration, and death could not have been difficult to make.[23]

Except this is not all the book has to say on the matter.

After Gordon's ECT and another failed suicide attempt, Esther is rescued from a miserable mental ward (this one in a city hospital) by her benefactress Philomena Guinea. She's taken to a "private hospital that had grounds and golf courses and gardens, like a country club." Here, she is treated to white tablecloths and fancy meals and is astonished to be placed under the care of a nurturing woman psychiatrist ("I didn't think they had women psychiatrists"). Doctor Nolan is "a cross between Myrna Loy and my mother," the very opposite of Gordon. The superintendent is also non-threatening, a "handsome, white-haired doctor" who amiably talks about Pilgrims and Indians and who plays no meaningful role in her treatment. Esther gets psychotherapy, occupational therapy, insulin therapy, and yet more ECT. In a stark difference, Dr. Nolan tells Esther that her last ECT experience "was a mistake . . . It's not supposed to be like that." "If it's done properly," Nolan explains, "it's like going to sleep." Though the treatment is similarly framed with a frightful trip to a "high bed with its white, drumtight sheet," this ECT renders Esther instantly unconscious. When she awakens, "All the heat and fear had purged itself. I felt surprisingly at peace. The bell jar hung, suspended, a few feet above my head. I was open to the circulating air." Like in *The Snake Pit*, this round of electroconvulsive therapy has its benefits despite its scares.[24]

In this country club asylum, Esther meets not zombies but friendly patients who share her sense of disconnectedness from the world. Joan is athletic and outgoing, though Esther finds her lesbian behavior disconcerting. Then there is Valerie who has had a lobotomy. Valerie tells Esther that she is "Fine. I'm not angry any more. Before, I was always angry." Hardly the image of a brain-damaged robot. But this asylum offers no happy ending. Valerie confides that she wants to remain here forever, and Joan commits suicide. Esther knows she must leave in order to make a real life for herself.[25]

Like Esther, Plath also went to a fancy mental hospital thanks to a wealthy benefactress. McLean Hospital was a well-regarded and well-funded affiliate of Massachusetts General Hospital in the 1950s. The real-life Philomena Guinea was Olive Higgins Prouty, the woman who wrote *Now, Voyager*. Plath is not kind to her in *The Bell Jar*, describing Guinea as a "weird old [woman]" who wanted to "adopt" Esther in order to make her "resemble" her. And yet Guinea delivers Esther to a place that is anything but a house of horrors. Explaining her own institutional experience in a 1953 letter, Plath wrote, "by fairy-godmother-type maneuverings, my scholarship benefactress at Smith

got me into the best mental hospital in the U.S., where I had my own
attractive private room and my own attractive private psychiatrist. I
didn't think improvement was possible. It seems that it is." Tellingly, in
the same letter, she cringes at her "shuddering horror and fear of the
cement tunnels leading down to the shock room." "Somehow, all this
reminds me of the deep impression the movie 'The Snake Pit' made
upon me about six years ago." In a later journal entry, she'd implore
herself, "Must get out SNAKE PIT." *The Bell Jar*'s shades of *The Snake
Pit* are not accidental. Like that movie, Esther has a scary asylum experience but also a kind doctor and a reasonable "cure." [26]

Though Plath took her life nearly a decade after her asylum and
ECT experiences, and though Dr. Nolan's treatment helps Esther recover, it is Esther's horrifying initial trial with ECT and Dr. Gordon's
condescension, fused to Plath's dreadful demise, that dominated
the popular Plath narrative. She became a pre–Women's Liberation
martyr to brutal patriarchal psychiatry, an inspiration to women who
would not settle.

For good reason, Plath is often paired with poet Anne Sexton. Both
Plath and Sexton grew up in Massachusetts and endured mental torments and institutionalization; both composed poetry that reflected
their battles; and both killed themselves. When Plath died, Sexton
asked why she had left her to "crawl down alone / into the death I
wanted so badly and for so long." Anne Sexton's relationship to the
feminine mystique was more ambiguous than Friedan's. She rankled
at society's restrictions while still buying into them, telling one inter-
viewer, "I wanted to get married from the age of thirteen on. I wanted
nothing else." In her letters, Sexton confesses she is just a "normal
American housewife." She chose not to go to college but rather to get
married and have kids, just as the mystique instructed her to do. But
she was profoundly unhappy; after the birth of her second child, she
became suicidal and landed in a mental hospital.[27]

Sexton was labeled with a number of mental monikers in her adult
life: " 'hysteric,' 'psychoneurotic,' 'borderline,' and 'alcoholic.' " She was
certainly a troubled soul, with destructive personal relationships and
serious chemical dependencies. She carried barbiturates in her purse
that she called "kill-me" pills. She went in and out of psychiatric institutions until the end of her days. She attempted suicide on a number
of occasions. In 1974, she succeeded. She also sought and received

psychoanalysis. In fact, it was a psychiatrist who first encouraged her to write poetry. Her early poems were intended to be merely therapeutic, but it was soon obvious that she had a special gift. Anne's poems expressed hidden longings, execrable torments, and occasional, sublime elucidations that enraptured readers.

Like Plath, Anne Sexton was known as a "confessional" poet. Confessional poetry aimed to tear holes through the fabric of Cold War conformity. Pioneered by Robert Lowell, John Berryman, Randall Jarrell, and others, this style addressed pains of the sort that could land you in an institution—depression, suicide, divorce, and substance abuse. The poet Elizabeth Bishop described confessional poetry as rooted in "the idea is that we live in a horrible and terrifying world, and the worst moments of horrible and terrifying lives are an allegory of the world." Mental hospital trips made for fine, honest poetry. Lowell, a major influence on both Plath and Sexton (both attended his writing seminar at Boston University), spent time in McLean.[28]

For Anne Sexton, the asylum would serve as something more than a metaphor for suffering. It became both a patriarchal panopticon and a space for reflecting on the impediments to living a complete life. In the words of Diane Wood Middlebrook, Sexton and her literary kin provided "a very important form of resistance" to the status quo.[29]

Sexton's first book, *To Bedlam and Part Way Back* (1960), established her as a poet of note. Not all of the poems are about madness and the asylum, but all sear with the intensity of one who has experienced institutionalization. Yet this is no forward charge against the system. It is more a heart's plea to join the poet on a journey through shadow territories. The book opens with, "You, Doctor Martin," addressed to the psychiatrist who encouraged her to write poems. The piece takes us into an institution with all of the trappings of the asylum genre. The doctor is all powerful, "the god of our block" whose "third eye / moves among us and lights the separate boxes / where we sleep or cry." This is the standard paradox of "summer hotel" with an "antiseptic tunnel" beneath, a place where "the moving dead still talk / of pushing their bones against the thrust / of cure." The narrator is "lost," a "large" child denuded of liberties like the others. In "Music Swims Back to Me," we travel deeper into the mind of the institutionalized. The author hears music from an unseen radio, is locked in a "chair," and asks, helplessly, "Which way is home?" The pathos is intensified right at the beginning: "There are no sign posts in this room, / four ladies, over eighty, / in diapers every one of them." In "Noon Walk on the Asylum Lawn," we read how the "summer sun ray" "sucks the air" and the grass "blades extend / and reach my way." This makes a pleasant stroll on parklike asylum grounds seem hideous. It recalls the way in which homelike asylums are not really safe. The poem ends, "There is no safe place."[30]

This last line well summarizes Sexton's work as a whole, including her poems about life outside the institution. Throughout her writings, the horrors of unreality, reminiscent of Friedan's argument about the "schizophrenic" nature of housewifery, reminds us of the restraints imposed on women and problems that no therapy can alleviate. In "Lullaby," the "night nurse" on the "best ward at Bedlam" serves up sleeping pills that function as a kind of ultra-layer of reality, floating her "out of myself / stung skin as alien / as a loose bolt of cloth." In "Flee on Your Donkey," from *Live or Die* (1966), Sexton reflects on landing once again in a mental hospital after six years "shuttling in and out." A new doctor advertising his "tranquilizers, insulin, or shock / to the uninitiated" makes no impression. Here is "the same old crowd, / the same ruined scene." Her ultimate desire is escape, hence the title's reference of Biblical flight. She begs herself to leave, "For once make a deliberate decision. / There are brains that rot here / like black bananas." She knows flight is her only chance: "Ride out / any old way you please!" But escaping doesn't resolve her problems. For home is also a horror. In "Housewife" (from 1962's *All My Pretty Ones*) the house is "another kind of skin" in which the woman "sits on her knees all day, / faithfully washing herself down." This ghastly, genuflected self-scrubbing brings to mind Friedan's argument about housework being an endless, mindless task filling all available time. In her life, Sexton was unable to be a good mother, unable to be a faithful wife, unable to enjoy the suburban dream. Neither institutions nor home could provide succor. She embodied Friedan's sense of "strange discrepancy" between reality and image and was unable to collate the two into a happy balance.[31]

Sylvia Plath and Anne Sexton both configured the domestic sphere as an asylum, while blurring the difference between suburban and institutional experiences. The home and the mental hospital worked together in a kind of seamless, inescapable horror. Their deaths put an exclamation point on their argument. Both would be hugely popular among the college crowd in the 1970s when women sought to liberate themselves.[32]

FROM YR TO ETERNITY AT CHESTNUT LODGE

Joanne Greenberg was just sixteen years old when her parents committed her in the posh Chestnut Lodge. It was 1948, the same year that Twentieth Century Fox released *The Snake Pit*. Diagnosed as schizophrenic, Greenberg heard voices, smelled strange odors, hurt herself, and spoke in a language she had invented. Four years later, she emerged from the Lodge cured, adjusted, and ready for the world. In 1964, a year after *The Bell Jar* debuted in England, Greenberg published a fictionalized memoir of her hospitalization experience under the pseudonym "Hannah Green." Like Plath's book, *I Never Promised You a Rose Garden* narrates events from a past era. Also like that book, it resonated with readers and became a huge seller. High schools and colleges assigned it, and nurses handed it out to institutionalized patients. By the late 1970s, *Rose Garden* had sold over five million paperback copies. It would eventually be translated into a dozen languages, spawn a movie, and inspire a number-one country song. The book's title burrowed into the culture, many people saying it even if they had no knowledge of the source. It was a cute way of saying, "Look, I never said that everything would be perfect."[33]

I Never Promised You a Rose Garden has a familiar ring to it. Here is a sensitive woman beleaguered by stifling familial and social expectations, who knew the feeling of profound unease, and who was pronounced unwell because of it. But unlike many others, her asylum experience helped her profoundly. This was all thanks to a female Freudian and her unique, loving treatment. In *Rose Garden*, an older woman frees a girl from the living death of incarceration and the belittlement of paternal rule. We might think of it as a more feminist *Snake Pit* or perhaps a *Bell Jar* with a happy ending.

Chestnut Lodge billed itself as a different kind of hospital. While most of America's leading psychiatrists were Freudians, the reality of institutionalization meant that drugs, confinement, and shock treatments were far more common than talk therapy. Investing years on a single individual was simply cost prohibitive. Psychiatrists knew that working in overcrowded state institutions dependent on public taxes was neither remunerative nor rewarding, and so they tended to work in offices treating the better off "worried well." At Chestnut Lodge, a small, for-profit hospital located in the suburbs of Washington, DC, a well-to-do clientele could afford analysis, and analysis is what they got. It was, in fact, the only hospital in the country to use psychotherapy exclusively.[34]

Chestnut Lodge started life as the Woodlawn Hotel, a luxurious, Second Empire–style retreat. Built in 1889, it featured gas lighting, indoor plumbing, and a lively ballroom. The hotel fell on hard times and went to the auction block in 1908. Purchased by Milwaukee surgeon Dr. Ernest Bullard, Woodlawn was reborn, after renovations, as Chestnut Lodge Sanitarium. It became a "spa"-style clinic to treat the "nervous" rich with hot baths and cold packs in a lavish setting. When Bullard died in 1931, his son Dexter took over and transformed it into a bold venture in Freudian methods. As he would explain, "We started with the idea that if analysis made sense for the neurotic, it had to make sense for the psychotic." In 1935, Dexter hired German émigré Dr. Frieda Fromm-Reichmann. It is ironic that Dr. Fromm-Reichmann, a Jew, found a welcome home here. Rockville, Maryland, like many parts of the country, had a restrictive housing covenant that prohibited Jews from owning homes. The Lodge was, in a sense, an asylum for her as well as for her patients. During the Great Depression, Chestnut Lodge survived thanks to her influence.[35]

Dr. Fromm-Reichmann presented regularly at conferences, served as President of the Washington Psychoanalytic Association, and wrote an influential text. Her main contribution was in the use of psychotherapy to treat schizophrenics. She believed that, because schizophrenia was caused by "traumas," it could be cathartically resolved with careful analysis. In her *Principles of Intensive Psychotherapy*, she argues that hallucinations are essentially a "bursting-through into awareness of an unbearable surplus of repressed or dissociated thoughts and feelings," and, thus, "it is feasible for them to yield when enough material is brought into awareness" by the psychiatrist. Her thesis was a controversial one, and she would come under attack by orthodox Freudians. Fromm-Reichmann would make a name for herself in the psychiatric community thanks to her writings, but she'd become world-famous as "Dr. Fried" thanks to Greenberg.[36]

I Never Promised You a Rose Garden centers on the experiences of Deborah Blau (a lightly fictionalized Greenberg), though the narrative also meanders through the perspectives of her parents and her psychiatrist, Dr. Fried. Chestnut Lodge is "Victorian, a little run-down, and surrounded by trees. Very good façade for a madhouse . . . There were bars on all the windows." This is pleasing to Deborah who expects to be tortured: "Deborah smiled slightly. It was fitting. Good." Her parents at first find the whole experience shameful and frightening. Her dad confides to his wife, "They call it a mental hospital, but it's a place, Es, a place where they put people away. How can it be a good place for a girl—almost a child!" Later, Deborah's mom wonders how to tell Deborah's sister Suzy about the "convalescent school" she is supposedly at.

> Who had not heard all the old-style high melodrama of insanity; of the madwoman in Jane Eyre, of bedlam, of the hundreds of dark houses with high walls and little hope; of lesser dramas in lesser memories, and of maniacs who murdered and passed on the taint of their blood to menace the future? "Modern Science" had given the official lie to much of this, but beneath the surface of facts, the older fears remained in the minds of the well no less than of the sick. People paid lip service to new theories and new proofs, but often their belief was no more than the merest veneer, yielding at a scratch to the bare and honest horror, the accretion of ten thousand generations of fear and magic.[37]

I Never Promised You a Rose Garden honestly deals with the family dynamics of coping with serious mental illness, and it adds a new character to the literature—the heroic, female asylum doctor. Prior to this, women asylum doctors in prose and film can be found, but they typically conform to standard formulae of femme fatale and/ or love interest. *A Thousand Faces* has a female physician, though her role is negligible. In *One Drop of Blood*, Dr. Harlow, a "girl doctor," offers mainly some light, Freudian insights and an attractive appearance. In the movie *Nightmare Alley* (1947), the immoral "consulting psychologist" Lilith Ritter tricks the protagonist out of the cash he had already swindled and even threatens to commit him. In *Spellbound* (1945), Ingrid Bergman plays a Freudian analyst who begins as a "sexually repressed automaton" and learns that falling in love with a patient makes her a better therapist. Winfred Van Atta's 1961 pulp novel *Shock Treatment* has Dr. Mary Haines, a friendly asylum doctor who, we learn, became a shrink after becoming suicidal when jilted. Her main help to the protagonist is having her car stolen as part of the hero's escape. In the 1964 film version, the sadistic male psychiatrist, Wolfgang Schierwagen, is a woman, Dr. Edwina Beighley, played by Lauren Bacall. Bacall coolly uses psychedelic drugs and ECT to demolish the brain of a man who would expose her plot to steal a million dollars from a patient. The same year *Rose Garden* was published, Natalie Wood played a "research psychologist" in *Sex and the Single Girl*. In this movie, she falls for Tony Curtis, who is actually just posing as a patient. In *The Bell Jar*, Dr. Nolan marks a step forward, though her role is scarcely fleshed out, her main descriptors being her stylish dress and caring attitude. Dr. Fried is something different. She is competent, authoritative, and her looks are not a factor. She does not change to suit the protagonist. Rather, the protagonist changes as a result of Fried's expertise.[38]

Dr. Fried is an almost mystically powerful shrink. She knows just how to handle Deborah's psychosis, helping her dig down to the roots of her problem. And she is no disinterested observer; she comes right out and tells Deborah what it will take to heal herself. This was an accurate representation of Fromm-Reichmann's real-life technique. In *Rose Garden*, Dr. Fried explains that Deborah's illness is a "desperate fight for health." If it were as simple as giving "a nice shot of this or that drug or a quick hypnosis and say 'Craziness, begone!'" then hers would be an "easy job." But true healing is not so easy. Fried must help Deborah "destroy" the "defenses or shields," through intensive psychotherapy. She helps Deborah to lay down a "firmer ground" for herself.[39]

First, Deborah must travel through the horrors of her mind. She has constructed an inner world, "Yr," which has its own gods, language, and mythos. Entities like "the Censor" stand in judgment of her. Dr. Fried accepts that Deborah believes in this world and helps her see that the real world can be coped with on its own terms, without recourse to fantasizing. In the meantime, Deborah lives among a cast of unusual patients, harms herself, and even spends time amidst "the un-dead" on the Disturbed Ward. Her final cure commences when Dr. Fried convinces her that she did not try to kill her baby brother years ago, thus freeing Deborah of the childhood guilt that sparked her insanity. Through analysis, catharsis occurs, allowing Deborah to put away her illness for good. The book perfectly illustrates Dr. Fromm-Reichmann's theory that schizophrenia can be treated effectively via talk therapy and that its origins lie outside of biology.[40]

This book is not the first to bring Chestnut Lodge to wide attention, nor even the first to offer a fictionalized version of Joanne Greenberg. The Lodge entered the wider discussion in 1954 with the publication of *The Mental Hospital* by Alfred H. Stanton and Morris S. Schwartz, a psychiatrist and a sociologist respectively. Based on a detailed, two-year research project centered on a close investigation of the disturbed women's ward of Chestnut Lodge, it was "the largest, most systematic study of a mental hospital ever conducted." *The Mental Hospital* would be a highly influential text for psychiatric residents for years. The main argument is that institutions matter when it comes to patient outcomes. Beyond the therapeutic offerings of psychiatrists, what happened during "the other twenty-three hours" was very important. The actions of the staff and the organization of the setting interacted with profound consequences. As Stanton and Schwartz explain, "In our experience, an acute crisis was always preceded by a period of less acute personal disorganization among the staff; a 'contagion' did not arise out of the blue, but out of recognizable conditions." The institution then, at an organizational level, became the most meaningful arena to implement mental health reform. Following Albert Deutsch, this study draws our attention away from horror stories and toward a more realistic investigation of patient needs and institutional requirements.[41]

In fiction, the Lodge appears to first show up in a throwaway line in *Lolita*, when Nabokov refers to "Chestnut Lodge" where a fleeing Lolita stays the night. It's an inn. In 1961, J. R. Salamanca published the novel *Lilith*, a book about a beautiful, delusional asylum waif who seduces a young occupational therapist at "Poplar Lodge" in the town of "Stonemont" (described exactly like Chestnut Lodge in Rockville). Poplar Lodge is "an old Gothic building, typical of the early part of the century, full of bays and towers and long dormers, surmounted by a slate mansard roof, through which five ivory-covered chimneys, their moist bricks showing between the leaves, projected comfortably." It is no horror house. "There was nothing grim or terrible about it; never were there faces peering from high barred windows, or the sound of screams or violence within. With its elaborate and spacious grounds and its air of age and dignity, it had, indeed, a peaceful, almost idyllic aspect." Salamanca uses a wise hospital manager, Bea Brice, to explain the therapeutic rationale at Poplar Lodge. She is not a psychiatrist like Dr. Fromm-Reichmann, but she plays the role of gentle guardian. Her discourse is right out of the Chestnut Lodge playbook:

> There are different theories about the causes of schizophrenia and the most effective way to treat it. Some people feel that it's an organic disease—that is, that there's something actually physically or chemically wrong with the structure of the brain—that it can be treated like any other physical illness. Other doctors believe that it's a functional ailment—that there's no actual physical damage or deficiency—but that the mind has become deranged functionally, through acute emotional problems, tensions, conflicts and so on. We tend toward the last interpretation, here; and we also use classical therapy—that is, analysis. This is so expensive, and usually so prolonged, that most state institutions can't afford it. They do a great deal with shock—electrical or insulin shock—and with drugs and surgery. But we don't feel that those methods are as thorough or permanent.

Psychoanalysis offers release from the prison of schizophrenia at Poplar Lodge. First, one must go "back to the old conflicts and tensions, and exploring them until he begins to gain insight into them. This takes years sometimes and requires enormous skill and experience on the part of the analyst."[42]

Unlike *Rose Garden*, in *Lilith* the asylum proves to be a tragic place. This follows from the fact that the narrator, an occupational therapist, believes that occupational therapy is better than analysis, and that actual chances for wellness are slim. Lilith herself is a beautiful schizophrenic who snares the narrator. She does not get well and she drags the narrator down with her. Ultimately, he opines, "There must be some way to defeat her . . . For some monstrous reason I want her more now than I ever did before! Whore, monster, oh, beautiful tender child!" The affair ends after another patient, also in love with Lilith, kills himself. Lilith descends into a catatonic state and her parents remove her to a Swiss sanitarium. There she drowns in an Alpine lake. The hero quits his job.[43]

Like Deborah Blau, Lilith has constructed a detailed, delusional world for herself. In a passage that seems to foreshadow Greenberg's book, Bea Brice describes Lilith's condition: "She doesn't just escape into a jumble of disorderly hallucinations; she's constructed an entire universe for herself, with its own history, its own cosmology, its own laws and art, even its own language." This is no accident. Salamanca had himself been an occupational therapist at Chestnut Lodge and he based Lilith off of Greenberg. According to Salamanca, Greenberg "was a brilliant girl, and after she was 'cured' as they called it, she wrote a rather celebrated novel called *I Never Promised You a Rose Garden*. She wasn't particularly beautiful, but she was fascinating." Salamanca's Lilith is not entirely Greenberg though. She is a seductress, an eternal mythical being, in full charge of her helpless suitor. More femme fatale than virginal innocent, Lilith shows the influence of pulp noir on asylum fiction, even when that fiction is grounded in fact.[44]

Salamanca's book was sufficiently popular (it was condensed in *Good Housekeeping*) for Hollywood to make a film of it. Starring a young Warren Beatty, the 1964 movie left audiences cold and flopped in the box office. It was simply too "art house" to break out into the wider culture. The asylum in the film is picturesque, the staff friendly and sympathetic, and the patients subdued or just quirky. Aiming for realism, the director had sent his actors to Chestnut Lodge to perform "psychodramas" with the patients. Beatty would remark that the Lodge had "a greater sense of reality than Madison Avenue."[45]

While *Lilith* is essentially a conventional love tragedy that paints madness as eccentricity, *I Never Promised You a Rose Garden* is different. It posits that insanity is a real and horrifying psychological condition. As Greenberg would later explain, "I wanted to say there is such a thing as real mental illness and it is not romantic." Yet *Rose Garden* works within the current of asylum narratives. Here is a Freudian rescue; the doctor, not the institution, saves Deborah. The fact that the hospital provides a caring and unique setting is essentially secondary. The cure feels "miraculous" with sanity teased out by a genuinely gifted master of the analytical art. If Dr. Fried becomes fantastical, the very title of the book, which tells us that happiness is no guarantee, also operates to obscure the real Fromm-Reichmann. The phrase "I never promised you a rose garden," is what Fried tells Deborah when Deborah asks her to report the physical abuse of a patient by an attendant. After Deborah pleads the case, Dr. Fried reluctantly agrees to report it, even though "I am not an administrative doctor." This is a bit shocking today—Fried admits she believes Deborah's story but does not particularly want to do anything about it. Then comes her wise explanation: "I never promised you a rose garden. I never promised you perfect justice . . . I never promised you peace or happiness. My help is so that you can be free to fight for all of these things." When read in full context, this sage advice seems tainted—what does helping a person cope with an unjust world have to do with reporting violence? Regardless, the takeaway seems to be a very useful message of empowerment. Interestingly, this phrase was not the title Greenberg originally wanted. She'd tried to title her book the more ambiguous *The Little Maybe*.[46]

Fromm-Reichmann would also gain some modicum of fame for her association with the "schizophrenogenic mother." This phrase, which appears only once in all of her writings, inspired much attention. Friedan's argument was that, in America, where mothers have more influence than they do in Europe, a child's "fear of his domineering mother" could lead to mental illness. The idea that mothers could make their kids schizophrenic corresponded with popular concerns about women in this period. Influential books like *Generation of Vipers* (1942) by Philip Wylie and *Modern Women: The Lost Sex* (1947) by Marynia Farnham and Ferdinand Lundberg argued that mothers were becoming monsters, afflicted with "penis envy" and taking out their frustrations on their kids. This argument did not just belong to anti-feminists. Though Betty Friedan noted in *The Feminine Mystique* that, after World War II, "It was suddenly discovered that the mother could be blamed for almost everything," she concedes that mothers, repressed and brainwashed by society, have a hand in "produc[ing] latent or overt homosexuality" in their sons, and even in creating "schizophrenic children." Regardless, in *I Never Promised You a Rose Garden*, a "schizophrenogenic mother" is not to blame for Deborah's illness, though the parents do not get off scot-free.[47]

Rose Garden gets a coda of sorts in Joyce Rebeta-Burditt's 1977 bestseller *The Cracker Factory*. In this novel, a young mother named Cassie gets committed to the psychiatric floor of a hospital after she has a breakdown in the supermarket and attempts suicide via aspirin. This hospital is no snake pit—in fact, she begins by referencing Olivia de Havilland, "wandering the Snake Pit being vague, an out-of-focus Dante in hell. I pictured myself tied to a bed while sadistic attendants forced gruel down my throat with a tube." But she finds instead a "private psychiatric ward artfully disguised as a Holiday Inn, done in soothing shades of green, with family-motel furniture, carpeting, and famous artists' prints on the wall." Here she receives gentle care from Dr. Edwin Alexander and ultimately comes to the awareness that she is an alcoholic. Dr. Alexander's recommendation that she join Alcoholics Anonymous pays dividends, and, in the end, she checks out and goes back to her husband and children. With an awareness of the domestic trap that forced her to a crisis point—Cassie has an overbearing mom, a distant and cold husband, and children who misbehave—the asylum is a place of rest and cure. It is even compared, not unfavorably, to an ocean cruise liner.[48]

What *Rose Garden* and similar works did was highlight the ambiguity of the mid-century asylum, even as it became a stand-in for the domestic prison. This ambiguity, in turn, reflects the internal struggles of the postwar female to liberate herself from a place she was supposed to love. And while Freud could be blasted as a patriarch, his method had room for redeeming applications, as Greenberg makes evident. Even for Plath and Sexton (and Friedan and Ward), psychiatry has its uses. McLean, for example, is no hellhole in *The Bell Jar*. Further, Plath and Sexton both had constructive, long-standing relationships with their analysts. Plath's "Doctor Norton," Dr. Ruth Tiffany Barnhouse in real life, was her psychiatrist and confidant even after she left McLean, helping her resolve her problems with her mother and even getting her into her first birth control device (though *The Bell Jar* turns this into a disastrous episode). Sexton was quite close with Dr. Martin Orne, who inspired her poetry and whom she distantly idolized. Under Norton's care, ECT helped Plath, and Sexton's psychiatrists often prescribed drugs that calmed her extreme manic states. In short, one must be careful not to consign the asylum to the status of unambiguous, patriarchal prison. If anything, with the popularity of *One Flew Over the Cuckoo's Nest*, the asylum could be viewed as a *feminine* trap for men.

OTHER VISIONS

Film, memoir, and fiction offered a wide range of application for the asylum in the early years of the Women's Movement. In *Valley of the Dolls*, Haven Manor seems to trap a talented singer, but its function is ambiguous, highlighting the tension between liberation and the desire for love and marriage. The talented, wild singer Neely O'Hara goes in for a "sleep cure" and gets trapped against her will. Her psychiatrist, Dr. Massinger (an apparent riff on Menninger), explains that the sleep cure wouldn't work on her since she is too "deeply disturbed." Only an extended stay can help. Like many a previous literary asylum, this "ivy-covered Tudor mansion" is really a prison. Neely learns this soon after she signs in, when she's told that there will be no sleep cure and no exit. Instead, she receives "deep psychiatric therapy," hydrotherapy, and occupational therapy. Her mail is monitored, she's thrust in windowless rooms and rooms with steel screens, and is refused simple liberties like lighting her own cigarettes. Other standard features are also included: burly attendants, "husky" women nurses, forced medicines, and a cast of fellow inmates railroaded by devious husbands. As another patient, Mary Jane (a nod to the *Snake Pit* author perhaps), explains, "You can't fight them. They show the record to your lawyer, or husband, or whoever is responsible for you." Neely loses her autonomy. Says the superintendent, Neely "is in no condition to make any decision about her future."[49]

Yet Haven Manor is not an old-style prison for the innocent. Neely is addicted and out-of-control, flirting with suicide and abusing those around her. As her stay continues, she realizes that the other women are not actually railroaded victims. One is an alcoholic, while another has invented children that do not exist. The hospital also houses "incurables . . . kept here for life on a custodial basis" in special "cottages" out back. Susann's message throughout the book is the simple, ironic warning that getting what you desire can prove disastrous. Neely's demand for fame demolishes her kind personality and poisons her relationships. She becomes a monster, a suitable denizen of an asylum.

Haven Manor is, above all, a convenient plot device, a cage of last resort for a woman incapable of handling the treacherous gift of fame. It even helps stabilize her. She exits in a peaceful state of mind. But it cannot save her. After she gets out, a new fame trip makes her again into a reprehensible human being.[50]

Valley's sanitarium reflects both the long literary history of asylum horrors as well as the more recent Freudian interposition. Like the fictionalized Chestnut Lodge in *Rose Garden*, Haven Manor channels the old mansions of doom while acknowledging that actual ill people are kept here and treated. Unlike Greenberg's book, here analysis is no answer. In fact, Neely's friend John mocks it in a pep talk: "I'm tired of all these fancy doctors who blame everything on the poor mothers of the world. So your old lady kicked off early. Did she do it purposely just to get even with you? Listen, Neely, you'll be a lot better off if you forget your headshrinker. You got where you are on your own."[51]

Haven Manor corresponds with other sensitive 1960s asylum representations. It looks pleasant and serves a population in need of serious help, despite it having insidious aspects. On the *Rose Garden* end of the spectrum, movies like *Splendor in the Grass* (1961) and *David and Lisa* (1962) served up downright positive asylum experiences. Both films feature mansions of healing and safety, where a lot of love and a little Freud go a long way. *David and Lisa*, based on a book written by a psychiatrist, is a low-budget, art house melodrama that became a surprise hit. It concerns a group of disturbed teens who live in a pleasant asylum that operates like a therapeutic day school. The protagonists come across as eccentric teens, whose peccadillos—Lisa rhymes everything and calls herself Muriel, and David is condescending and can't stand to be touched—are cured when they fall in love. This love process, which typically occurs *despite* adults in typical teen romances, happens *because of* the fatherly guidance of their psychiatrist. Alan is not the standard Freudian master. He talks to the kids on their own level while eschewing psychological terminology. His asylum works because the youngsters are kept isolated from the originating problem—their parents. The film (but not the book) makes it clear that David's overbearing mom has caused her son's paralyzing awkwardness. She's a smothering, intrusive harridan who tries to control David's life (and she pushes around dad as well). Ultimately, catharsis is achieved, thanks to Alan and the love he facilitates. This pleasant sanitarium for disaffected youngsters clearly was not "too much" for audiences to believe.

Similarly, *Splendor in the Grass* offered a Freudian exercise with Natalie Wood playing Deanie Loomis, an impressionable, young girl tortured by the conflict between her hormones and her Viper Mother. She's eventually driven to a suicide attempt which in turn inspires an asylum stay. The *Splendor* asylum is a stately mansion where folks sit around in rocking chairs looking out picture windows or doing pleasant occupational therapy. Deanie meets Johnny, a boy driven to madness by his demanding parents. Together, they make a connection that will end in marriage, though, as the movie tells us, it is no burning love like Deanie's original flame, Bud (played by *Lilith*'s Warren Beatty). Like *David and Lisa*, the *Splendor* asylum is a quiet place to recover from bad parenting. Here youngsters learn to accept badly dealt hands—at one point, a doctor tells Deanie, "We blame our parents for everything these days," when instead we should just "accept" them. Acceptance is the bittersweet message of the film, ending, as it does, with Wordsworth: "Though nothing can bring back the hour / Of splendor in the grass, glory in the flower, / We will grieve not; rather find / Strength in what remains behind."[52]

In the same period, however, darker asylum visions can also be found. Another Natalie Wood vehicle, *Inside Daisy Clover* (1965), is a black comedy that rings similar tones to *The Bell Jar* with its portrayal of a sensitive, talented girl overrun by life's events who attempts suicide. Unlike Plath's book, here it is mother who is institutionalized. When Daisy breaks down, she decides she cannot wind up institutionalized like mom, so she puts her head in the oven at her beach house. Played, jarringly, as a comedic scene, Daisy turns on the oven, puts her head in, and then gets interrupted by the phone, then the doorbell, and then by the oven itself, which doesn't seem to cooperate. She decides against doing herself in, choosing instead to use the gas to blow up the house in the movie's final scene. She walks away from the wreckage, happy in her liberating act of domestic demolition.[53]

By the end of the sixties, feminists regularly conceptualized homes as akin to asylums, places where control took concrete architectural form, and where Freud represented the superintendent. As historian Mari Jo Buhle notes, "The repudiation of Freud [a feminist

theorist] affirmed, was a basic principle of second-wave feminism."
Anne Koedt argued that Freud assumed that women were "an inferior appendage to man." Kate Millett connected him to fascism. Ger-
mane Greer blasted Freudians for devaluing women as sexual objects.
Even female analysts, whose numbers grew in the 1960s, sparred with
Freud's retrograde Victorian attitudes. Notably this had begun well
before Friedan's battle cry; as early as 1932 famed Neo-Freudian Karen
Horney quietly took down the great old man's portrait from the wall
of her home.[54]

Unfortunately, the Women's Movement, like the rest of America,
also had a racism problem. The African American experience was
often devalued and ignored. One Black writer, Gayl Jones, used the
asylum to communicate how whiteness irreducibly informed patriarchy. In her short story "Asylum," the nameless but clearly African
American narrator finds herself in an institution after having urinated
in front of her nephew's first grade teacher. This place is sparsely described. We know there is a nurse, "a big black woman," along with a
patronizing series of white male doctors. The woman refuses to let
a doctor examine her genitals, telling him, "I ain't got nothing down
there for you." The story ends with her trying to figure out how to
escape. The doctor asks, "You should tell me what you are thinking?"
and she responds, "Is that the only way I can be freed?" Escape from
this white-controlled prison can only be attained by playing the psychotherapy game, one in which the protagonist relinquishes power
under the gaze of the doctor. One critic intoned, "Beneath the asylum
tale lies the slave narrative."[55]

"Asylum" appeared in a collection of short stories Jones published
after her second novel, *Eva's Man*, which also made a powerful asylum
statement. In *Eva's Man* (1976), the protagonist finds herself in a "psychiatric prison" for poisoning and then biting off the penis of her
lover. The reason for Eva's crime has to do with the sexual brutality
and poor treatment she's experienced all her life. But we are left in the
dark as to what specifically made her commit the crime. Eva doesn't
tell us, and she does not play by the rules of the asylum either. She
simply puts up a wall of silence. As in "Asylum," it is a defense strategy against a system that seeks to quarantine, define, and dissect
her. *Eva's Man* troubled reviewers. It was called a "sad, dark chant"
and a "squalid appraisal of the souls of Black folk." Eva's nightmare,

once situated in the context of asylum literature, however, takes on familiar hues. There is a protagonist who offers a disjointed story; it is unclear what prompted her actions; there is an abusive superintendent named Miss Floyd, who gropes a female patient; and the treatments are worthless. Eva's cellblock neighbor Elvira refers to all of the shrinks as "Dr. Fraud." She explains, "I call em all Dr. Frauds. You know. But that's all they do. Nothing. And get ten, twenty dollars an hour for it too. Except the state pays em. If I had to pay em, I wouldn't pay em. I just stay crazy."[56]

While it is clear that Eva committed a horrible crime, we also know that her life experiences are weighted with burdens almost impossible to carry. Hers is the life of the disenfranchised and dismissed. She manifests what Afro-Caribbean psychiatrist Frantz Fanon called the mind-set of the colonized, "prepared for violence since time immemorial." Eva makes her own rebellion, and once institutionalized, she enacts her own Marcusean Great Refusal. She is willing to negate all social expectations and defy all who would control her. Eva's is the feminism of the subaltern.[57]

By the 1970s, refusing psychiatric authority was a much more tenable proposition than it had been in the past. The struts holding up the state hospital system were being kicked away, one by one. The high walls of the asylum were about to come down.

CHAPTER 8

ASYLUMS DON'T WORK

Then the gates swallowed the ambulance-bus and swallowed her
as she left the world and entered the underland where all who were
not desired, who caught like rough teeth in the cogwheels, who
had no place or fit crosswise the one they were hammered into,
were carted to repent of their contrariness or to pursue their mad
vision down to the pit of terror . . . She was human garbage carried
to the dump.
—Marge Piercy, *Woman on the Edge of Time* (1976)

tarting in the late 1950s, the state mental hospital system began
to collapse. By 1980, the patient population was at less than
a quarter of its mid-century level, despite a huge expansion in the
overall US population. This process would be called deinstitutionalization.

This chapter explores deinstitutionalization via books, articles,
films, and art that served as a kind of background soundtrack to the
demolition of the mental hospital. I highlight the 1970s here, because
this was when the anti-asylum critique became most sustained. William Peter Blatty's *The Exorcist* (1971), for instance, tells us that America
was a sick country and that institutional medicine was a frightening
failure. Milos Forman's *One Flew Over the Cuckoo's Nest* (1975) served
up a banal and terrifying institution that captured psychiatric disillusionment and laid out a terrifying blueprint for future asylum films.
The resurrection of silver screen star Frances Farmer brought to light
a vast conspiracy of psychiatrists aimed at reducing freedom.

All of these projects, and many more, collected around a single
theme: The asylum didn't work.

DECLINE

In 1949, a French naval surgeon experimented with a synthetic anti-histamine called promethazine in an effort to mitigate shock in his patients. The drug turned out to have an unexpected and remarkable calming effect. A derivative of this compound, chlorpromazine, was synthesized in December 1950, and it went on to become the world's first successful antipsychotic. After sweeping Europe, drug company Smith, Kline & French renamed it Thorazine and broke into the American market by targeting state governments overburdened by escalating health-care costs. Nicknamed the "chemical lobotomy," the affordable drug helped to bury psychosurgery and was soon prescribed to some two million Americans. As hospitals began to empty out, most believed that the drug was working its magic.[1]

A second factor of decline is arguably even more important: laws. The creation of the National Institute of Mental Health in 1949, a result of Truman's National Mental Health Act of 1946, led the charge, inspiring a variety of community treatment options. In 1954, the Governors' Conference on Mental Health pushed hard for such centers, with New York and California first in requiring their construction. The community centers signaled a profound shift in the treatment of mental illness, from full service live-in facilities to outpatient centers. This notably predates the widespread acceptance of Thorazine. In 1963, the federal government stepped in when John F. Kennedy signed the Community Mental Health Act into law. While this law provided new monies for outpatient care, budgetary constraints and problems in prioritizing serious mental illness quickly undermined it. Regardless, knowing that Uncle Sam was involved prompted states to start unburdening themselves of their responsibilities. The end of the state hospital system was in sight.[2]

The biggest blow came ironically with the biggest federal boost to mental health care spending. Part of President Johnson's Great Society, Medicaid was designed to end the horrific imbalances in health-care coverage between rich and poor. Thanks to the new law, the government would now cover between 50 percent and 80 percent of state mental health-care costs. But there was a catch. Funds could not be used on patients in psychiatric hospitals. The purpose was to maintain the state-funded asylum status quo. However, because nursing homes *were* covered by Medicaid, the law incentivized shifting the aging mentally ill there. And this is exactly what happened. While census numbers began to decline slightly in 1955, after Medicaid the numbers plummeted at an absolute rate of about 8 percent per year (with the elderly having a higher rate). In 1972, Nixon tried to plug the holes with the Social Security Amendments, which created Supplemental Social Security Income (SSI) for the Aged, the Disabled, and the Blind. Unlike Medicaid, SSI was a fully federally funded allowance for the mentally ill. But because there was no provision as to how the allowance was spent, states could essentially remove themselves from direct responsibility for treatment. On came a hodgepodge of services, community centers, and residences, all effectively disconnected from the state hospitals and many operating for-profit. In 1980, Jimmy Carter signed a law aimed at covering rising psychiatric costs for more vulnerable populations, but this was rescinded by Ronald Reagan in 1981. Reagan's budget supplied block grants to states rather than specific spending requirements. The effect would be a continued decline in expenditures on people suffering mental illness.[3]

Drugs and legislation go a long way toward explaining deinstitutionalization, but there are other factors as well. Kennedy pushed for community mental health when state institutions were under sustained attack in the press and academia; his solution was a political expedient that did not improve the lives of the stigmatized patient population. When Johnson launched Medicare, the nation was rent by urban disorder, countercultural revolutions, and an increasingly unpopular war. Then, in the late 1960s, an economic slowdown kicked in characterized by declining manufacturing profits, flattening wages, and a corporate assault on the middle and working classes. All this had the effect of undermining shared responsibility for the needy. Twinning the eras of deinstitutionalization and deindustrialization helps us to see a moment of uncertainty and blight. Hubert Selby Jr.'s 1978 novel *Requiem for a Dream* graphically illustrates this.

Selby's book is about a junkie named Harry and his mom, Sara, plus his best friend Tyrone and his girlfriend Marion. The title refers to the death of the American Dream. Sara lives alone in her apartment, overeating and watching TV, while her son Harry hustles to become a "free man." There is no hope for either of them. Harry wanders the streets, which resemble "a battleground of WWII." Abandoned buildings, trash fires, empty blocks, and dope fiends are everywhere. His entrepreneurial dream of opening a coffee shop crashes against the reality of economic stagnation. Sara's dreams die too. She wants to be on a TV show, and, in her effort to prepare herself, she gets hooked on diet pills and descends into delirium. She winds up in Bellevue. Here, a callous doctor puts her on Thorazine and sentences her to round after round of ECT. As per literary convention, this procedure is done unethically. Sara is zapped without any sedation, totally aware of her surroundings. In one long, magnificent sentence, we get what must surely be the most grandiose electroconvulsive event in all of American letters:

> . . . something jammed between her teeth and people were talking and laughing, but the voices were a blur and it seemed like there were many faces leaning over her and she could feel her eyes opening wider as they looked, peered, and she could hear laughter and then the faces seemed to recede and drift away in a haze and suddenly fire shot through her body and her eyes felt like they were going to burst from their sockets as her body burned then stiffened and felt like it would snap apart and pain shot through her head and stabbed her ears and temples and her body kept jerking and bouncing as the flames seared every cell of her body and her bones felt like they were being twisted and crushed between huge pincers as more and more electricity was forced through her body and her burning body arched and slammed itself down on the table and Sara could feel her bones snapping and smell the burning of her own flesh as barbed hooks were thrust into her eyes yanking them out of their sockets and all she could do was endure and feel the pain and smell the burning flesh unable to yell, to plead, to pray, to make a sound or even die, but stay locked in the torturous pain as her head screamed AAAAAAAAAAAAAAAHHHHHHHHHHHHHHHHHHHHHHHHH hhhhhhhhhhhh . . .

Suffice it to say Sara loses her mind and winds up among the living dead at the State Mental Hospital. Her friends find her here, but they don't recognize her. "Bones stuck out everywhere. Her hair hung dead from her head. Her eyes were clouded and didn't see. Her skin was gray." The tragedy is especially sharp in Sara's case because, before she undergoes ECT, a conscientious doctor tries to save her and fails. He is told by an administrator that what really matters is that the hospital "functions smoothly." The abandonment of human feeling coincides with the abandonment of the American Dream.[4]

Hubert's novel speaks to the ongoing institutional critique that would be called anti-psychiatry. This represented the view that institutional medicine, and the field of psychiatry itself, were deeply flawed, even malicious. The history of this dim view predates the Cold War, it was in this period that rebellions against authority and conformity combined to create social resonance. From Beat declarations that institutions were "isolation chambers rather than hospitals in the usual sense" to right-wing suggestions that mental health was a "Marxist weapon," the stage was set for a truly massive backlash.[5]

Anti-psychiatry took many forms. It could be seen in the protests of shaggy-haired, young patients in art house movies like *Lilith* and in Herbert Marcuse's declaration that psychiatry is "an engine of suppression." Ken Kesey's *Cuckoo's Nest* expressed it, as did Edward Kienholz's graphic, mixed media installation *The State Hospital* (1966). In this piece, two figures with fishbowl faces lie on a bunk bed, strapped by the wrist to their beds, filthy bedpan just out of reach, bare bulb dangling from the ceiling. Kienholz himself had worked at a state hospital. Musicians joined in, as in James Taylor's 1969 single "Knockin' Round the Zoo." The Zoo in question is McLean, where Taylor had spent time as a younger man: "There's bars on all the windows / And they're counting up the spoons, yeah. / And if I'm feeling edgy, / There's a chick who's paid / To be my slave, yeah, watch out James. / But she'll hit me with a needle / If she thinks I'm trying to misbehave." Taylor would later describe modern psychiatry as being little better than the Zoo: "Now they lock you up in a chemical jail."[6]

The most influential wave of criticism came from the pens of social theorists and renegade psychiatrists. Thomas Scheff, Erving Goffman, August B. Hollingshead, Robert Perrucci, and J. K. Wing argued that institutionalization embodied capitalist control, that it was dependent upon social inequality, and that it encouraged patients to make "careers" of mental illness. Sociologist Kai T. Erikson took the argument to one logical conclusion in a much-quoted 1962 essay in which he asserts that "agencies of control," such as asylums

and prisons, gathered social deviants together and gave them "an opportunity to teach one another the skills and attitudes of a deviant
career." In other words, asylums manufactured deviants who would,
in turn, go on to play the important social role of showing the rest of
us "what evil looks like" and hence what the "norm" should be.[7]

The most radical argument was proffered by a Thomas Szasz, a
psychiatrist whose *The Myth of Mental Illness* is a landmark in institutional criticism. Szasz never met a demonizing psychiatric metaphor or analogy that he didn't like. In this book and other writings,
he argued that mental hospitals are "mirror images" of concentration camps, and "prisons" too. Treatments are "torture," psychiatrists
played a "leading role" in developing Nazi gas chambers, and Karl
Marx was actually a "therapist." According to Szasz, the ultimate aim
of mental health is to "enslave man." He assigned psychiatry, along
with "chattel slavery, the Inquisition, National Socialism, and Communism" to the "pantheon of man's inhumanity to man."[8]

Thomas Szasz's arguments had an enormous appeal for many,
for a variety of reasons. His libertarian insistence that the welfare
state should stay off our backs and that the mad be held accountable
for their actions made him alluring to conservatives like William F.
Buckley, Jr. His arguments that homosexuality was not a mental illness, that a woman had a natural right to abortion and birth control, and that patients were victims of "stigmatizing labels" made him
appealing to many on the New Left and in the Women's Movement.
His conspiratorial theory that psychiatry was part of an encroaching
Communist program tapped widely held Cold War paranoias.[9]

Szasz is often grouped with another iconoclastic psychiatrist,
R. D. Laing. Laing rose to fame in the late 1960s and 1970s with a series
of books and lectures that questioned the validity of psychiatric diagnosis and treatment. Essentially, he accused society of being insane.
He believed that schizophrenics, reacting to the utter alienation of
our present world, are on a "voyage" worth learning about. In his way,
Laing addressed the same set of concerns and paranoias that Szasz
did. We had entered *1984*: "Exploitation must not be seen as such. It
must be seen as benevolence. Persecution preferably should not need
to be invalidated as the figment of a paranoid imagination; it should
be experienced as kindness . . . Orwell's time is already with us." But
unlike Szasz, Laing recognized that the mentally ill experienced

something tangible and could be therapeutically helped. Further, his politics were firmly on the Left. For him, the "industrial-military complex" was a cause of insanity, as was our drive to "live in relative adjustment to a civilization apparently driven to its own destruction." Such wisdom produced gems like, "The perfectly adjusted bomber pilot may be a greater threat than the hospitalized schizophrenic deluded that the Bomb is inside him." Though anything but close, (Szasz would write that Laing's aim "was not to expose the nature of psychiatric power but to seize it"), both men, along with Goffman, Foucault, and the labeling theorists, captured the seductively ironic argument that supposedly benevolent institutions were in fact malevolent.[10]

By the 1970s, the attack on asylums had become mainstream and integrated. In a shattering 1973 article published in *Science*, "On Being Sane in Insane Places," psychology professor David L. Rosenhan sent eight "pseudopatients" into the mental health-care system and instructed them to say that they were hearing voices. After they were admitted, they were to act completely normal. They were kept in the hospital for an average of nineteen days, and all but one was diagnosed as schizophrenic. Later, Rosenhan made mental hospitals look even worse. He told a research hospital that over the next three months, one or more fake patients would make their way in. The hospital indicated 193 patients as possibly faking insanity. In fact, no fake patients had been sent.[11]

One did not have to deny mental illness to be in the mainstream of thinking that something was radically wrong. Even back in 1958, Dr. Harry Solomon had argued in his presidential address to the American Psychiatric Association that mental hospitals were "bankrupt beyond remedy" and needed to be "liquidated as rapidly as can be done in an orderly and progressive fashion." In 1963, President Kennedy, whose own sister had been lobotomized by Dr. Freeman, told Congress, "Breakthroughs have rendered obsolete the traditional methods of treatment which imposed upon the mentally ill a social quarantine, a prolonged or permanent confinement in huge, unhappy mental hospitals where they were out of sight and forgotten." Finally, the era of long-term institutionalization was coming to an end. Drugs, Medicaid, community treatment, and laws (such as the 1967 California Community Mental Health Services Act, based on a study quoting Szasz, Laing, and Goffman, which capped the maximum stay for involuntary committal to seventeen days), plus the investigations, plowed the old system under. One radical, commenting on the lack of provision for aftercare, wrote, "When you have Buchenwald, you do not worry first about alternatives to Buchenwald."[12]

Rhetorically, the attack on asylums was meeting the wildest dreams of critics. All at once, the past evils were being purged: "Railroading" was to be ended with patients' rights cases and legislative limits to involuntary commitment; "slavery" was stopped by ending patient peonage; "torture" would end by demanding the abolishment of ECT, psychosurgery, and other "extreme" measures; and, finally, "imprisonment" itself would end with the closing down of state hospitals. While psychiatry did not end (a biological-pharmaceutical model fit well with the politics of expedience), the landscape had irrevocably changed.

EXORCISING THE ASYLUM

Horror is an appropriate genre for investigating this evolving landscape. The most notorious example from the 1970s serves quite well. *The Exorcist* (the 1971 novel and 1973 film) is about a girl possessed by the Devil. Starting at a dig in Northern Iraq, where elderly Father Merrin comes across a statue of the demon Pazuzu, evil travels to Georgetown where young Regan lives with her actress mom and the household help. We then track a lengthy process that begins with Ouija board tricks and ends with full-blown telekinetic, mind reading, blaspheming gruesomeness. William Peter Blatty's novel devotes considerable space to the various medical investigations of Regan's symptoms. Regan first gets diagnosed with "hyperkinetic behavior disorder" and is put on Ritalin. When she continues to decline, she's taken off Ritalin and put on Librium. Still no help. Neurologists examine her. Then come spinal taps, EEG, hypnotherapy, x-rays, and brain probes. The nonplussed doctors debate hysteria, neurasthenia, psychasthenia, multiple personality, split personality, thanatophobia, schizophrenia, and old-fashioned divorce guilt. Eventually, Regan is sent to the "Barringer Clinic" (an apparent riff on the Menninger Clinic), but no succor is to be found. Treatments fail because the problem is not biological—it's moral. Ruminates the detective on the case, "The world—the *entire world*—is having a nervous breakdown." The Vietnam War serves as corroborating evidence. In a prefatory quote before a section of the book, titled "The Abyss," we read the following quote between two Biblical passages: "... *A [Vietnam] brigade commander once ran a contest to rack up his unit's 10,000th kill; the prize was a week of luxury in the colonel's own quarters ... Newsweek, 1969.*"[13]

Help comes in the form of a skeptical Jesuit priest named Damien Karras. He wants to believe that the problem is secular and psychological, even telling Regan's mother that exorcisms are passé, "Since we learned about mental illness; about paranoia; split personality; all those things that they taught me at Harvard." But Karras comes around as evidence for Satan piles up. Through the priest, we travel from confidence to utter disbelief in mind science. The contemporary public, having lived through political assassination, riots, and failed promises, was primed for such cynicism. By 1971, Americans had recently endured the end of JFK's New Frontier, an expanding war into Cambodia, the coming to light of the massacre of Vietnamese civilians at My Lai, the Manson murders, and an economy that seemed to be slowing. *The Exorcist* became a number-one bestseller as disillusionment with the American promise rose to new heights.

Directed by William Friedkin, the movie of *The Exorcist* visually elaborates on Blatty's bleak worldview, including his take on institutional medicine. Bellevue is shown to be a depressing place filled with staring or self-chatting unfortunates. Father Karras visits his mom here and sees her tied to a bed. She's released, only to be found dead in her apartment. At the Barringer Clinic and Foundation, referenced but not described in the book, we see Regan through a TV monitor, lab-coated doctors closely observing her. Her frustrated mother tells this crew, "I'm not going to lock her up in some goddamn asylum." Once Regan returns home, her bedroom becomes the asylum. The bedposts are covered thickly in white (or beige) sheets, the room is stark white, and drugs are pumped into her. But in this universe, priests, not Freud, rescue the waif from her confinement.[14]

The Exorcist demolished box office expectations and embedded itself deeply within popular consciousness. Amazed by the size and diversity of the crowd showing up to see it on a weekday morning, film critic Vincent Canby ruminated that if it were not for its incredible popularity, this "claptrap" "wouldn't be worth writing about." Stunningly, it had become "the biggest thing to hit the industry since Mary Pickford, popcorn, pornography and 'The Godfather.'"[15]

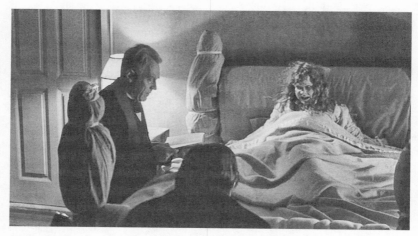

The bedroom as asylum and the priest as doctor in *The Exorcist* (1973)

In 1978, Blatty published *The Ninth Configuration*, his first "sequel" to *The Exorcist*. A hybrid of "Dr. Tarr and Professor Fether" and *Spellbound*, the novel follows an insane doctor running an asylum and catering to the wild fantasies of his patients. The doctor slowly learns that he is not who he thinks he is, and that he is facing a crisis of theological proportions. The asylum in this book is literally imported from the Old World, shipped brick by brick by the eccentric American wife of a German Count. The 1980 movie version, directed by Blatty, was shot in an actual castle in Hungary. For good measure, he threw in a large poster of Bela Lugosi on one wall and includes a scene with a patient in a Frankenstein mask. And his castle asylum is also modern. It's part of a secret government program, "Project Freud," created to figure out why so many soldiers are going insane in Vietnam.[16]

The Ninth Configuration opens with the arrival of a new psychiatrist, Dr. Vincent Kane. The obvious Biblical reference is par for the course. He's a man lost to God. Kane's primary patient is Cutshaw (apparently the astronaut featured in the party scene in *The Exorcist*, where Regan tells him, "You're not coming back"), who must be convinced that God exists in order to be cured. As the plot develops, Kane figures out that he is not a doctor but Special Forces legend "Killer" Kane, who, through a computer mix-up à la *Catch-22*, has been sent here to treat psychotic Marines. His brother is the real superintendent, but for therapeutic reasons he allows Kane to think he's in charge. His plan is to allow Kane to come to terms with his war sins so he can "wash away the blood" and "do penance for the killing—by curing." Kane builds a therapeutic community and eventually accepts who he really is, and, after saving another patient from a biker gang (and killing a bunch of bikers in the process), he kills himself.[17]

In *The Exorcist*, the Devil is defeated through the "shock treatment" (as a Barringer Clinic doctor actually describes it) of exorcism. In *The Ninth Configuration*, Satan is beaten via the shock treatment of Kane's suicide. Writes Kane in a final letter to Cutshaw, "I am taking my life in the hope that my death may provide a shock that has curative value." It works. Cutshaw is cured, and so are the other inmates, who proceed to go back to normal (and non-military) lives. Cutshaw makes sure to tell us that Kane is "a lamb." Kane's martyrdom saves his patients and his soul, just as Father Karras's suicidal act saves Regan. *The Ninth Configuration* is less a "sequel" than a variation on *The Exorcist*. Or, rather, a longer dialogue that Blatty is having with himself—this book is an updated version of one he wrote in 1966. In any case, all explain madness as something not within the provenance of psychiatry to deal with.[18]

In 1983, Blatty published *Legion*, starring detective William Kinderman from *The Exorcist*. In this novel, the Devil inhabits the resurrected corpse of Father Karras, who now resides in a padded cell on the disturbed ward at Georgetown General Hospital. His body also happens to host a deceased serial killer. The Gemini Killer's backstory is also asylum-based. He had an abusive father who tormented his mentally disabled twin brother, and, after they locked him up in the San Francisco State Mental Hospital, a careless nurse caused him to die of fright when she turned off his night lamp. The trauma of losing his brother birthed the Gemini Killer. After he is killed, he takes up residency inside Karras's undead body, his spirit leaping into other patients who then go forth to kill. Their weapon of choice is a sedative drug used for ECT, with which they paralyze their victims before chopping them up. Blatty has fully asylumized his *Exorcist* universe.[19]

Blatty wrote and directed the film version of *Legion* under the title *The Exorcist III*. (*The Exorcist II: The Heretic*, written by William Goodhart and released in 1977, is not a Blatty product.) In *The Exorcist*, Regan's room became a metaphorical asylum after a real one failed. In *The Ninth Configuration*, an actual asylum does the job. In

The Exorcist III, the battle takes place in an asylum cell. Kinderman finally ends things by shooting Karras with his revolver. Reminiscent of Marx's dictum that history goes from tragedy to farce, first Karras dies after taking Regan's un-asylum-treatable illness onto himself, then dies again after instructing a cop to shoot his re-possessed corpse in an actual asylum. Between the two events, a Marine liberates the inmates of an asylum, thanks to his divinely inspired suicide.[20]

A CZECH MOVIE

In 1975, Milos Forman logged a new kind of horror into the cinematic register—the well-run hell. *Cuckoo's Nest*'s voyage from page to screen began in 1962, when Kirk Douglas purchased the rights for $47,000. Douglas hoped to produce and star in the movie, and he began by commissioning scriptwriter Dale Wasserman to convert it into a play. Opening on Broadway on November 13, 1963, it tanked. Seats went unfilled and critics were unkind. The *New York Times* sarcastically wrote, "Do you find the quips, pranks and wiles of the inmates of a mental hospital amusing? If you do, you should have a merry old time at *One Flew Over the Cuckoo's Nest*." Nine days later, Kennedy was killed in Dallas. As Marc Elliot puts it, now, "Nobody wanted to go to the theater to see a play about crazies." The show closed a few months later. For his part, Kirk Douglas did not blame Lee Harvey Oswald for his failure. According to him, people just did not want to see the bigshot actor on Broadway. The play didn't vanish either. Kirk's son would remember how his father was saddened to see it being "revived on both coasts with great success." In 1972, the aging star tried to sell the property but found no takers. After some legal wrangling with Wasserman, he turned the rights over to his son Michael.[21]

Michael Douglas was a young Hollywood player who currently starred in the TV show *The Streets of San Francisco*. He was excited about his new property, feeling that it spoke to the times, "an individual man fighting the system . . . trying to overpower the establishment." Interestingly, director Milos Forman was actually Kirk Douglas's inspiration first. Unbeknownst to Michael, Kirk had once tried to give him a copy of Kesey's book after meeting him on a goodwill tour behind the Iron Curtain in 1966. A customs inspector had impounded the book and Forman never received it. Kirk Douglas did not know this and assumed a snub. Funny how a critique of American institutions was assumed to be bad for World Communism. Years later, Kirk's son chose Forman. The director read the book and suddenly realized that he'd be making "a Czech movie. This is a movie about [a] society I just lived twenty years of my life [in]. You know, it's about everything I know. And I know how these people feel." Forman had grown up under oppressive circumstances. His parents had died in Nazi concentration camps, and he'd been raised in an environment he'd nickname "Kafkarna." His was a gray world of ubiquitous "surveillance" so pervasive that it became "boring." *Cuckoo's Nest* would be his second American film.[22]

Unlike previous asylum films, *Cuckoo's Nest* would be shot almost entirely within a real institution. This was only partly to do with its small budget. They wanted veracity. The actors lived on the campus of the Oregon State Hospital (OSH) and absorbed their surroundings. They were also assigned to watch *Titicut Follies*, an infamous mental hospital documentary. Filmed at the Bridgewater State Hospital in Massachusetts, that 1967 film would be tied up in litigation and not widely seen until the 1990s. One reason OSH turned out to be such a good shooting location was that there was space on the ward. Thanks to deinstitutionalization, rather than having over a thousand patients like in its 1950s heyday, there were only two to three hundred inmates.[23]

Dr. Dean Brooks felt the filming would be "therapy" for his patients, and over ninety of them worked behind and in front of the camera. In the most remarkable casting decision in all of asylum film, Brooks was asked to play Dr. Spivey. The superintendent played the superintendent. Forman had Brooks improvise with Nicholson when their characters met for the intake interview. Forman had given Brooks a realistically prepared patient "report" just before the scene started, instructing him to "just do your job as if this is your new patient." The scene rings true. The filmmakers were sad to cut down the footage to just six minutes.[24]

Legendarily, Jack Nicholson was nobody's first choice for R. P. McMurphy. Kirk Douglas wanted the part, but his son told him he was too old. Both Gene Hackman and Marlon Brando were offered it, but they reportedly turned it down. Nicholson, on the other hand, was very interested. He'd had a recent hit in *Chinatown*, and, in *Five*

Easy Pieces and *The Last Detail*, he showcased what one journalist dubbed "that Nicholson energy and hatred of authority." Kesey didn't approve—he called Nicholson a "five-foot six-inch wimp"—but he'd become so estranged from the production at this point that this must be taken with a grain of salt. Kesey's script had been discarded, and because he'd sold the rights, he had to sue the studio to get a slice of the returns. Seeing Jack's face on the cover of his book made his rage rise, even as the actor helped rocket paperback sales to over seven million copies. Regardless, Nicholson was an inspired choice. He played McMurphy as a funny roustabout, a young man gleefully bucking the system as much of the 1970s audience would have liked to do. Even his unintimidating size helped; the little guy was tweaking the monster's tail. The small budget helped too. As Forman explained, because Nicholson was "known to us," we identified with him as he entered "a world unknown to us" peopled by unfamiliar, low-paid actors. When McMurphy realizes he is under the absolute control of Nurse Ratched, the audience's sympathy for him makes for a profound impact.[25]

The ECT scene symbolized Forman's approach. After brawling on the floor with attendants, Cheswick, Bromden, and McMurphy are sent to wait on a bench like misbehaved children outside the Principal's office. Cheswick is taken in first, screaming as he gets dragged off. In a touching scene where McMurphy learns Chief Bromden can talk, he suggests breaking out together. "What are we doing in here Chief?" he asks. "Huh? What's us two guys doin' in this fucking place?" Next, we see Cheswick wheeled off on a gurney, incoherent. Cut to McMurphy and Bromden watching. Out comes a nurse with two big attendants: "Mr. McMurphy? Please follow me." Our fears are rising, and we can see anxiety in McMurphy's demeanor. Into the ECT room he goes, an attendant on each arm. What is most effective about all this is Jack Nicholson's performance. He's clearly terrified, yet he presents a forced nonchalance and whimsicality. He flashes a big, cheesy smile, and two thumbs up, to Chief before going in. McMurphy visibly shudders at the sight of the crew gathered in the ECT suite but again reverts to his carefree stance. As they lay him down and take off his boots, he jokes, "Light shine, boys." He startles when the nurse puts conductible gel on his temples. "A little dab'll do ya," he says. Then comes the mouth guard. The nurse explains that it will keep him from biting his tongue.

He struggles with the mass in his mouth, coughs. Next come the white headphones. The familiarity the staff has with the apparatus, the lack of soundtrack, the firm hands holding down his shoulders, and the group's businesslike dismissal of McMurphy's antics makes for an excruciating buildup. He still resists, humming a song now that he can no longer speak. But his face betrays his fear. Then comes a clicking sound, no Hollywood blaring horns. He goes into a massive convulsion, back arching as the attendants struggle to hold him down. An extreme close up of his face shows unbearable agony.

This ECT event marks the start of a new epoch in film asylum treatments, though it clearly builds on what has come before it. The first cinematic ECT, in *The Snake Pit*, has us suffer with Olivia de Havilland as she sits on a hallway bench watching the previous victim getting carted off before a nurse comes out and tells her, "You're next." Virginia admits to the patient next to her that she's "terribly afraid." She enters as a crew sets up the bed like a house cleaning service. The camera closes in on the machine as she eyes it across the room. It is black with dials and a glowing, circular gauge at the center. Virginia tells Dr. Kik that she's going to be "electrocuted," and Kik replies, "Just trying to make you well." He gently lifts her onto the bed. As they swab on the conductible gel, she wonders if they "dare to kill me without a trial?" She decides to get a lawyer, but when she opens her mouth she only gets out "I want—" before the mouth guard goes in. We watch as Kik's hand turns the dial, the loud, blaring horns telling us the shock is happening. We next see Virginia lifted off the bed, disoriented. In *Fear Strikes Out* (1957), where another Freudian helps another young person (in this case ballplayer Jimmy Piersall), we only see the door to the ECT room. Like *The Snake Pit*, this treatment, while scary, helps the hero. The most jarring ECT scene prior to *Cuckoo's Nest* is in *Shock Corridor* (1962), in which the hero gets blasted in full view of the camera. As the music intensifies, coupled with a high pitch electronic sound and screaming from elsewhere, we see him writhe about, a double exposure superimposing other scenes to disorienting and alarming effect.[26]

One Flew Over the Cuckoo's Nest elaborates on this cinematic language, with the hallway anticipation, the jammed-in mouth guard, the crew of attendants and nurses, the seizing, and the sense of disorientation. Its main innovation is its documentary style and the context

of watching an individualist's defenses ground down by a bureaucratic disciplinary process. It feels genuine. We know we are in a real
place. As Forman demanded, "It must be real." The reality he gives us
is consistent with pre-sedation treatments of the 1950s, but less so for
the ostensible 1960s date of the film (based on the 1963 World Series
footage used).[27]

Even more notorious is the lobotomy scene. Lobotomy had been
scarcely treated in film prior to *Cuckoo's Nest*. It is only a threat in
Suddenly, Last Summer. In *A Fine Madness*, we get an explanation (if
comedic) of the procedure and later a post-op moment when we are
not sure if Sean Connery is a goner (he isn't). There's also the *Planet
of the Apes* silliness, and one might add for fun 1973's *Don't Look in the
Basement*. Shot by the director who would go on to make *Don't Open
the Door!* and *Keep My Grave Open*, this movie makes lobotomy an
inane plot mover, warning us that both psychosurgery and Aquarian
mind healing methods are equally suspect.[28]

In *Cuckoo's Nest*, we don't see the procedure at all, nor do we get
a description. After nearly strangling Nurse Ratched and getting
struck down by an attendant (the film does without the tearing-open
of Ratched's blouse), we fade to a scene of the patients playing cards.
They start talking about McMurphy's whereabouts. Has he escaped?
No, says Harding. He is upstairs, "meek as a lamb." We learn the horrible truth when Bromden watches as a pair of attendants bring in a
zombie McMurphy late at night into the dorm. Bromden unties himself from his bed and walks over. He lifts Nicholson's head and we can
see two small scars in the moonlight, one on each side of his forehead.
The scar symmetry and blank stare evoke Frankenstein. Bromden
smothers the sad monster with a pillow.[29]

Thanks to these and other powerful scenes, *Cuckoo's Nest* earned
over $108 million domestic, not including later video, streaming, and
cable revenues. Adjusted for inflation, the tally is more in the neighborhood of $400 million. The biggest coup came on Oscar night, when
it took home all five major awards, including Best Picture, Actor, Actress, Director, and Adapted Screenplay. The press hailed it as a classic
of "pop-mythology."[30]

The media's celebratory tone reflected the contemporaneous and
somewhat jaded temper of film criticism and social activism. Vincent Canby in the *New York Times* wisely noted that Forman's film was

part of a longer tradition in which "mental institutions are popular as metaphors for the world outside." The patients are "the sanes, while all of us outside who have tried to adjust to a world that accepts war, hunger, poverty, and genocide are the real crazies." Rex Reed in *Vogue* similarly commented that this hospital "is a metaphor that symbolizes the plight of the individual caught up in a computerized and inhuman system of incarceration where humans are numbers and lives are filing cabinets." Forman's innovations were also singled out. Canby thought the film's success lay in its resistance to the old madness clichés evident in *The King of Hearts*, which was still "playing almost continually around the country." While it is "one more epic battle between a free spirit and a society that cannot tolerate him," it was also real. It went along with the prevailing sentiment that mental hospitals destroyed healthy minds. Wrote Ruth McCormick, thanks to the revelations of abuses and "the work of such leftist psychologists as Reich, Laing, Cooper, Szasz, Fromm and others," we can have a film that tells it straight. But for McCormick, metaphor trumped documentary realism. She asserts that "neither the novel or the film are really *about* mental illness." They are about battling the establishment.[31]

One of the lasting contributions of *Cuckoo's Nest* was the Nurse Ratched archetype. Clearly, the brutal asylum female was a long-standing literary figure. Even in film, domineering asylum nurses could be seen in *The Snake Pit* (1948), *The Cobweb* (1955), *The Caretakers* (1963), even *The Disorderly Orderly* (1964). But Forman's vision is different. In not making her a cartoon, Louise Fletcher evokes the bureaucratic nightmare. Ironically, Fletcher's depiction of female power would be used against her sisters, slamming women who strove to assert themselves in the workplace. To be a "Nurse Ratched" was to be a "ball buster" who bullied and emasculated the men beneath her. This was not Fletcher's intention, nor did most reviewers take this message from the film. Many were relieved that the movie did not display the "rampant sexism" of the novel. Wrote Pauline Kael, Fletcher's Ratched is not "the big white mother that she is in the book. That part of the symbolism has been stripped away. She's the company woman incarnate." As Fletcher herself would explain, "I see her as a human being. She's not a medieval witch." Wrote Marsha McCreadie, this was someone "we've all known," a "'well-meaning' but destructive [type]." In a recapitulation of Foucault's argument that

power controls by insinuating itself throughout mundane bureaucratic structures, this Ratched dominates by politely yet ruthlessly
exercising institutional authority. Her gender might be incidental to
the Combine, but to an America wrestling with the Women's Movement, it mattered a great deal.[32]

The film also reflects post–Civil Rights changes. The African
American attendants are dignified. Even when Scatman Crothers's
character lets McMurphy have his night party, we see a kindly gentleman who cares for his charges. The African American attendant
who physically battles McMurphy evokes not servitude but rather the
forthrightness of a man who knows and accepts his occupation for
which he earns a deserved wage. Ruth McCormick noted that, unlike
the book, the "orderlies are no longer seen as malevolent; they're just
doing their job, and without much enthusiasm. The fact that they are
black is a fact of reality; the work they do is one of the most oppressive, thankless and poorly paid of jobs, just the kind of job often held
by minority people."[33]

Perhaps the most oft-heard accusation of the film is the role it
played in advancing anti-psychiatry laws. Not since *The Snake Pit*
had an asylum movie created such a negative stir. One psychiatrist
confirmed that it had "a major impact on the lack of availability of
ECT, despite the development of much safer delivery systems and
its potential for lifesaving quick benefits." A spokeswoman for the
Royal College of Psychiatrists would comment that it (and similar
films) "did for ECT what *Jaws* did for sharks—the depiction of treatment in that film is completely over the top, with the patient being
held down, writhing in pain, as he is electrocuted." There is truth to
this, but it also, without a doubt, overstates the case. ECT was already gaining criticism well before the film's unfavorable publicity
had plagued the treatment. Negative portrayal of ECT on film was
at least as old as *The Snake Pit*, and according to Edward Shorter
and David Healy, it was Kesey's novel that was "the primary source
of information on ECT for most of the liberal intelligentsia." Ernest
Hemingway's and Sylvia Plath's suicides were imaginatively wedded
to their ECT experiences before Forman's film, and writings by Szasz,
Phyllis Chesler, and Doris Lessing, not to mention articles in major
newspapers and magazines, had been bashing away at the treatment
for years. *De rigueur* is the description of ECT in Millen Brand's hit

1968 novel *Savage Sleep*, where it is shown as something that physically damages the brain.[34]

But Forman's film undoubtedly had a major effect. In her 2008 memoir *Wishful Drinking*, actress Carrie Fisher talks about her decision to receive electroconvulsive therapy. She had suffered for many years with mental illness before finally deciding that it was either "ECT or DOA." Though a number of psychiatrists had already recommended it to her, "I couldn't bring myself to consider it as it seemed too barbaric. My only exposure to it was Jack Nicholson in *One Flew Over the Cuckoo's Nest*, which wasn't exactly an enticing example. From the seizures to the biting down on a stick to the convulsions, it looked traumatic, dangerous, and humiliating. I mean what do we know for certain about it? Aren't there a bunch of risks? What if something goes wrong and my brain blows up?" Ultimately Fisher decided to "ride the lightning."[35]

Interestingly, psychiatrists did not uniformly condemn Forman's movie. The 1976 American Psychiatric Association's annual meeting praised it for its "timely relevance" and expressed "hope that it will break down some of the barriers that have made mental illness a hidden quality [*sic*] in American culture." The staid medical journal *The Lancet* even asked psychiatrists to give it a chance. *Cuckoo's Nest* may have all the old asylum trappings, such as the "watchtowers, high fencing, and straight-jackets," but it offers an important lesson for psychiatrists. It can teach humility to practitioners falsely certain that their "authority is self-evidently and unquestionably incorruptible."[36]

Cuckoo's Nest deeply influenced the screen asylum. After 1975, we could expect Fletcher-style Big Nurses, Nicholson-style rebels, clean-but-frightening institutions, authentic-looking dayrooms filled with loveable casts of misfits, and graphically depicted psychiatric horrors, especially ECT. For instance, in a 1977 episode of the hit TV show *Starsky and Hutch*, the two detectives go undercover to get to the bottom of the frighteningly high death rate at Cabrillo Mental Institution. Starsky gets committed as "Skyler," whose illness seems to be his outlandish goofiness. He shakes things up in the rec room by getting the patients to join in a cockroach race. The Big Nurse is a dour, heavy-set woman who administers shots to shut down Starsky's antics. In a twist, she ends up saving him when he's about to be eliminated by the evil superintendent, who is killing off the patients in a mad effort to create a cure for insanity. This hospital, in sum, offers no treatments, incarcerates the eccentric, is lorded over by an evil superintendent and a brutal nurse, and it functions as a disciplinary space. The show even hired an actor from *Cuckoo's Nest* to play a patient.[37]

THE SAD BALLAD OF FRANCES FARMER

Perhaps nobody embodied the damage of the asylum as much as Frances Farmer. A silver screen star who had once starred with Bing Crosby, Cary Grant, and Ray Milland, her posthumous 1972 autobiography *Will There Really Be a Morning?* marked a landmark in asylum horror. In her afterlife, we can trace the new, hostile anti-institutional climate.[38]

According to her autobiography, Farmer received insulin treatments in a private sanitarium in LA following a series of run-ins with the law, after which she was released to her mother's care in Washington State. A big fight caused her mother to send her to the state hospital at Steilacoom. What she describes next takes us beyond all previous descriptions of asylum horror. A sadistic nurse forces her to eat her own feces. She is physically assaulted by orderlies and staff. She witnesses the rape of a young woman by a brutal, older female patient, an event described over multiple pages of lurid detail. In hydrotherapy, she's trussed into canvas bindings and left to totter before falling on her face, her teeth badly cutting her lower lip. She's picked up and tossed into an empty tub, injuring her back. She screams and struggles, blood gushing from her mouth, when the "icy crash" of water sends her into shock. She's left this way for ten hours. After three weeks of this, "All personality was washed away and all that was left was a water-clogged robot."[39]

After Farmer's release, more fighting with her parents result in their "railroading" her back inside. As a "recidivist," Francis gets sentenced to the lowest rung of asylum hell: the back ward. Her head is shaved, her nails cut down to the quick, and she's shoved with a pole into a "screaming, milling mob of naked women."[40]

This experience is extreme. Food is "thrown into the pen" where it is "pounced upon by the strongest." "Epidemics of vomit" are "lapped up by the human scavengers." Rats are eaten "as a matter of course," and when a cat sneaks in, it is torn apart, clawing and howling "as its eyes were pulled loose and eaten." At night, Farmer is molested by fellow patients and "strange men" are let in at night to rape "every" patient. She is beaten with soap wrapped in towels until she passes out. The inmates become "living skeletons, threadbare leftovers" who suffer a "relentless and deathless death. Living parts of their spirits were buried as each moment sluggishly passed. Segments of their souls, the most intricate part, subsided, never to be reborn." Nothing like this had ever been articulated in print. There is almost no way to imagine a worse asylum experience.[41]

The press was astounded. The *New York Times* called it "a ghastly tale, not easy to forget." One reviewer wrote, it "reaches the limits of readable; only a few years ago it would have been unprintable." According to *Women's Wear Daily*, it was "worse than any horror movie that Hollywood ever turned out." Yet, it "could not have been invented." This critic concluded that the extremeness of the horrors, which "for all we know" are still going on, prove its veracity. Other critics agreed that Farmer brought something new and important to light. Clarence Petersen of the *Chicago Tribune* thought the chapter in which she is sent to the back ward "ought to be reprinted by every organization interested in reform of these Bedlams." Perhaps most significantly, some were already connecting it to the longer stream of women's asylum narratives. Kevin Kelly of *The Boston Globe* wrote that Farmer's experiences "recall 'The Snakepit,' 'The Bell Jar' and 'Faces in the Water.' " Kelly concludes, "It's clear, I think, that she was never insane, should never have been committed."[42]

Farmer's autobiography came out the same year Phyllis Chesler published *Women and Madness*. This landmark study argued that women had been pathologized by a chauvinistic mental health industry. Using the insights of Goffman, Szasz, and others, Chesler made the case that it is all about control: men have it and they don't want women to share it. Thanks to psychiatry, sane women are regularly hospitalized and then made mad by their treatment. Chesler's most important contribution is her powerful indictment of Western culture as being at the root of the evil. Women have historically been "impaled on the cross of self-sacrifice." When they show independence, they are duly "punished in patriarchal mental asylums." Chesler updated and upgraded Packard's critique, even calling out Packard for her devotion "to a (male) Godhead." The book sold more than three million copies. Later, she'd write the foreword to *Women of the Asylum: Voices from Behind the Walls, 1840–1945*, a work that includes an excerpt from *Will There Really Be a Morning?*[43]

This new feminist argument soon got a sci-fi twist. In Marge Piercy's 1976 novel *Woman on the Edge of Time* (she thanks both Chesler and the Mental Patients Liberation Front in her dedication), Consuela "Connie" Ramos is psychiatrically incarcerated by a patriarchal, racist system. Connie's only chance lies with her ability to communicate with enlightened twenty-second-century beings. In the future, gender and race are no longer "stigmata." People refer to each other as "per" (for "person"). Everyone recycles and eats local, fresh foods, no one is on drugs, and children are "comothered" by three parents (and men can breastfeed too). In stark contrast to the asylum where Consuela is consigned, future mental institutions are Laingian fantasies, "open to the air and pleasant," places "where people retreat when they want to go down into themselves—to collapse, carry on, see visions, hear voices of prophecy, bang on the walls, relive infancy—getting in touch with the buried self and the inner mind."[44]

Connie's journey begins when she smashes a bottle into the face of her niece's brutal pimp. For this act, she is subjected to ECT, drugs, restraint, attendant abuse, and physician neglect. She discovers the underlying logic of ECT: "A little brain damage to jolt you into behaving right," to get you "scared" enough to want to go home and do "the dishes and [clean] the house." When patients do not conform, they are sent back "for more barbecue of the brain" until they are reduced to "shock zombies." Ultimately, Connie decides to rebel against the institution by poisoning four doctors. Afterward, she washes her hands, telling the mirror, "I killed them. Because it is war."[45]

Piercy's institution is a machine of gendered control, built to punish those not cowed by sexist, racist, social structures. For example, Piercy tells of one inmate incarcerated for "being a practicing witch, for telling women how to heal themselves and encouraging them to leave their husbands." Another, Skip, is homosexual, and he recounts how doctors tried to "cure" him by attaching electrodes to his genitals and showing him lewd images of men, shocking him when he got aroused. This reference to aversion therapy marks an early, literary critique of the then-current psychiatric practice of treating homosexuality as an "illness." (Perhaps the most famous episode of this in pop culture is when Alex is forced to watch scenes of sex and violence in Kubrick's 1971 film *A Clockwork Orange*.) Aversion therapy often involved electric shocks deployed while the patient gazed upon "bad" sexual imagery, with pleasant music played for hetero, that is, "good," imagery. Skip eventually kills himself.[46]

As Piercy's book built a following, Farmer's autobiography gained wider notice. In 1973, Dell put out the first paperback edition, with another to follow. More fame came with the 1975 American publication of *Hollywood Babylon*, Kenneth Anger's steamy, photo-filled exposé of Tinsel Town. Anger's book has an entire chapter devoted to "Daughter of Fury: Frances, Saint." Clearly, the recent autobiography is used as a source; his 1965 version only has a fleeting reference to her. Making the horror message of *Will There Really Be a Morning?* into dark, daft legend, Anger portrays Farmer as the "patron saint" of the "Hollywood Magdalenes who have drunk at the well of madness." Hers is the ultimate Hollywood tragedy, "the most gruesome ordeal any screen personality was ever forced to endure." In a book that included a photo of Jane Mansfield's dead dog and Marilyn Monroe's lifeless corpse, a shot of Farmer standing in baggy jeans with a rope belt is par for the course. Then came *Shadowland*.[47]

William Arnold's 1978 biography mainstreamed Frances Farmer fully into the deinstitutionalization narrative. *Shadowland* begins with a remarkable paragraph tying Steilacoom to national shames of Indian subjugation and white imperialism:

> In the State of Washington, at a remote spot near the southern end of Puget Sound, there is a large complex of buildings known as Western State Hospital at Steilacoom. It is situated in what is the oldest white settlement in the state and, during the Indian skirmishes of the 1850s, had actually been a frontier army post. Before the turn of the century the post was converted into a huge public insane asylum, but people still called it "Fort Steilacoom" and, shrouded as it usually is in the fog and mist that continually roll in from the Sound, its massive presence continues to evoke that name—fortresslike and forbidding.

One might wonder what Arnold could possibly add to the autobiography. His answer is that Farmer never wrote one. *Will There Really Be a*

Morning?, he tells us, was actually composed by the woman to whom the book is dedicated.[48]

Like *The Exorcist*, *Shadowland* is a detective story. Arnold sifts through the clues to figure out why, at the height of her fame, a movie star "had suddenly gone violently insane, was mysteriously committed to a public mental institution, and seemed to disappear forever." The answer takes him deep into a mire of secrets and lies. Arnold hears "stories of the FBI and the CIA, of psychiatric abuse and medical atrocities and high governmental cover-up." Dalton Trumbo tells him that "they wanted to bust that kid wide open" for her leftist activism, "and they finally had the opportunity." Arnold travels to all of the locations Frances visited and speaks to everyone still living who she would have known.[49]

The first bombshell of the book is Farmer's lobotomy. On page two, we learn that, at Steilacoom, the most "famous psycho-surgeon" in the world came here armed with a secret weapon—an icepick. This is Dr. Walter Freeman, who claims here that he can jab his pick into the brain of "the most defiant maniac" and transform them into "a reasonable citizen." He's testing out his new device, and, as fate would have it, "one of the most famous patients in the history of America's public mental hospitals" is in residence. Thus far, ECT, insulin shock, hydrotherapy, and "experimental drugs" have all failed to "break" Farmer. But the icepick will do the trick. Afterward, she "would no longer be a threat to anyone."[50]

In Arnold's telling, Farmer is the victim of a nefarious plot. The judge who puts her away is a powerful, right-wing figure on the Seattle scene. His hand-selected neurologist had already "personally committed thousands of people to Washington State insane asylums, many of whom were obvious psychotics; but others more plainly criminals, anarchists, Wobblies, and other social undesirables." Moreover, this doctor had previously attended the 1930 International Congress on Mental Hygiene. "It sounds incredible today," writes Arnold, but, at this meeting, psychiatrists had determined that "they should run the world," intending to make their profession "an indisputable part of the everyday functioning of government—Communist, fascist, democratic, it didn't particularly matter what kind of government . . . and to a very large extent over the next forty years, they did."[51]

Arnold knows how this sounds. He disarmingly wonders whether he might just be imbibing the "all prevailing theme of the '70s," Water-gate-fueled paranoia. His hedge is less-than-convincing: "Whether or not there was actually an overt conspiracy between Seattle politicians and specific psychiatrists to incarcerate Frances Farmer in 1944, I do not know. Given the political climate and the people involved, it seems very possible." Later, he writes, "It seemed to me that the real conspiracy against Frances Farmer was the conspiracy of psychiatry against any individual who happens to be different." The Psychiatric Power has engineered Farmer's downfall.[52]

Arnold is not satisfied with the horrors described in the autobiography. He ups the ante. There was not even a floor in the back ward, just "dirt." Not only did they give Farmer drugs, but "practically every experimental drug that came along in that period was tested on her." Not only was she raped, but she was raped by "drunken gangs of soldiers" "hundreds of times." Not only was she disobedient, but "was very likely the most rebellious patient in the history of Steilacoom—she was so resistive that she became a kind of Ken Kesey heroine to many of the patients." Just like with McMurphy, when they learned they couldn't "break her," they go the lobotomy route.[53]

Arnold is clever about this part. He tantalizes the reader at the start with the icepick vignette, then lets the thread go. Much later, he wracks his brain about how Farmer could have been possibly brought to heel. It is not until he speaks with a journalist named Alan Dobson that he gets a clue. The powers-that-be "wanted to demonstrate how effective psychiatry could modify the behavior of even the most notorious troublemaker—essentially part of the now famous CIA psychiatric program of the same period." Arnold at first thinks the reporter is off his rocker. Then he hears him say "something or somebody called 'Freeman.'" Suddenly, everything clicks.[54]

Arnold portrays Walter Freeman as a physician of the Dr. Mengele persuasion. The founder of the lobotomy, "Dr. Egar [*sic*] Moniz," attended the infamous 1930 International Congress on Mental Hygiene and then created a procedure to crush "schizophrenics, alcoholics, homosexuals, and even political radicals"—in other words, deviants. Freeman's dream followed Moniz, his ambition to "control" every "deviation that has ever plagued society." Arnold tells us that Freeman examined Farmer "at least three times." On one visit to Steilacoom in 1948, he gave her ECT and then had all the nurses and orderlies vacate the room. Though "no one will ever know exactly what happened next," the "overwhelming conclusion drawn by the people of Steilacoom at the time was that the doctor lifted her right eyelid and stuck a needle into her brain." Arnold's evidence? After this, Farmer "was not the same person she had been, and she would never be the same person again." Note that Arnold has removed the witnesses and then goes with an "overwhelming conclusion" rather than a simple declaration of fact. He later similarly writes that she had "*almost certainly* been surgically tampered with."[55]

After *Shadowland* came out, Frances's sister Edith vehemently denied the lobotomy. In the years to come, doctors and nurses at Steilacoom would make the same proclamation. Freeman himself never mentioned this famous patient in his memoirs, and his biographer notes that there is no evidence he even met the actress. Keeping in line with Arnold's hedged assertions, even favorable book reviewers ceded that the lobotomy evidence was not definitive.[56]

Movie talk was almost immediately in the works. At a press conference sponsored by the Scientology-funded Citizens Commission for Human Rights (Scientology had long been waging a war against psychiatry; the CCHR was a co-production of L. Ron Hubbard and Thomas Szasz), Arnold announced he had sold the movie rights to Noel Marshall. Marshall had previously been an executive producer on *The Exorcist*. Arnold was happy that a film was happening, but he was also wistful: "I find myself feeling guilty, like I'm cashing in on a tragedy."[57]

As it happened, Arnold need not have been worried. A different production company would make the biopic and cut him out of all royalties. Universal Pictures' *Frances* (1982) clearly built on Arnold's book (and the autobiography), but the producers did not pay for any rights. They claimed that solely the known public record of Frances Farmer inspired them. It is hard to sue for non-fiction, so Arnold tried a novel strategy. He argued that his was not a pure work of history. In a remarkable statement, Arnold's lawyer stated, "*Shadowland* is not purely factual. It has certain things in common with a work of fiction, which *is* protectable." Arnold and producer Noel Marshall sued for five million dollars. They lost.[58]

According to journalist Jeffrey Kauffman, Arnold's work is riddled with errors, including such mundane facts as the number of films Farmer made and her correct birth date. As for the lobotomy, Kauffman asserts, "Archival data clearly show all of Freeman's surgical subjects, and Frances was not among them. Indeed, Frances was not operated on by any doctor for any reason whatsoever during her stay at Western State."[59]

In the movie, Jessica Lange plays the bedeviled actress. She had wanted the role ever since she read the autobiography in 1974 but hadn't been able to convince anyone to produce the film. She felt she could relate. As she told *Time* magazine, "The movie is a statement about women's independence, and how frightening it can be. Politically, Frances was a radical. But she didn't have a generation backing her up. The Hearsts hated her, and Hollywood raped her. L.A. is a tricky place—there are a lot of killers here." With the Women's Movement ten years in, Farmer had finally found her moment. Explained the *New York Times*, "The differences between 1938, when Frances Farmer defied Hollywood, and 1982 are instructive. Jessica Lange's life style [she currently lived with and had a child with a man with whom she was not married] would not have been tolerated for a minute forty years ago."[60]

Frances clearly owes much to *Shadowland* and to the antipsychiatry movement. Farmer is a social rebel and is not insane. The asylum unhinges her, making her a drug guinea pig, a gang-rape casualty, and a lobotomy victim. The movie also adds a new character to the mythos, Harry York, a savior/love interest. According to Arnold, York is modeled after him, a final insult to his unremunerated contribution. The movie pulls back from Arnold's psychiatric conspiracy theory while fully embracing his argument about how the mental health system controls women who do not embrace the submissive feminine role.[61]

The movie's lobotomy scene differs from Arnold's description. It is less the smashing of the will than the transformation of a broken human into a robot. It begins with a demonstration by the Freeman character, who illustrates to a room full of witnesses and photographers how his "icepick technique" works. When he blasts Frances with ECT, she does not protest. Then he wiggles his probe-like device over her face. Writes one scholar, "As if the lobotomy were not evil enough, it is presented as a virtual rape, complete with diagrams of remarkably long instruments." The scene ends with a close-up of the doctor, leukotome pointing down and off-screen in one hand and what appears to be a small judge's gavel in the other, boasting, "Lobotomy gets 'em home." Then tap, blackout. Afterwards, Lange becomes an automaton version of Frances, who repeats herself and dully tells York, "Things are going to be slow from now on, know what I mean?" She has essentially become a pod person from *Invasion of the Body Snatchers*.[62]

Like *Spellbound*, *Frances* is obliged to give us a disclaimer. The producers let us know at the end of the credits that "there have been major advances in the care and treatment of the mentally ill" since the 1940s, and that "the reprehensible conditions experienced by Frances Farmer are not typical of mental health treatment today." This disclaimer is preceded with what can only be called a disclaimer-disclaimer: "In exchange for the use of certain facilities and per agreement with the California Department of Mental Health the producers have agreed to the following." Regardless, this information probably does not matter to an audience that just sat through a rape scene in which a soldier brags, "Best deal I ever made. Twenty bucks to fuck a fucking star?"

The real Frances Farmer, whoever she might have been and might have experienced, was gone and buried, but in the world of popular culture, she lived on. She appeared in novels, a TV movie, plays, music (i.e., the song "Lobotomy Gets 'em Home" by The Men They Couldn't Handle), and art. Probably the most famous ode is "Frances Farmer Will Have Her Revenge on Seattle" by alt-rock legends Nirvana. Lead singer Kurt Cobain was deeply versed in Farmer mythos. As he explained, "My way of letting the world know that bureaucracy is everywhere and it can happen to anybody and it's a really evil thing . . . Judges and heads of state were part of this conspiracy to put her in a mental institution, give her a lobotomy, and she was gang raped every night she was there and she had to eat her own shit . . . They just fucked with her all the time."

When Kurt married Courtney Love in 1993, his bride wore a silk dress formerly owned by Farmer. Incidentally, Cobain's own grandfather had been committed to, and had died in, Steilacoom.[63]

CHAPTER 9

BREAKOUT

> When a shattered and deserted half-deranged Thing effects Its
> escape, the people of the county for miles around turn out like
> bloodhounds to recapture the fugitive. "It's such a real sport, you
> know; better than a fox-hunt, any day," I once heard a country
> swain remark in the presence of his sweetheart.
> —Julius Chambers, *A Mad World and Its Inhabitants* (1877)

On November 4, 1980, America elected Ronald Reagan president
in a landslide. A politician more hostile to the mental institution
could scarcely have been found. As governor of California (1967–1975),
he had waged a war against state hospitals with the aim of shutting
them all down. In his first gubernatorial term, state hospital cen-
suses dropped from 26,567 to 7,011. In practice, this meant "liberating" people suffering mental illness to live on the streets, in prisons,
in shelters, in run-down hovels, or at home with overburdened families. The disheartening, new reality of disturbed persons roaming
alleys or occasionally getting involved in spectacular crimes (such
as the schizophrenic John Hinckley firing shots at Reagan in order
to impress actress Jodie Foster) caused some to worry that deinstitutionalization was a mistake. As early as 1981, the *New York Times* editorialized, "The vogue word 'deinstitutionalization' once signified the
most humane reform in caring for the mentally ill ... [It] has become
a cruel embarrassment, a reform gone terribly wrong, threatening not
only the former mental inmates but also the quality of life for all New
Yorkers." Fear percolated.[1]

Enter the new Hero from Hell: the escaped psycho maniac.

THE NIGHT *HE* BROKE OUT

Halloween (1978) has an unforgettable opening scene. It is Halloween night, 1963, in the town of Haddonfield, Illinois. A four-minute-long subjective tracking shot takes us on a murder rampage through the eyes of the killer. First, he stalks a house from the bushes, watching as two teens make out and then go upstairs for sex. He comes in through the kitchen, and we see a small costumed arm grabbing a big knife. He waits for the boyfriend to leave before going upstairs to the girl's room. The arm reaches out to put on a clown mask, and then, through the restricted vision of the eye slits, we watch as he stabs the girl to death before exiting. Out front, a car pulls up. The tracking shot ends and we finally see the killer for ourselves—a young boy in a clown costume. Flash forward to October 30, 1978. On a dark and stormy night on a country road, psychiatrist Dr. Loomis rides in a car with a nurse. Loomis asks, "You ever done anything like this before?" She replies, nervously smoking, "Only minimum security." The headlights illuminate a sign on a chain link fence up ahead: The Illinois State Hospital.[2]

The two are on their way to retrieve the now-grown boy, Michael Myers, whom Loomis refers to as "it." The nurse scolds him, "Don't you think we could refer to *it*, as *him*?" Yet her voice is void of compassion. She is bothered by patients' "gibberish" and how "they start raving on and on." Loomis intends to put this patient on Thorazine prior to seeing the judge. The nurse says that this will make him incoherent. For Loomis, that is the idea. This patient must never get out. The nurse wonders why they are even going through the charade. "Because," replies Loomis, "that is the law." Frustrating bureaucratic legalities and misplaced notions of patients' rights have forced him to parade a monster before a judge in order to keep him confined. As they pull up to the hospital, we see in the headlights a group of white-gowned patients aimlessly milling about on the lawn.

The asylum breakout scene in *Halloween* is telling of the age of deinstitutionalization. Carpenter does not show Michael Myers forcing himself out of the institution, nor does he show Myers being brutalized or mistreated. In fact, in this scene, we don't see the asylum at all, and we will never get a glimpse of its interior. What we see is a field full of zombies. As the headlights illuminate the mad on the lawn, one is reminded of the "Thorazine shuffling" cannibals in George Romero's 1968 *Night of the Living Dead*. That movie introduced a new cinema monster—the pale, flesh eating, vacant-eyed undead who inexorably rend the living. Though he was not meaning to do it, Romero created the perfect model for the horror-film deinstitutionalized, the mindless escapees incapable of participating in society, deadly by virtue of their past confinement. In the case of *Halloween*, Myers is at once a released patient—he too wanders in a gown—and something more. Unlike the zombies on the lawn, he is fast, leaping on the nurse's car and smashing his way in. He steals the car and spares the nurse. Dr. Loomis immediately recognizes the significance, lamenting, "The evil is gone."[3]

Michael Myers is, as Loomis says, The Boogeyman. He is pure evil, at once familiar and unknowable. We repeatedly hear that asylum medicine hasn't changed him. After the breakout, there's an acrimonious conversation between Loomis and the superintendent in front of a hospital that looks like a public office building. The superintendent, who resembles an officious manager, tells Loomis, "I'm not responsible, Sam." He even blames the psychiatrist for not making Myers's meds "strong enough." Loomis yells back, "I told everybody! Nobody listened." We gather that the primary function of institutional medicine is to dope monsters into submission in order to contain them. As Loomis says directly, Myers isn't even "a man." This doctor is not here to heal but is rather more akin to his literary forebear, Dr. Abraham Van Helsing, who also recognized the limits of Western science. Destroying evil is their game.[4]

Film distributor Irwin Yablans dreamed up the basic plot of *Halloween*. Having worked with John Carpenter to produce the surprise hit *Assault on Precinct 13*, Yablans wanted to make a suspenseful shocker like *The Exorcist*. His idea was of a killer stalking babysitters on Halloween night. After he communicated this to Carpenter, the director reportedly said, "Don't tell me any more. I know exactly what to do." What he did was create a stylish, ninety-minute tour of terror. Myers lurks, stabs, and even takes a moment at one point to observe his ghastly handiwork. The film culminates with the remaining babysitter Laurie Strode (Jamie Lee Curtis) battling Myers, stabbing him with a variety of objects in an effort to slow him down. Loomis ends it by unloading six rounds into Myers's chest, sending him flying out the bedroom window. When we look out the window, however, the body is gone.[5]

There are lots of interesting stories attached to *Halloween*. Michael Myers was the name of the man who worked with Yablans on *Assault on Precinct 13* in England. The mask he wears, a cheap Captain Kirk simulacrum spray painted bluish-white, was selected almost randomly from a shop on Hollywood Boulevard by art director Tommy Lee Wallace. Haddonfield is the name of co-writer Debra Hill's hometown. Perhaps of greatest significance, Carpenter had once taken a field trip to a "mental institution" as a student at Western Kentucky University. It stuck with him. "The kid I saw the day I went," he recalled, "had the Devil's eyes, and he stared at me with a look of evil and it terrified me." Carpenter would "utilize the experience" in creating Myers.[6]

While Myers's breakout is not an overt allegory of deinstitutionalization, it speaks to the social forces that wiped out the big state hospitals. The year *Halloween* hit theaters, the press brimmed with negative stories about the recently released. A March 1978 article in the *New York Times* reported on "smoldering community resentment," and how deinstitutionalization had turned formerly safe neighborhoods into "bedlams." Another piece told how some New Yorkers lived in a state of terror, confusing "their fear of crime with their fear of insanity." The tagline of *Halloween*, "The Night *He* Came Home," brings to mind the purported threat of the ex-patients. Myers escapes a hospital that can't fix him and is pursued by a doctor convinced that there is no cure except a bullet. Regardless of the agenda of the film, which Carpenter acknowledges as a purely "stylistic exercise," we are presented with an unfixable, homicidal monster unleashed from an ineffective institution who goes on to terrorize his community.[7]

Perhaps an even more obvious horror response to deinstitutionalization is 1979's *When a Stranger Calls*. Directed by Fred Walton, this movie also features a babysitter under siege by a maniac. Inspired by urban legends (and by "caller in the house" films like the 1972 short *Foster's Release* and Walton's own 1977 short *The Sitter*), it concerns a murderer who phones a babysitter from upstairs in the same house. In the tense, twenty-one-minute opening sequence, the young sitter (Carol Kane) gets repeated crank calls from a man asking, "Have you checked the children?" As the night wears on, he makes increasingly vile comments. Eventually, the cops trace the call and find it's coming from inside. The killer, who has butchered the children, is upstairs covered in their blood. We aren't shown this, but a policeman explains it to detective John Clifford. We then fast-forward seven years. Detective Clifford is now a private investigator, and he's being told by the father that the killer, Curt Duncan, has just escaped "a state mental institution where the security is less than perfect." Clifford is hired to track down the monster. His first stop is the hospital, a prison-like place where a prim and dismissive female psychiatrist explains that Duncan is not going to "run right out and kill more children." She explains he has been under "continuous therapy, some of it rather forceful," including "drugs, tranquilizers, depressants, lithium." Duncan had also received ECT thirty-eight times, a point that clearly unnerves the detective. In later flashbacks, we see Duncan strapped into a straitjacket, huddled in the corner of a padded call. When Clifford tells her that Duncan would still be here if "you'd done your job right," she admonishes, "This is a hospital, Mr. Clifford, not a penitentiary." She then concedes that doctors know little about "the human mind." The escape is merely a sad event in the life of an essentially worthless institution that can neither hold nor understand its charges.[8]

The movie then takes an unusual tack for a horror film, following Duncan as he tries to survive outside. He pathetically hits on a woman in a bar, gets beaten by a customer, and, after following the woman home and being rejected, spends the night in a flophouse. He is on his way to becoming another homeless ex-patient living in a trash-strewn alley. He's nicknamed "Crazy Curt." Scenes of Duncan talking to himself, muttering nude in front of a public restroom mirror, sweating, and nervously looking about make for a pathetic sight.

The remainder of the film mainly involves detective Clifford tracking Duncan down, while Duncan becomes increasingly disturbed. Eventually, we arrive back with the original babysitter, now married with kids of her own. She's living in a cozy suburb and preparing to go out to dinner with her husband. She puts the kids to bed, and then the babysitter arrives. As might be expected, Duncan is on his way. He found her by reading an article about her in a gutter newspaper. At dinner, a waiter comes by and tells the woman she has a phone call. She hears the familiar old voice: "Have you checked the children?" The parents dash home and find everyone safe. But Duncan is already there. He jumps out of bed right next to her, playing the role of husband (whom he has beaten and stuffed in the closet). The detective shows up in the nick of time and shoots Duncan repeatedly in the chest, killing him.

The context of *When a Stranger Calls* is deinstitutionalization. A maniac without rational motive murders children, gets committed to an ineffective institution, and then breaks out to kill again. On the streets, he becomes an anonymous, homeless person. Though we begin to sympathize with him, Duncan cannot escape his narrative function. He returns to the suburbs to kill. Tracked by a detective who understands that death is the only "cure," Duncan is executed before he can murder more children. Like Dr. Loomis, Clifford is a wise Van Helsing character filled with experientially earned pathos, the only one who understands that the monster must die. Duncan is, incidentally, killed in virtually the same manner as Michael Myers—a revolver to the chest at close range. This kind of gun is a weapon of home defense, a nod to the save-yourself individualist backlash of the increasingly conservative times. While Duncan's body does not vanish, the closing shot features the superimposition of his eyes over the house, implying that his spirit is still alive. As Carpenter would say about *Halloween*, "Your house is supposed to be a sanctuary. Nowadays, maybe because of conditions beyond our control, there is no sanctuary."[9]

ASYLUM SPAWN

The outrageous financial success of *Halloween* inspired a raft of films featuring robotic psychopaths butchering nubile teenagers. Most conspicuous was the *Friday the 13th* cycle, with its hockey-masked killer who cannot be destroyed. Jason is not an asylum escapee (and in the first film, his mom turns out to be the killer), but . . . the madhouse is coming. In *Friday the 13th Part III*, the girl who re-kills Jason is taken away in a cop car, laughing wildly. It is implied that she's going to an institution. In *Part IV* (*Friday the 13th: The Final Chapter*), the boy who re-kills Jason gives the camera a crazed stare in the film's final moments. We learn in *Part V* (*Friday the 13th: A New Beginning*) that he has spent the next seven or so years at the Unger Institute of Mental Health. Early on in this film, a crude attendant takes him to the Pinehurst Youth Development Center in a white van. Pinehurst is a halfway home for disturbed youths, where he can prepare for his life outside the hospital. The doctor that runs the place is a kind of younger, hipper Dr. Alan from *David and Lisa*. Looking over the boy's chart, Dr. Matt ruminates, "Boy they've given him every treatment, every therapy they can think of. It's a wonder his mind isn't fried with all the drugs they've given him." A shot of the "Treatment Record" reveals he's been given, among other things, Thorazine, Ritalin, Darvon, Valium, and even Percodan ("To ease anxiety"). This all casually recapitulates the popular view of asylums as worthless, even hazardous places for patients. Pinehurst, however, seems to be different. Dr. Matt explains, "You'll find we're very different from the State Institution. We don't have any guards here. Nobody's going to tell you what you can do or what you can't do. Basically you're your own boss." Our sympathy for this Laingian community treatment center is reinforced by the distasteful remarks by a crude, poor, white neighbor who calls it a "loony bin" and a "fuckin' crazy farm" and threatens to shut it down. Consistent with the moral economy of the slasher film, she is murdered along with the fornicating teens and inept authority figures. Sadly, Pinehurst does not protect its residents from Jason (in a twist, "Jason" in this movie turns out to be a demented paramedic).[10]

In *Jason Lives: Friday the 13th Part VI*, Tommy (the boy) has escaped from yet another mental hospital, having been apparently reinstitutionalized since *Part V*. Tommy then ironically resurrects Jason after digging him up with the express purpose of stabbing him with an iron spike. The spike becomes a Frankenstein-style lightning conduit during a storm and brings Jason to life. When the mayhem starts, the town sheriff is convinced that the asylum escapee Tommy, "a very sick boy," is behind the killings. But of course it's Jason, and Tommy ultimately manages to chain him to a boulder dropped to the bottom of Crystal Lake. In *Friday the 13th Part VII: The New Blood*, we meet Tina, a girl with telekinetic powers, who vacations on Crystal Lake with her parents. After we see her send her father to the bottom of the lake (he'd been abusing mom), we fast-forward to her teenage years. Like Tommy, she's been institutionalized in the interim. She returns to Crystal Lake with mom and Dr. Cruz, an asylum psychiatrist who explains how the hospital has been unable to help her. At the lake, he hopes to cure her. Dr. Cruz is a creepy Freudian who is trying to get Tina to "overcome" her "guilt" about killing her dad. Wishing her

father back, Tina unwittingly releases Jason from his watery tomb.
While Jason executes all the teens in the next bungalow over, we learn
that Dr. Cruz had been conducting a malicious experiment on Tina
at the institution, keeping her "trauma and stress levels high" so as
to "induce huge psychokinetic reactions." When her mom discovers
this, Dr. Cruz threatens to recommit Tina. The power of the psychiatrist to strip liberties is paralleled with Jason's villainous strength, as
both men are after Tina. Dr. Cruz's depravity gets reinforced when he
thrusts Tina's mom in front of Jason's blade in order to save himself.
He still gets killed by Jason, who is in turn re-killed by Tina.

For the *Friday the 13th* series, the asylum serves various functions:
a repository for Jason's victims who've survived but have lost their
minds; a storage house where his victims gestate and sometimes
become evil themselves; and a place where evil doctors try to create
superhuman monsters. What all of these references have in common
is the idea that asylums are useless at best, harmful at worst. They
steep the killer's crimes in another layer of degradation.[11]

Other horror films made the connection between robotic "psycho"
and failed asylum in a more straightforward manner. In 1982, New
Line Cinema released *Alone in the Dark*, starring *Halloween*'s Donald
Pleasance in another turn as a madhouse doctor. This film might be
described as the "Tarr and Fether" for the most cynical of the anti-
psychiatry set. In the movie, an idealistic, young psychiatrist named
Dr. Potter gets a position at The Haven, a mansion-style institution
run by Dr. Bain (Pleasance). Dr. Bain believes that psychotic patients
are just sensitive and misunderstood "voyagers." He tells Potter, "We
don't lock people up here and fry their brains with electricity." Puffing
a ridiculous feathered peace pipe, Bain expounds, "What the medical
gang calls schizophrenics are people who've taken a journey into the
inmost reaches of the psyche." The Haven will not be "a jail house."
There are no bars but rather an electricity-based security system.
Then a blackout occurs.[12]

What happens next is not unexpected. A group of four psychotics,
including a war vet (Jack Palance), a deranged preacher (Martin
Landau), a huge pedophile, and a man called "the Bleeder," erupt into
the community and commence a murderous spree, specifically targeting the house of Dr. Potter.[13]

One critic called *Alone in the Dark* "a spoof." Indeed, it broadcasts

its commentary so loudly that it's hard to take it seriously. Psychiatry is roundly mocked, with Bain as a silly R. D. Laing who, when told
that the escapees have killed three people, responds, "Alright they're
crazy. Isn't everybody?" Dr. Potter is little better, an ineffectual man
who tells his besieged family, "Breathe deeply. Hopefully, we'll never
have to go through this kind of stress again." The asylum is a dismal
failure not only due to psychiatry's incompetency in the treatment
of psychoses, but also thanks to Dr. Bain's misguided decision to use
electricity rather than bars to contain the mad. We gather that real
prison was needed.[14]

The film's cynicism runs yet deeper. When the blackout occurs,
the whole town runs riot, with random fires set and people running
through trash-strewn streets with appliances they'd recently looted.
Authority is a mirage, and only the newfound, rugged individualism
of Dr. Potter saves his family. Holding a maniac at bay, he yells at his
wife holding a butcher knife, "Do it!" She stabs him to death. Potter
goes on to kill another one. In a society that cannot be relied upon to
provide for the safety of its members, the only redoubt is to be found
in man's primal instinct for violent, familial defense. The Haven is no
haven, nor is it even a penitentiary. It is just a failure.

One of the biggest horror franchises, *A Nightmare on Elm Street*
series, also utilizes the asylum. The villain is Freddy Krueger, a child-
murdering misanthrope burned alive by a gang of vengeful parents.
The first film tells the story of Freddy's posthumous return via invad-
ing the dreams of the surviving kids of the parents. There is no asylum
per se in this first installment, but there is plenty of asylum-style
action. It opens with a sequence in a subterranean, industrial setting
in which Freddy tracks a blond teen in a flowing, white nightgown
running through a long, concrete hallway and into a boiler room. She
awakens safe in bed just as Freddy grabs her. As Freddy begins knocking off the de rigueur cute and hormonal youths, the Final Girl (the
trope in which a spunky, virginal girl is the last to survive and who
often slays the psycho) is treated to therapy at the Katja Institute for
the Study of Sleep Disorders. A sleep drug, Hypnocil, is said to be a
possible solution to nocturnal, teen torments. The idea of misguided
(and in this case dangerous, since you don't want to sleep) hospital treatment combines with the underground tunnels and Woman
in White sequences to graft an asylumized quality to this slasher.

Nightmare was a huge success and spawned lots of sequels, as well as the inevitable reboot. Most important here is the third movie of the cycle, 1987's *A Nightmare on Elm Street 3: Dream Warriors.*

Dream Warriors takes place in a mental institution for young people. The Westin Hills Psychiatric Hospital is a forbidding brick structure filled with bleak hallways, "quiet rooms," and grated windows. A patient jokingly calls it "the snake pit." Showing *Cuckoo's Nest* influence, *Dream Warriors* includes a cast of scrappy misfits, ineffective therapies, a domineering female medical authority named Dr. Elizabeth Simms, and a street-smart, African American attendant. The patients at Westin Hills are tortured by Freddy dreams, which their Freudian psychiatrists dismiss as a "group delusion" and "byproducts of guilt" stemming from "overt sexuality." Dr. Simms even accuses the kids of "blaming your dreams for your own weakness" and demands that they take sedation, which of course dooms them to yet more Freddy visits. Fortunately, the sympathetic Dr. Neil Gordon and the now-grown-up Final Girl from the first film, Nancy Thompson, are here to help. Nancy has become a therapist and is interning at Westin. She also takes Hypnocil regularly, which apparently helps her. We eventually discover that the Westin Hills kids were made mentally disturbed by Freddy, since they are "the last of the Elm Street children." Through teamwork, they learn to fight Freddy together in their dreams, and with the help of Nancy, who sacrifices herself, Freddy dies (again).

Dream Warriors also tells us that Freddy is the product of an asylum. Back in the 1940s, Amanda Krueger was a young staffer at Westin. Just before Christmas, she had been accidentally locked into the wing for the criminally insane. The inmates kept her hidden over the holidays, raping her "hundreds of times." The result was Freddy. He is thus genetically evil, the seed of quarantined monsters. This explanation conforms to the eighties sensibility that psychopaths are not made but rather are born evil, thus absolving society of any structural guilt. In Freddy's case, he is a cumulative product, "the bastard son of a hundred maniacs."

Mark Edmundson makes the argument that Freddy evokes the deinstitutionalized homeless. He's "a dingy bum dressed in a broken fedora and football hooligan's cast-off sweater." Freddy has a deranged laugh, and he lives in a boiler room, the sort of place where a destitute person suffering from mental illness might find shelter from the elements. One could also add that Freddy's mode of attack mimics sensational reports of slashings by the homeless, that his face recalls historical, bestial visages of madness, and that his misbegotten parentage evokes genetic arguments of insanity.[15]

Of course, the best homages to *Halloween* would be the long train of *Halloween* sequels. No other horror franchise makes such carnivalesque out of the breakout. In *Halloween II*, set immediately following the events of the first film, Myers continues his rampage as newscasters warn of the "escaped mental patient." Loomis is again blamed for "let[ting] him out." In this film, we also learn that, while in the asylum, Myers was "the ideal patient" because he "didn't talk . . . didn't cry. Didn't even move." This notion of the "ideal" mental patient being comatose speaks to a deep scorn for hospital therapeutics—ineffectual psychiatrists are happiest when they need only babysit catatonics. In the big twist, we also learn that Michael Myers is Laurie Strode's brother, adopted away after her Myers birth parents died. As Loomis summarizes, "He killed one sister fifteen years ago, now he's trying to kill the other!" Loomis also extends his critique of bureaucratic hurdles by using his gun to force a reluctant marshal to take him to protect Laurie. The film eventually turns into a Woman in White event with a hospital-gowned Laurie stumbling through the antiseptic halls of Haddonfield Memorial as Myers slaughters everyone in his path. The film culminates with Laurie shooting Myers in the eyes. Then she and Loomis turn on the gas, and Loomis, in his final therapeutic act, says, "It's time, Michael" and uses his lighter to explode the room with them both inside. The killer lurches out aflame and collapses, burning to a cinder. One senses this was supposed to be the end; the next *Halloween* movie was a stand-alone tale that has nothing to do with Myers. But that movie flopped. Thus *Halloween 4: The Return of Michael Myers*.[16]

Halloween 4 begins with Myers back in a mental institution, his body apparently surviving the conflagration of the sequel. Deep in a subbasement of the Ridgemont Federal Sanitarium he lies, in a complete coma for the past ten years. Ridgemont is fortified and secure. Explains one guard, "This is where society dumps its worst nightmares." Their mistake is to transfer him back to Smith's Grove. In transit, Myers revives and escapes, ushering another round of carnage, this time in pursuit of Laurie's daughter Jamie. Once again, Loomis stalks around with a pistol sending up lines like, "You're talking about him as if he were a human being. That part of him died years ago." Notably, Loomis, now with a scarred face from the hospital explosion he set off, is becoming something of a monster himself. He's a monomaniac with murder on his mind. One doctor even tells him, "I've said this before. I think you're the one who needs mental help." This film ends with Michael absorbing another hail of gunfire and tumbling into a deep mineshaft. In the final twist, Jamie, who survives, puts on a mask and grabs a sharp pair of scissors, suggesting a hereditary factor to Michael's madness. In *Halloween 5: The Revenge of Michael Myers*, we find young Jamie in the Haddonfield Children's Clinic, mute and institutionalized. Still scarred and limping about in his trench coat, Loomis lovingly cradles an automatic pistol and offers his wisdom: "I prayed that he will burn in hell but in my heart I knew that hell will not have him." He also tries some talk therapy on Michael, explaining that the rage "won't go away" and that he must "fight it." But Loomis is ultimately not interested in fixing Myers. He uses Jamie as bait to kill the maniac. The film ends with a captured Myers getting rescued from a police station by a mysterious man in black. In *Halloween 6: The Curse of Michael Myers*, the filmmakers go beyond psychiatry and into the occult to explain Myers. Michael is apparently part of a long, druidic line of killers who sacrifice their next of kin on Halloween night to spare the "lives of the entire tribe." So Michael, in a bizarre twist, is now the hero, murdering siblings to save humanity. Chasing him is a cult that wants a new era of evil to begin. The cult leader, appropriately, is the superintendent of Smith's Grove Sanitarium. Michael kills him and his staff before being bashed apart by a metal pipe.[17]

Halloween 6's supernatural backstory is dropped in the sequels to follow. In *Halloween: Resurrection*, the eighth movie in the franchise, an adult Laurie Strode (Jamie Lee Curtis again) lives in the Grace Anderson Sanitarium, a big, gothic structure with long hallways and basement tunnels. When Myers breaks in to kill her, she turns the tables and traps him, but he kills her before she can finish him off. She exits with the line, "I'll see you in hell." In the most recent addition to the franchise, 2018's *Halloween*, Strode is alive (the film presumes the post-1978 sequels did not happen) and kills Myers once again, after he breaks out of a transport bus taking him from one asylum to another.[18]

For those keeping track: Michael Myers breaks out of an asylum in the first film, is seen rotting there as a child in part two, lands back in one and escapes in part four, breaks into his niece's institution in part five, invades the original asylum to get at a demonic cult in part six, breaks into Laurie's institutional residence in part eight, and escapes one yet again in the eleventh film of the series (films nine and ten are part of Rob Zombie's reboot sequence and not discussed here). No other series comes as close to Asylumland.

An epic sequence of atrocious asylum horrors waded alongside Myers on celluloid. In films like *A Night to Dismember* (1983), *Splatter University* (1984), *Night Train to Terror* (1985), *Sorority House Massacre* (1986), and *The Last Slumber Party* (1988), escapees hack their way through paper-thin plots to terrify kids.[19]

HANNIBAL LECTER AND COMPANY

In 1982, Robert Bloch published a sequel to his 1959 classic novel of horror, *Psycho*. In *Psycho II*, Norman Bates escapes an asylum for the criminally insane after decades of incarceration. Though he's been "buried alive" for decades, Norman's mind is intact. This is because his psychiatrist, Dr. Claiborne, has elected not to use ECT or psychosurgery but rather intensive analysis. Norman's murderous escape coincides with both deinstitutionalization and the rise of a new, cultural villain, the serial killer. Writes Bloch, this was the age of "the Skid Row Slasher, the Hillside Strangler, the Freeway Killers, and all the other mass murderers glamorized by the media's fancy labels." Norman Bates fits right in.[20]

Mass murderers had periodically sparked widespread unease and hand wringing, though explanations for their actions changed over time. In the early twentieth century, they were often defined as atavistic echoes of our darker, collective past. The Age of Freud offered a psychosexual framework that found twisted, oedipal factors involved. After World War II, mass killers could be construed as having "expertise" in their chosen field, making them nightmare versions of the Men in Gray Flannel Suits. The rise of pop-psychology added a new medical vocabulary that previously had been the provenance of doctors' offices and universities. Deinstitutionalization helped make serial killers into a national panic. As Leonard Cassuto argues, "The emergence of the serial killer *story* in America . . . parallels the movement towards outpatient care and the gradual withdrawal of federal funds to pay for it." Emptying hospitals seemed to signify society's inability to properly quarantine evil.[21]

Coinciding with the collapse of the state hospitals, newspapers in the early 1980s suddenly declared that serial killings were pandemic, accounting for upward of a quarter of all murders. The serial killer panic, in turn, helped reinforce the technologies of control that the anti-welfare, religious Right banked on. Obsessing over these beasts buttressed the emergent paradigm of conservative individualism. They walked to center stage just as Freud, the Great Society, world socialism, and the Hippy Generation's ethos exited.[22]

An exemplar of the new killer is Hannibal Lecter. Introduced by Thomas Harris in his 1981 novel *Red Dragon*, Lecter blasted into international stardom with Anthony Hopkins's shocking performance of him in 1991's *The Silence of the Lambs*, a movie based on Harris's second Lecter novel. Lecter lived in the basement of a mental hospital, controlled the unfortunates around him, and eventually erupted into the outside world.

In *Red Dragon*, FBI special agent Will Graham is on the hunt for a serial killer called the Tooth Fairy. The Tooth Fairy likes to sneak into suburban houses at night, massacre whole families, bite them (hence his *nom de carnage*), and then position their bodies with mirrors in their eyes. His behaviors stem from his tormented background. He was born with a hideous lip deformation, was raised by a sadistic grandmother who threatened him with castration, and he never received love. One doctor posits that he has an "unconscious homosexual conflict." The Tooth Fairy fits in with standard Freudian ideas and Robert Bloch's pathologizing *Psycho* format. But the other killer in the novel, Dr. Hannibal Lecter, is something much different.[23]

"Hannibal the Cannibal" Lecter is a psychiatrist who killed at least nine people and performed "unspeakable practices" on their bodies. He had been declared criminally insane after being tracked down by Graham, whom he savagely wounded. Lecter now lives in the "maximum-security section" of the hospital, in a unique room:

> Steel bars covered the entire cell. Behind the bars, further than arm's reach, was a stout nylon stretched ceiling to floor and wall to wall. Through the barrier, Graham could see a table and chair

bolted to the floor. The table was stacked with softcover books and correspondence.

Lecter is nothing like the Tooth Fairy. He is motiveless. In the words of the institution's chief of staff Dr. Chilton, he is "impenetrable." Too intelligent and powerful to be categorized by ordinary methods, he's an "enigma" to every psychiatrist who has tried to diagnose him. His eyes are "maroon and they reflect the light redly in tiny points." He once tore out the tongue and eye of a nurse who briefly let her guard down. His very presence makes one's hair stand on end. Graham tries to get Lecter to help him find the Tooth Fairy, but Lecter only wants to toy with the agent. He gives the Tooth Fairy Graham's personal address. Eventually, Graham and his girlfriend stop the killer. Lecter remains incarcerated.[24]

The asylum serves several telling functions in *Red Dragon*. For Lecter, it is little more than a holding tank. He is kept under permanent surveillance in a special room, never to be released or treated, only quarantined. As for the Tooth Fairy, agents think that he might have once been institutionalized. Graham doubts it, since serial killers are typically "just like the rest of us" and undetectable. After a wheelchair is discovered to have been in his possession (he uses it to kill a journalist), Graham is ready to postulate that he might have once been a patient. He speculates, "If you spend time in a mental hospital you pick up the drill. You could pass as an orderly, get a job doing it when you got out." This notion of the killer having learned to make a "career" of his illness echoes anti-psychiatry arguments about the career of the patient, though in this case the career has murderous ramifications.[25]

Agent Graham is personally familiar with mental institutions. His special capacity to enter the minds of serial killers had once rendered him deranged and committed to the "psychiatric wing" of a hospital. When his stepson learns about this, he gets nervous. Graham makes it clear to the boy that he wasn't put in a regular "mental hospital," since at this place, "they treat everything." For Graham, "The distinction seemed important." This relates an interesting juxtaposition. Asylums can be holding tanks or even career-makers, or, in their more beneficent, "hospital wing" mode, they can be sanctuaries from the consequences of dealing too closely with psychosis. In later books, Harris becomes much more skeptical of anything mental-health related.[26]

The first filmed version of *Red Dragon*, Michael Mann's 1986 *Manhunter*, focuses on Graham's monomaniacal search for the Tooth Fairy. While it gives us some Lecter time (spelled "Lecktor" here), the evil doctor is a sideshow to the main event, the cat-and-mouse game between serial killer and tortured cop. Notably, Mann (who also wrote the script) chose not to provide the Tooth Fairy's sad background, establishing him as the "motiveless" one. Played by Tom Noonan, this serial killer is a force of nature, born without a starting place. The film also includes some classic slasher elements, including an opening first-person subjective killer sequence. Unfortunately, the film was a financial failure.[27]

In 1988, Harris published a follow-up novel, *The Silence of the Lambs*. This book is something of a retread—an FBI agent, with the help of Lecter, races to track a serial killer with a tortured past. In this case, the agent is a young trainee named Clarice Starling. She's sent to interview Lecter about Buffalo Bill, a killer who skins his victims in order to make a girl suit for himself. Like the Tooth Fairy, Buffalo Bill is conflicted sexually and is trying to transform into something greater via murder. Whereas the Tooth Fairy was packed off to live with his grandmother after a stint in an orphanage, Buffalo Bill was adopted by his grandparents after first his dissolute mother and then a foster home failed him. After killing his grandparents, he'd been committed at a mental institution. That failed him too, getting shut down six years after his arrival. Released into society, Bill has only the skill he's perfected in occupational therapy: sewing.[28]

Harris expands on Lecter in *The Silence of the Lambs*. He's even more enigmatic, telling Clarice, "Nothing happened to me, Officer Starling. *I* happened. You can't reduce me to a set of influences. You've given up good and evil for behaviorism, Officer Starling. You've got everybody in moral dignity pants—nothing is anybody's fault. Look at me, Officer Starling. Can you say I'm evil?" Like other serial killers, Lecter is motiveless and unknowable. He mocks behaviorism because he understands that psychology can't account for his behavior. In tune with Reagan-era diatribes about unredeemable criminals who deserve harsh punishment, Lecter's message is that mental health policy has no role to play in fixing the baseness of the world. This is not to say that mind science has no use for Lecter. In fact, he's a Freudian, carrying out his analysis of Starling as part of a "quid pro quo" setup wherein she gives him her personal history in exchange for his detailed workup of Buffalo Bill. This process mimics the Freudian method, in which the doctor helps the patient recall original childhood traumas in order to facilitate cathartic release. In this case, however, the catharsis is not intended for Clarice but for the vampiric Lecter. She discloses pain and he consumes it. Hardly a more damning indictment of Freud can be conceived.

Lecter is the ultimate monstrous psychiatrist, dwelling in his institutional lair and controlling those who stray into his path. He betrays the confidentiality of his clients, recounting the sexual peccadillos of one former patient before explaining that he had to kill him. "Best thing for him, really," explains Lecter. "Therapy wasn't going anywhere. I expect most psychiatrists have a patient or two they'd like to refer to me." While Dr. Chilton ostensibly is in charge of Lecter's treatment, he's also at his mercy. Lecter taunts him in the professional literature. Chilton embodies the sad endgame of the mental institution—the doctor as bureaucratic caretaker. In the film, he even whines to Starling that he has "rights," and that he's "not just some turn-key."[29]

Lecter manifests evil in other ways. His hair has a "widow's peak." In his blank white cell, the only colors "were his hair and eyes and red mouth, in a face so long out of the sun it leached into the surrounding whiteness; his features seemed suspended above the collar of his shirt." He's even given a hockey mask to wear when he travels, recalling Myers's blank white disguise as well as Jason Voorhees's hockey mask. It mimics Lecter's own face, his skin "as pale as the mask." Lecter's humanity is almost entirely extinguished in this book, replaced by superhuman traits. His sense of smell is wolf-like. He can read minds. He can cause death via suggestion (he talks the inmate next door into swallowing his own tongue). He does not sleep at night. Even when his eyes are closed, he is completely aware of his surroundings. His hands, like Stoker's beast, are monstrous (in his case not hairy but six-fingered on his left hand). He's immensely strong for his size. Although he is not denoted as foreign, his elegant taste alludes to a European sensibility, which Welsh actor Anthony Hopkins taps. (Harris, in his next book, will tell us that Lecter was born Lithuanian.) Lecter is essentially Dracula. The film reinforces this with the black, slicked hair, the widow's peak, the focus on his eyes, and even, in one promo shot, a tight lit still of Hopkins's eyes. Hopkins admitted he based his performance on Lugosi. A guard even wonders if it's true that Lecter is "some kind of vampire." In the subsequent book, *Hannibal*, Harris adds to his list of powers the ability to control man-eating pigs and the capacity to elicit labels of "Shaitan, Son of the Morning" from the lips of passing gypsies. In *Hannibal,* Harris informs us, "There is no consensus in the psychiatric community that Dr. Lecter should be termed a man. He has long been regarded by his professional peers in psychiatry, many of whom fear his acid pen in the professional journals, as something entirely Other. For convenience they term him 'monster.'"[30]

The asylum in *Silence of the Lambs* is a dungeon that has no discernible therapeutic value. Clarice Starling's visits to Lecter are described in no uncertain terms: "Descending through the asylum with Alonzo toward the final keep, Starling managed to shut out much of the slammings and the screaming, though she felt them shiver the air against her skin. Pressure built on her as though she sank through water, down and down." The 1991 movie communicates this visually, with a long sequence wherein Starling (Jodie Foster) travels down multiple flights of stairs, through arcane hallways, and into a glowing red anteroom before entering an even gloomier zone in which there is not even paint to cover the rough, irregular, bare brick walls. Director Jonathan Demme describes the scene as a "journey to Hell." We meet Hopkins's Lecter standing in his cell, as if waiting for Starling's arrival. Explains Hopkins of his decision to do it this way, "He's omnipotent; he can smell her coming."[31]

Like *Manhunter, The Silence of the Lambs* movie omits the background information in the novel, making Buffalo Bill a motiveless monster who can only be cured by a bullet. Unlike the bright and modern institution in *Manhunter*, Lecter's home in this movie is a gothic, red-brick structure. *Manhunter*'s asylum was shot at Atlanta's High Museum of Art; Demme chose the Western State School and Hospital for *Silence of the Lambs*. Western was a dilapidated, nineteenth-century relic inhabited by a shrinking population of severely developmentally disabled persons. For the interior shots, Demme used the Alleghany County Jail in Pittsburgh, impressed by its "very, very old Gothic" look and "strange passageways." Lecter's cell set was built in an old factory. Demme chose to place a Plexiglas barrier with air holes instead of bars, allowing a therapeutic closeness between Starling and Lecter. The movie was a massive hit and became the first film since *One Flew Over the Cuckoo's Nest* to take home the "big five" Academy Awards (Best Picture, Actor, Actress, Director, and Screenplay).[32]

It is a hard thing to leave a popular enigma alone. Just as the *Halloween* franchise felt compelled to tell us that Michael Myers was afflicted with an ancient druidic curse and *Elm Street* told us that Freddy was bred from asylum denizens, so did Harris have to account for the evil of Hannibal Lecter. In *Hannibal*, the third book in the series, he fills us in. To summarize, the Nazis did it. In the last years of World War II, an eight-year-old Hannibal survives the destruction of his Lithuanian family estate along with his two-year-old sister Mischa, only to fall victim to a marauding band of "deserters." The deserters kill and eat his little sister. Up until this moment, Lecter had "not been bothered by any considerations of deity, other than to recognize how his own modest predation paled beside those of God, who is in irony matchless, and in wanton malice beyond measure." Now, he becomes unhinged. Plot-wise, the bulk of the story centers on Lecter again helping Starling, this time dueling a psycho named Mason Verger. Verger is himself a survivor of Lecter, having fed his own face to his dogs at Lecter's bidding prior to being paralyzed by him. Sequestered in the family estate and sustained by machines, Verger plots his revenge. His soul reflects his exterior—he is a child molesting, dictator-helping, corporate villain. Verger is so bad that he makes Lecter look good. This, coupled with unfair internal FBI attacks on Starling, opens up a new dynamic. We can root now for Lecter without guilt, especially since we know his tortured past. We are even satisfied when he saves Starling, destroys Verger, and then lobotomizes the corrupt Justice Department hack who colludes with Verger to ruin Starling's career. When Starling joins Lecter to feast on the man's prefrontal lobes and subsequently flees to Argentina with him, though, it seems a bit much.[33]

The most interesting asylum aspect of *Hannibal* is its reference to deinstitutionalization. Lecter's former home, the Baltimore State Hospital for the Criminally Insane (which Harris changed from the

Chesapeake State Hospital for the Criminally Insane in *Silence of the Lambs*; in the movie it's the Baltimore Forensic Hospital), has been shut down. The "old brown building, house of pain, is chained and barred, marked with graffiti and awaiting the wrecking ball." It had been "going downhill for years," and after its chief, Dr. Chilton, vanished, investigations disclosed "revelations of waste and mismanagement and the decrepitude of the building itself." The patients had been either sent off to other institutions or simply cut loose, and now "wandered the streets as Thorazine zombies in an ill-conceived outpatient program that got more than one of them frozen to death." This sad, little, deinstitutionalization story provides the background for a haunted house scenario in which Starling enters the ruins to retrieve Lecter's medical records. She sifts through the empty drawers, rotten sandwiches, crushed Alka-Seltzer tablets, condoms, fast food boxes, crack pipes, and feces. She ends up in the "dungeonlike basement level" where Lecter had once been imprisoned. Here she finds Sammie, a former patient, who is clearly deranged. Sammie lives with a homeless woman whom he protects in exchange for her caretaking prowess. Programs, says the woman, are useless: "You go out in the world and do all that shit and come back to what you know." Society has failed them.[34]

This short section, a single chapter in a 103-chapter book, is telling. Starling cannot get Lecter's medical records. Lecter's asylum is a rotting wreck, habituated by vagrants who have been abandoned by the system. While the asylum at least contained the dangerous in the previous books, deinstitutionalization has rendered it even less socially useful. This section is not included in the film version of *Hannibal*. Neither is the childhood explanation for Lecter's behavior.[35]

Harris was not done with Lecter. In *Hannibal Rising*, he goes back and fills in more blanks. We discover that Lecter ate some of his sister Mischa too. Thus, his first act of cannibalism was essentially foisted upon him, staining his soul but absolving him of agency for the initiation of evil. Once he's implicated in that horrendous event, he is transformed into an unfeeling fiend. Not only does Harris humanize and "explain" Lecter here, he adds further, sympathetic details like how his intellect was cultivated by a Jewish academic fired from his post under Nazis. The only asylum reference in *Hannibal Rising* is a small but telling one. The policeman who pursues him tells another, "I don't want a conviction, I want him declared insane. In an asylum they can study him and try to find out what he is." In the next paragraph, he answers his own question: "The little boy Hannibal died in 1945. His heart died with Mischa. What is he now? There's not a word for it yet. For lack of a better word, we'll call him monster."[36]

Hannibal Lecter was but one killer in a crowded field of post-deinstitutionalization psychopaths. No summary could do them all justice. I'll give just one example. In the controversial 1991 novel *American Psycho*, Bret Easton Ellis created Patrick Bateman, a Wall Street trader obsessed with the accoutrements of upward mobility. We get pages and pages on skin care products, hi-fidelity stereo equipment, bespoke clothing—and human dismemberment. So graphic is the carnage that many thought it revealed Ellis's own unredeemed misogyny. Many called for a boycott, and some critics labeled the book perverse. Ellis and his defenders contended that the over-the-top horror is precisely the point of the novel, which is satire. In the book, Patrick Bateman cannot discern the difference between materialism and murder. It is all a kind of consumption, a processing of commodities through an amoral filter. Seen in this light, *American Psycho* becomes an indictment of the endless consumerism touted in Reagan's epoch. Bateman's obsession with the acme-capitalist of the day, Donald Trump, is a case in point. He is perpetually worried that he might not like something that Trump likes, or that he might miss being where Trump is. At one point his girlfriend complains, "Not Donald Trump *again . . .* This obsession has *got* to end!"[37]

There's no whiff of an asylum for Bateman. Such institutions do not exist in his selfish, atomistic world. The only reference is in regards to a homeless, African American woman who is out of her mind. This seems to allude to Joyce Patricia Brown, a woman who lived on a hot air vent grate in New York City and successfully contested Mayor Ed Koch's program to forcibly commit the disturbed homeless in an effort to protect them from the elements. Says Bateman's friend Timothy Price, "We get some crazy fucking homeless nigger who actually *wants*—listen to me, Bateman—*wants* to be out on the streets." He concludes, "*Let* the fucking bitch *freeze* to death, *put* her out of her own goddamn self-made misery." Such is the logic of Reagan's welfare state—give the mad the freedom to die exposed while the rest of us consume.[38]

CHAPTER 10

STANDARDIZATION

Do you know about the shit they do to us in the basement?
—*The Jacket* (2005)

n the 2008 film *Changeling*, a single mother returns home from work one day to discover that her young son is missing. Christine Collins (Angelina Jolie) frantically scours the neighborhood, fearing the worst. Weeks pass, and then to her relief, she learns that her son has been found in Illinois. Accompanied by press and the chief of police, she goes to the train station to meet her boy—only to realize that he is not her son. This being 1928, the authorities choose to act as though this stranger is her son, thus avoiding political embarrassment. When Collins enlists the help of a crusading preacher, she's confined in the LA County General Hospital Psychopathic Ward. She receives the full complement: burly attendants, firehose shower, black rubber-gloved cavity search, miserable cell. Collins learns that many of her fellow inmates are sane women like herself, whose only crime is to have resisted police brutality. As a prostitute explains, "If we're insane, nobody has to listen to us." When the prostitute challenges the head doctor in Collins's defense, she is sent to Room 18, where attendants pin her down and a stone-faced nurse cranks up a big ECT machine. It is a powerful moment, all the more worrisome because, "This is a true story."[1]

The only problem is that ECT did not exist in 1928.

Changeling is based on shocking real events in Jazz Age Los Angeles. A woman named Christine Collins endured her son's kidnapping, his replacement by a different boy, and then a subsequent commitment to the psychiatric ward of the LA County General Hospital for

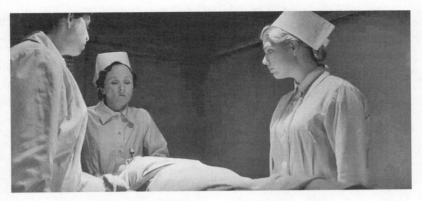

Anachronistic ECT in *Changeling* (2008)

one week. A notorious serial killer named Gordon Stewart Northcott, who was later found to have molested and murdered some twenty children at his ranch in Wineville, California, had probably abducted and murdered her real son. (The boy's survival in the film is a bigger embellishment than the ECT part.) Collins's story has everything Hollywood likes—a gutsy hero, murder, corruption, and a bizarre twist. The theme is the struggle of one woman against a vast conspiracy of medically sanctioned, masculine power. Reviewers had no problem catching on. As Andrew Geoff noted in *Sight and Sound*, "Northcott's crimes serve as a nightmarishly distorted and deadly reflection of both the LAPD's self-serving exploitation of the boy they claim is Walter Collins, and of the medical establishment's use of incarceration and electric shock treatment against women deemed troublesome. We're still perhaps not very far, after all, from the kill-or-be-killed ethos of the old West." Most critics, however, were less kind. One thought it was too simplistic and preachy, noting, "Most viewers today already agree that it's bad to lock up innocent mothers in loony bins, so *Changeling* doesn't have a lot to prove when it threatens Collins with sedatives and shock treatments." Another saw her asylum for what it was—a blatant Hollywood stereotype. Explained Ryan Gilbey in *New Statesman*, "When she refuses to accept her son's return, Captain Jones commits her to a mental institution, and you know just what's coming: the naked hosing-down scene, the smattering of Nurse Ratched types, the shock treatment accompanied by amplified thunder claps." This critic is versed in the film asylum.[2]

The construction of the celluloid asylum accrued over the history of narrative film. As early as 1904 (*The Escaped Lunatic*), we see a dungeon-like institution. Tall, iron gates date at least to 1917's *The Woman in White*. Frightening psychiatric treatments date to the 1920s. Factory-style, brick edifices and prison-appropriate, high fences come into play in the 1940s. By the late 1970s, audiences could reasonably expect to see, in some combination: loveable misfits, dire treatments, straitjackets, brutal attendants, and malicious superintendents/doctors/nurses. They could also anticipate long, stark corridors and antiseptic white rooms, padded cells, and dayrooms stuffed with drugged-out zombies. Rainy nights are common for establishing shots. Victims might be taken in strapped to a gurney, with a tracking shot intercutting a series of overhead hallway lights. Aurally, audiences could expect to hear screams, frenzied laughing, unnervingly placid music, and crying. As the critic of *Changeling* notes, they knew "just what's coming." This is a familiar place.[3]

Whether or not this corresponds to reality is perhaps not the most interesting question to ask. After all, Hollywood is a dream engine. But movies, one can argue, do help inform our real-life experiences and thus impose on our reality. Writes Neal Gabler, thanks to the soaring success of film, "Where we had once measured the movies by life, we now measured life by how well it satisfied the narrative expectations created by the movies." Movies and TV shows offer a parallel, substitute world, one bestowing vicarious pleasures while reinforcing social expectations. The fact that many asylum movies are presented as being "true" or "real" also means that accepting them is an act of complicity. For instance, *One Flew Over the Cuckoo's Nest* was filmed in an actual asylum, with real patients as inspiration and extras, and it is based on a book written on a mental ward. Yet it is filled with cartoons. McMurphy is hardly believable, his Native American sidekick is magically powerful, and the treatments are exaggerated and obsolete. Fantasy and reality mix. Symbols become "truths."[4]

One might reasonably note that there have always been plenty of factual accounts against which to check such fantasies. But I'd argue that when we read true accounts, we think about movies, and vice versa. We might tell ourselves we can differentiate, but episodes such as the tremendous backlash against ECT following *Cuckoo's Nest*, or the acceptance of ECT in *Changeling*, suggests otherwise.

Doctors seem to know this. In her 1997 memoir of institutionalization, Daphne Scholinski reflects, "The only movies we weren't allowed to watch were *One Flew Over the Cuckoo's Nest* and *King of Hearts*; the staff thought the films would give us ideas." This chapter will explore how modern films, through a process I call standardization, create a place we are all familiar with. Having screened well over two hundred movies and TV shows with asylum themes, I must be highly selective here, offering what I consider representative examples.[5]

SCARY AND DYSFUNCTIONAL

The idea that the asylum is a scary and dysfunctional place dates back at least to the Early Republic in America. Paintings by William Hogarth were common referents in the nineteenth century, as were images of massive, gothic asylums. Poe needed only remind us of the "very usual horror at the sight of a lunatic" and describe the *Maison de Santé* as an isolated, spooky manse to evoke the appropriate level of disquiet. The visuality of cinema took us yet deeper, *showing* us the Women in White and the monsters, depicting the horrific treatments in action.[6]

Working in such a malleable medium, filmmakers have many ways of showing us that we're entering a forbidding place, and this allows them to create locales for plots of mystery or trampled genius. Gothic, brick structures are common, as are barred windows and chain fences. *Cuckoo's Nest* brought the asylum into the daylight. Forman's use of natural light and daytime shoots created a bright, "real" space. Other films follow his pattern, shooting in actual institutions and using natural light. Penny Marshall shot *Awakenings* (1990) in the Kingsboro Psychiatric Center in Brooklyn. James Mangold filmed *Girl, Interrupted* (1999) in the Harrisburg State Hospital in Pennsylvania. Other directors envisioned asylums more as postmodern hells. Michael Mann put Hannibal Lecter's asylum in *Manhunter* in Atlanta's High Museum of Art. In *Brain Dead* (1990), the asylum is the ultramodern Donald C. Tillman Water Reclamation Plant, a metaphor for the corporate villain driving the plot. John Carpenter used a block-like reclamation plant on Lake Ontario to communicate the prison feel he wanted for *In the Mouth of Madness* (1994). In *The Fisher King* (1991), Terry Gilliam used a real warehouse, making celluloid truth of the warehousing of those suffering mental illness.[7]

Most film asylums are not modern-looking nor are they fantastical. They are bleak and gothic, inheritors of a long tradition of despotic nightmares. One impact of the decline of the state hospitals (more on this next chapter) is the numerous, tawdry depictions of overcrowded and blighted asylums one finds in post–*Cuckoo's Nest* movies. In 2001's *Don't Say a Word*, for instance, the establishing shot of "Bridgeview Psychiatric Hospital" reveals a vast, fog-shrouded, stonework structure at night. Inside, we see a graffitied elevator, one of the more legible scrawls being "Sigmund," as if to emphasize the (un)death of the old master. For the exteriors, the director chose the old Bellevue building in New York City since converted into a men's homeless shelter. For the interiors, he used an abandoned section of the Whitby Psychiatric Hospital in Ontario, Canada. In this location, the production designer added paint, lights, and fixtures, plus some bars for more celluloid "authenticity."[8]

Heartbreaking asylums often operate as metaphors for themes of persecution and personal growth. Actor Geoffrey Rush's filmography offers at least two good examples. In *Shine* (1996), he plays piano prodigy David Helfgott, a troubled yet brilliant man who lands in an asylum after succumbing to the pressures of an abusive father and the next-to-impossible Rachmaninoff Piano Concerto no. 3. After a kindly piano teacher rescues him from the Glendale Psychiatric Hospital (a place both bright and gothic), inappropriate behavior gets him sent to a community care establishment, Eden Lodge. Here he stays under the benign gaze of a housemaster until he's again rescued by an older woman (Lynn Redgrave). Thanks to the love of women, the artistic prodigy is saved from quarantine in sad mental facilities. In *Quills* (2000), Rush is the rascal Marquis de Sade, writer of salacious adventures, persecuted by Napoleon and thrown into the madhouse. At the Charenton Asylum for the Insane, he becomes a kind of Revolutionary Age McMurphy. He livens up the place with plays and he tweaks the nose of authority by sneaking out obscene works for popular consumption. His Ratched is the cruel, new superintendent, Dr. Royer-Collard, played by Michael Caine. Royer-Collard tries to break de Sade's will with psychiatric torture devices, but to no avail. The Marquis inspires the inmates to rebel. Prior to his inevitable martyrdom, he leaves the gift of inspiration to the other patients. In this case, the main beneficiary is the generous Abbé de Coulmier, who ends up as a patient writing his own manifesto to be secreted out by a washerwoman. While the institution can crush the man, it cannot crush freedom.[9]

The idea of the psychiatrically incarcerated genius gets a post-modern twist in Ron Howard's *A Beautiful Mind* (2001). This true-life movie is about a brilliant mathematician named John Forbes Nash who suspects that he's being tracked by a shadowy government agency. Unlike many other asylum films, we are not quite sure if the hero belongs in or out. Howard shoots from Nash's perspective, and though he becomes more unhinged as he goes, his enemies appear legion. The tall, gray-haired psychiatrist (Christopher Plummer) is mysterious and frightful. Director Ron Howard quips, "Would you trust anyone who is lit that way?" Events come to a head when Nash is tackled, sedated, and taken into the asylum. We get the institution we expect—burly, white-coated attendants, screams, blank, white-tiled rooms with one-way mirrors, grilles covering windows, meandering corridors, and naturally lit dayrooms. Nash suffers a terrifying and stereotypical experience, finally learning that what he needs is to be off his meds so that he can be brilliant again. Nash received the Nobel Prize in 1994, an event that the movie crowns with a beautiful speech about love that he never actually delivered in reality. *The Guardian* gave the film a "history grade" of C-.[10]

Imposing asylums containing patients "who know too much" have been around since the first filmed adaptations of *The Woman in White*. One modern example is *Terminator 2: Judgement Day* (1991), in which Sarah Connor (Linda Hamilton) knows that the world will end when Skynet becomes self-aware. But saying so makes her sound insane. At "Pescadaro State Hospital," "A Criminally Disordered Retention Facility," shot in a converted office building, we get everything we'd expect—blank walls with white-on-white décor, brawny attendants who shock patients with an electric prod, surveillance cameras, and a creepy doctor who makes sure Sarah gets her "Thorazine." Sarah breaks out with the help of the Terminator himself, who is the good guy in this film. And, thus, does James Cameron give us an asylum breakout that saves humanity.[11]

Some films offer asylums that quarantine the mad but really shouldn't. Sometimes, a patient who appears completely out of touch with reality might actually be accessing a superior reality. Two films that do this are *Don Juan DeMarco* (1994) and *K-PAX* (2001). In *Don Juan DeMarco*, Johnny Depp is a young man who thinks he is the world's greatest lover. Dressed as a seventeenth-century Castilian, he is shipped off to Marlon Brando's hospital following a suicide attempt. Depp's unstoppable charm convinces Brando not only to not give him any medications, but also to rekindle his own relationship with his wife. Depp "escapes" by pretending to be non-delusional; Brando goes along with the ruse, and next thing you know, they are all on an exotic island to reunite the young man with his lover. This fable is situated in an asylum, albeit an innocuous one filled with incompetent doctors and lovestruck nurses, as a place that tries to crush a young man's romantic vision of himself. Psychiatry does not fix him; rather, he fixes the psychiatrist. Brando closes the film with a voiceover: "Sadly, I must report that the last patient I ever treated, the great lover, Don Juan DeMarco, suffered from a romanticism which was completely incurable. And even worse, highly contagious."

In *K-PAX*, Kevin Spacey plays "prot," a person claiming to be from the planet K-PAX. When he does not respond to medication, a sensitive psychiatrist (Jeff Bridges) must try to understand him before stronger, somatic methods are applied. Like *Don Juan DeMarco*, the rebel-oddball in *K-PAX* ends up teaching a doctor valuable life lessons while being shielded from drastic, asylum treatments. At one point, Bridges tells prot that if he does not work with him, he'll get, "A trip to a place where they'll stick a needle in your ass every morning which may or may not leave you with a stupid grin on your face for the rest of your days here on Earth." Though the director aimed to be realistic and to create a "sympathetic" view of the mental institution, tradition inexorably looms. The head doctor (Alfre Woodard) threatens to send prot up to "floor three," where, it is implied, more serious treatments await. We root for analytic success to save the sensitive soul.[12] In *A Beautiful Mind, Terminator 2, Don Juan DeMarco*, and *K-PAX*, filmmakers tell us that the odd and the eccentric are wrongfully committed simply because they are different. These movie asylums symbolize social intolerance, escaping represents heroic agency. One might wonder if there might be heroes who are better off within institutional settings. This is the question posed by the Academy Award–winning film *Rain Man*.

Rain Man (1988) is an unconventional road movie in which two estranged brothers, Charlie (Tom Cruise) and Raymond Babbitt (Dustin Hoffman) get to know each other. Raymond is a high-functioning "autistic savant" who has spent most of his life in a genteel sanitarium for the developmentally disabled. His arrogant brother Charlie discovers his existence only after he learns that their recently deceased father left everything to Raymond. Charlie decides to break Raymond out in order to ransom him back for his share of their father's fortune. Because Raymond refuses to fly, they have to drive to Charlie's house in California. En route, Charlie learns some life lessons, such as family is more important than money, and he decides that he wants full custody of Raymond. He gets a hearing in front of a lawyer and the asylum doctor. In an unexpected twist, it appears that Raymond really belongs in the institution. He is just not capable of independent living. The bittersweet ending has Charlie sending his brother back, because after all, his disability does exist. We are taught two things: (1) a caring brother and the open road can reach a patient better than a lifetime of asylum care, and (2) that might not be enough. In high Hollywood style, a strange man, wise and yet unable to conform, teaches a worldly cad life lessons before retreating back to his mansion of madness.[13]

Despite its haven-like function, the *Rain Man* asylum still manages to evoke unease. Its name, Wallbrook, references another, very disturbing place—Willowbrook State School, where, in 1972, investigative reporter Geraldo Rivera went undercover with a camera crew and filmed a level of squalor that resulted in a class action lawsuit and the passage of a new civil rights law for institutionalized persons with intellectual and developmental disabilities. The fact that even the benign Wallbrook could evoke such dark insinuations replays a metanarrative of tyranny and dysfunction.[14]

In one movie, the problem is that the asylum is too innocuous. In *Death Wish II*, Charles Bronson is faced with a worthless asylum that only protects a sneering villain from a prison sentence. The pleasant-looking McLarren State Hospital is a haven for the bad guy, a place where treatments are "all done with kindness now." Bronson goes undercover as a doctor and electrocutes him via a massive ECT machine.[15]

On the more farcical end of the spectrum, there is Mel Brooks's 1977 *High Anxiety*. Its setting, "The Psycho-Neurotic Institute for the

Very, VERY Nervous," might be called California Gothic. It is a big, white compound boasting lovely lawns and arched porticos, perched on the edge of a high Pacific cliff and with a strong gate bearing the sign "Keep In." Brooks includes film noir–inspired shots of shadows on walls, long, blank hallways, and a "Violent Ward" with the requisite iron doors. The cast includes a Ratched-style nurse named Charlotte Diesel, played with ruthless abandon by Cloris Leachman. Nurse Diesel is a brutal sadomasochist with a pale visage, tight black bun, and faint black mustache. She first appears in a starchy nurse uniform with jarringly pointy breasts. In *Cuckoo's Nest*, Kesey describes Big Nurse as having a "precision-made" face with "skin like flesh-colored enamel . . . A mistake was made somehow in manufacturing, putting those big, womanly breasts on what would have otherwise been a perfect work, and you can see how bitter she is about it." Nurse Diesel is a cartoon of a cartoon. Her authoritarianism is reinforced by the S&M outfit that she occasionally dons, a shiny, Nazi-inspired number with a built-in brassiere, leather skirt, truncheon, and Gestapo-style cap.[16]

Other post-Forman comedies accessed a broad palette of themes, moods, and models with which to critique asylum medicine. In 1976's *The Pink Panther Strikes Again*, Inspector Clouseau's nemesis and ex-boss Charles Dreyfus escapes from the genteel sanitarium where he's lived since Clouseau drove him insane. We find him trying hard not to act enraged whenever the inspector comes up—his analyst even has a dummy Clouseau in his office for practice. In *Annie* (1982), Carol Burnett's cruel Ms. Hannigan sings about how the little girl orphans are driving her crazy, crooning, "Some day I'll land in the nuthouse / With all the nuts and the squirrels (giggle) / There I'll stay / Tucked away / Until the prohibition of / Little girls!" In *Airplane II: The Sequel* (1982), Captain Ted Stryker has been railroaded into an asylum after being blamed for the crash of a poorly designed spacecraft. At "The Ronald Reagan Hospital for the Mentally Ill," with its slogan, "We Cure People the Old Fashioned Way," a gang of attendants beats a bedridden patient with clubs while yelling, "For your own good!" Across the room, a man diagnosed as "Anal Retentive" fights with a nurse over his bedpan. Stryker manages to break out, hopping a high wall while spotlights zigzag and sirens wail. *Good Burger* (1997) gives us "Demented Hills," complete with a Ratched-type yelling, "It's medication time!"[17]

The most complete post–*Cuckoo's Nest* comedic vision is *Crazy People*. This 1990 movie stars Dudley Moore as an advertising executive who has a nervous breakdown, with Daryl Hannah co-starring as the asylum waif he falls for. Moore's character gets committed to the stately Bennington Sanitarium after he has a breakdown and writes ads that are too honest. Once his company learns that his new ads sell, they employ him and the other patients to write copy, to hilarious results. For instance: "Amalfi Super Thins [cigarettes]. Pulmonary cancer? Perhaps . . . Flavor? For sure!" In *Crazy People*, the cosseted, peaceful world of Bennington is juxtaposed with "insane" Madison Avenue. However, as might be predicted, all is not what it seems. This sanitarium is not designed to heal. When the patients begin to improve thanks to the advertising work, the superintendent resists it, and then, once their production benefits him personally, pushes them to work harder under threat of being sent off to a place "that doesn't get too much sunlight." Dudley Moore ultimately saves them by swooping in on an Army helicopter piloted by Hannah's brother. They go on to create their own ad company. Bennington Sanitarium is both a critique of a crazy world and a despotic, if soft, prison lorded over by a greedy master. The breakout allows the zany crew to escape institutional rot and elevates the rest of us too, thanks to honest advertising.[18]

Some films evoke the asylum without even having an asylum. So familiar is the stereotype that directors and screenwriters can insert asylum elements to trigger appropriate emotional responses. Underground, cement tunnels laden with steam pipes, white rooms, evil doctors, straitjackets, endless hallways, crackling headphones, and other cues tap a deep cultural wellspring and drive plots. In *The Amityville Horror*, a hit 1979 movie about a family that moves into a haunted house, for example, we watch as a good father slowly loses his marbles. What drives George Lutz to make threatening gestures with his axe is the fact that the house is built over a place where the Shinnecock tribe once "put all the crazy people" and then "left them here to die." The ancient Indian ground is asylum ground. In *The Princess Bride* (1987), the hero gets tossed into a subterranean chamber and then tortured with "The Machine," a familiar set of headphones connected to a big device. The hero writhes about in a familiar way.[19]

THE DAYROOM

Nearly every film asylum features a dayroom. This is a place where the patients congregate, hatch plots, receive humiliations, get surveilled, and spy on their peers. In some older offerings like *Now, Voyager, The Cobweb,* and *David and Lisa*, this space is a pleasant, living room area, where troubled youngsters read books, play checkers, and contemplate their lives. In others, such as *The Snake Pit* and *Suddenly, Last Summer*, the dayroom is a waiting room from hell.

Cuckoo's Nest gives us the modern cinematic dayroom. Forman's bright and utilitarian space with nondescript furniture and plenty of light pouring in would become traditional afterward. The Forman dayroom gives directors the opportunity to introduce the cast all at once, allowing audiences to see them quarantined and medicated. After *Cuckoo's Nest*, we can expect things like unwatched TVs, glassed-in nurse's stations, clean floors, perhaps some board games that are either unplayed or cartoonishly played. For example, in a recent update of institutional insouciance, in *Unsane* (2018), a nurse plays on her cellphone instead of observing patients in the dayroom. The protagonist will use the dayroom to get the lay of the land and to dissect the dynamics of their fellows in order to best formulate an escape. Cluttering all the patients together allows the filmmaker to juxtapose personalities and physiognomies to suit the story. Forman wanted his characters to have an institutional "look," and yet each to be distinct from the other. Later directors transposed established "looks" onto their characters or, more lazily, just hired the same actors and changed the names.[20]

Standardization begat variation. In *12 Monkeys* (1995), a time traveler named James Cole (Bruce Willis) is sent back to 1996 to learn who is responsible for a plague that has devastated the planet. Arriving in 1990 by mistake, Cole is locked up in a psychiatric hospital, his rantings about time-traveling making him mentally suspect. Its dayroom is white on white with linoleum floors and light pouring in from small, barred windows. Within, we find hallucinating patients waving their arms or just staring off, a locked-up game cabinet, and an ancient black-and-white TV bolted to the wall playing cartoons, animal experimentation documentaries, and old films. The room is also in a state of deterioration, with missing tiles, peeling paint, and an air of

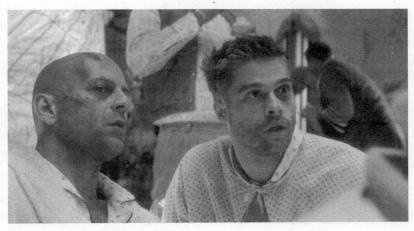

In the dayroom, *12 Monkeys* (1995)

neglect. Cole meets Jeffrey, played with manic urgency by Brad Pitt. Jeffrey appears to be deeply institutionalized, with his crazy haircut, pajama-jacket combo, and off-kilter eyes. Jeffrey tells Cole that most of the people here are not "mentally ill." They are here "because of the system." A nurse warns Jeffrey that if he doesn't stop raving, he'll "get a shot." Gilliam's dayroom lets us explore the dynamic between the two leads. Jeffrey later helps Cole break out, and then he goes on to introduce the plague that Cole was sent back to locate in the first place. In a classic, time travel plot twist, Cole unintentionally gave Jeffrey the idea while they were incarcerated together.[21]

THE CORRIDOR

A long hallway, with doors on either side, extending off into the distance under a line of overhead lights, is a mainstay of the celluloid asylum. It is a feature that pulls the viewer in, floating them downriver to the land of total control. The opening sequence of Sam Fuller's 1963 *Shock Corridor* is the classic, beginning with a slow iris wipe onto an endless corridor. This space is a tunnel of surveillance, a long, fixed passageway wherein one is monitored while descending into the depths of hell. *Shock Corridor*'s corridor also serves as a kind of dayroom, a place the inmates call "the street," where they congregate if well-behaved. Ultimately, this corridor becomes a hell for the hero. In the end, he imagines that a storm outside is now inside, and he stumbles along the corridor in a deluge, knocking on the closed doors but unable to escape.[22]

Asylum corridors evoke dread in a variety of ways. In *Awakenings*, Robin Williams's sensitive doctor character gets taken down one lined with wheelchairs carrying lolling chronic patients. Williams asks the attendant what these people are "waiting for." "Nothin'" responds the attendant. "But how are they supposed to get well?" "They're not. They're chronic." As Williams walks, we travel with him into a sad place in need of fixing. In *Terminator 2*, Sarah Connor flees down a corridor in slow motion, escaping the abominable treatments and abuse of the place.

The scariest celluloid corridor is in Stanley Kubrick's *The Shining*. At the Overlook Hotel, ghosts haunt young Danny through long halls, with Kubrick's pioneering Steadicam following the boy as he furiously pedals his big wheel. The hotel evokes the movie madhouse with its massive dayroom where Jack types nonsense, a green corridor of the confusing hedge maze, an institutional kitchen and storeroom, cruel ghost employees, and a ghastly superintendent in the form of the house itself. We watch Danny as he navigates the corridors that lure and then trap him. The audience already "knows" Kubrick's corridor. It is a place where madness is manufactured and monitored, where one is dragged into an inescapable nightmare. It is a mythical asylum space.[23]

A subcategory of the corridor shot is the "gurney shot." Nothing communicates the helplessness of the asylum patient so much as a trip down a hallway strapped to a gurney, overhead lights scrolling by. We transport from outside life into the kind of horrible in-betweenness theorized by Poe and Freud. An early example of the asylum gurney shot can be seen in the 1947 film noir *Possessed*. Many would follow. There's one in 1963's *The Caretakers*. Frances Farmer (Jessica Lange) gets carried off in a gurney to her lobotomy in *Frances*. Bill Pullman is wheeled around in a gurney through Lakeside Sanitarium in *Brain Dead*. There are gurney shots in multiple *Halloween* films (numbers 2, 5, and 6). In the horror film *Candyman*, a woman who uncovers the monstrous spirit behind an urban legend is pushed down a hospital hallway in a gurney before getting strapped onto a bed. No gurney is ever good.[24]

THE WHITE ROOM

The blank, windowless room is another movie asylum staple. It isolates and metaphorizes the character—they are helpless and alone. Sometimes, there is a one-way mirror or portal through which we watch them. Often the patient wears something institutional, a white jumpsuit, johnnie, scrubs, or even straitjacket. The white room can also help "unmask" evil psychotics, serving as a kind of window through which we discern a dark presence within a human exterior.

The paradigm model is a scene at the end of Hitchcock's *Psycho*. Norman Bates (Anthony Perkins) is in a blank room at the jail house. We know he is insane and likely headed to an asylum. As we hear Mother's voice berate him, the camera moves in on Perkins. He's draped in a police blanket, his face reacting to his mom's voice. Finally, the camera settles on Perkins's face, cutting to a fly landing on his hand before going back to his face. Staring at the camera, he smiles, and, as the shot fades into the scene of the murdered girl's car getting towed out of the mud, a skull flashes over his face. In the blankness of the room, his horrid true self, a death's head covered by a boyish appearance, is finally revealed. In the white room, evil is exposed.[25]

In *The Boston Strangler* (1968), a similar event occurs. When Albert DeSalvo (Tony Curtis) is finally caught and placed in the mental

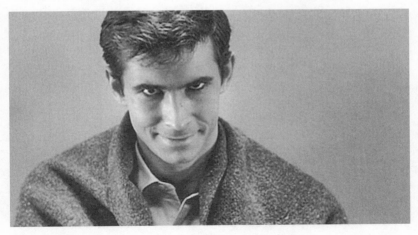

Norman Bates in the white room, *Psycho* (1960)

hospital, he's put in a white jumpsuit and locked in a stark white room with a two-way mirror. With a tape recorder and a microphone at hand, Detective Bottomly (Henry Fonda) interrogates him, eventually getting DeSalvo to face the darkness within. He ultimately reenacts his stranglings, eyes orgasmically closed. In the white room, he can no longer hide, even from himself. Closing text warns us, "The film has ended, but the responsibility of society for the early recognition and treatment of the violent among us has yet to begin." As the credits roll, the camera pans back, revealing the cavernous white room and DeSalvo standing catatonically in the corner, everything slowly fading to white.[26]

The white room can also be a damning symbol of modern society. In George Lucas's *THX 1138* (1971), everyone takes drugs to keep them mindless and sexless, and everyone wears identical white outfits with identical haircuts—bald. The hero, THX 1138, has an illicit affair with a woman named LUH 3417 after she switches out his drugs. He gets duly convicted of "drug evasion" and "sexual perversion" and is placed in a vast, blank white space to be "conditioned and held in detention." Lucas's bright, Orwellian hell reveals the framework of control supporting the surveillance state. The film ends with the expected escape from the institution. THX discovers that the whole society is underground and witnesses his first sunset as the credits roll. Like other films that use asylums without literally doing so, *THX 1138* taps into a storehouse of fears and anxieties. Six years later, Lucas would give us yet more sparse corridors, mindless servants, and mind control in *Star Wars*.

The Reagan era witnessed a plethora of white rooms. Popular music, evoking messages of social estrangement and alienation, found useful imagery in the white room, often coupled with straitjackets. Pat Benatar's 1982 album cover for *Get Nervous* features her in a straitjacket sitting in a padded cell, a look of shock on her face. In 1983, Quiet Riot released *Metal Health*, which soared on the hits "Cum on Feel the Noize" and "Metal Health (Bang Your Head)." The album cover features a man in a white room wearing a red leather straitjacket and a metal mask reminiscent of *Friday the 13th*. The video for "Metal Health (Bang Your Head)," which received a lot of airtime on MTV, begins with the lead singer dressed in the album cover outfit. He's trapped in a white padded cell, and he thrashes around until he breaks out, tearing off the jacket and running down a long corridor while fleeing a group of attendants. He erupts through a trapdoor and onto a concert stage, finally tearing off the mask and singing the hit song. The video ends with a gang of youngsters in institutional uniforms fleeing down the corridor, tackling staff along the way. Heavy metal rebellion becomes asylum breakout; school becomes a padded cell.[27]

The white room was simply irresistible to eighties rockers. Ozzy Osborne, Alice Cooper, Metallica, Iron Maiden, Mötley Crüe, Guns 'n Roses, Van Halen, KISS, and Aerosmith all featured straitjackets and/or padded cells in their visual work in this period. Van Halen even named an album *5150*, inspired by the California Welfare and Institutions code that authorizes the state to involuntarily confine a person. Metallica's "Welcome Home (Sanitarium)," from their 1986 album *Master of Puppets*, provides perhaps the most iconic message. In this song, the protagonist was "Just labeled mentally deranged." But he dreams of a place with "No locked doors, no windows barred / No things to make my brain seem scarred." The chorus, "Sanitarium, leave me be / Sanitarium, just leave me alone" evokes the blank white room of society closing in. Lead vocalist James Hetfield implores us, "Sleep my friend and you will see / That dream is my reality / They keep me locked up in this cage / Can't they see it's why my brain says Rage." Ultimately, violence is the best tool of escape. Growls Hetfield, "They think our heads are in their hands / But violent use brings violent plans / Keep him tied, it makes him well / He's getting better, can't you tell?" If society is the asylum, why not break the walls and destroy those in your path? This is, of course, pure fantasy, a fantasy of ruination built upon the metaphor of our asylumized existence. Hetfield evokes the pressures felt by many teens, disillusioned by the inconsistencies of the American promise, with little more than the word "sanitarium."[28]

Even cute, little aliens could get the white room. In the massive 1982 hit *E.T. The Extra-Terrestrial*, the diminutive creature gets captured by government agents in hazmat suits, and the suburban home where he is hiding gets converted into a plastic-coated, antiseptic hell. E.T. dies surrounded by lights, machines, and covered humans. He's packed into a white box. Then he comes back to life and is freed by Elliott, who proceeds to strap him onto the handlebars of his bike and soar over a police blockade. His breakout brought audiences to tears.[29]

The white room is especially appealing for the horror filmmaker. In *The Ring* (2002), a film that contains only minutes of asylum time but cannot seem to resist any asylum cliché, there is a scene in which Samara is hooked up to electrodes in a blank, windowless chamber covered with light green tiles and a smooth linoleum floor. It is hard to imagine a less comforting space for interviewing a mentally disturbed child. Of course, it's also totally appropriate; Samara is pure evil. She even explains to the interviewing doctor that she wants to hurt people, and that "it won't stop."

Hannibal the Cannibal also gets the white room in *Manhunter*; the bars that separate him from his guests are pure white, as is his outfit. In *The Silence of the Lambs*, Jonathan Demme went for the dungeon look in which to incarcerate Hannibal, with oozing, gray stone walls and a matching floor. But when Lecter travels, he gets a white outfit, which Anthony Hopkins supposedly wanted to wear for its evocation of the dental profession. In *Red Dragon*, the filmmakers split the difference with scenes of the *Silence* dungeon and another one (not in the book) in which Lecter prowls around a painted oval in a big recreation room while leashed to a metal cord. This space is massive and empty, with white walls, a white floor, and white light bathing Hopkins in his white outfit.

The padded cell continues the white room idea. These rooms are typically small and claustrophobic. The padding, often combined with the straitjacket, communicates to us that the patient is a threat to themselves and others and has also become a spectacle for those outside looking in.

Filmmakers use padded cells to suit various narrative ends. Victims might be here because they are monstrous, or a threat to power, or because they have been driven mad by events. A few examples suggest the possibilities. In the 1975 comedy *The Return of the Pink Panther*, bumbling Inspector Clouseau's rival Charles Dreyfus tries to assassinate him and winds up in a white padded room in a straitjacket, writing "Kill Clouseau" on the walls and floor with a crayon between his toes. He then becomes the only character to "see" the cartoon Pink Panther, who saunters in and sets up a camera to film him. Dreyfus also "sees" the scrolling credits. The padded cell becomes a portal to the bizarre, higher reality of the movie itself. In *Brazil* (1985), the protagonist winds up in a padded cell that seems

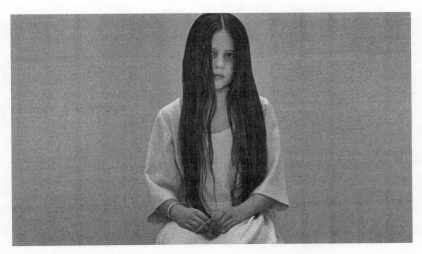

Samara in the asylum, *The Ring* (2002)

to go on vertically forever thanks to a high angled shot, an exagger-
atedly tall set, and a special, wide angle lens. The fantastical space
reflects the hyper-fascist reality of Terry Gilliam's *1984* parody. In the
1979 version of *Dracula*, Lucy, once made into a vampire by the Count,
gets locked up in a padded cell in Seward's asylum. She nearly bites
her betrothed Jonathan Harker and is contained at the last minute by
Van Helsing's judicious cross-wielding intervention. Dracula breaks
her out, tearing a hole in the wall and leaving the padding in shreds.[30]

Padded cells can also be final, sad destinations. In *Scrooged* (1988),
an update of *A Christmas Carol*, a padded cell is the depository for
the Tiny Tim character. In the Dickens original, Tim dies in a future
where Scrooge continues his mendacious ways. In this version, Cal-
vin's "doom" is the padded cell, where he sits hugging his knees and
staring off into space. Speaking of final destinations, in *Final Destination 2* (2003), Clear Rivers, the girl who cheated Death in the first
film, commits herself to an asylum for personal safety. Down at the
end of a long corridor she waits, disheveled and washed out. In her
bright white padded cell, Rivers has made herself into a prisoner. Her
television shows a closed circuit shot of the hallway, allowing her to
monitor all incoming visitors. The girl who has the premonition in
this movie visits Rivers to enlist her help. When Rivers declines, she
tells her, "In my opinion you're already dead." Asylum life being living

death, Rivers has not really escaped the Reaper after all. She decides to rejoin the living, getting out easily because she has committed herself. Sadly, she does perish in the end.[31]

Padded cells protect, confine, and punish, even all three at once. In John Carpenter's 1994 *In the Mouth of Madness*, a padded cell confines the protagonist, incarcerated after killing a man in a fit of insanity caused by a horror novelist. But then the cell protects him while the whole world implodes thanks to said novelist. In *The Green Mile* (1999), a "padded room" helps guards working death row punish a sadistic fellow employee. An overnight stay in the cell wearing a jacket reduces him to a babbling puppy. The padded cell can even be "Disneyfied." In the live-action version of *Beauty and the Beast* (2017), we get a padded cell wagon that carts off Belle's poor father. In these instances, and more, the padded cell itself needs no explanation. It is a well-established disciplinary space for the wayward, the dangerous, or the reckless. Given this rubric, a filmmaker's creative license can generate endless variations.[32]

THE SUBBASEMENT

Here's an old one. In "Tarr and Fether," the keepers become monstrous in "underground cells." In *Dashington*, the barbaric Mrs. Wainwright tells Langley, "You shall be removed to a loathsome dungeon—you shall be made acquainted with hunger, and cold, and nakedness, and stripes—you shall be converted into a *madman*, and die like a beast!" There is just something about sequestration beneath a structure of living death. Movies do this visually, whether getting us there by elevator (*Halloween 4*) or by taking stairs (*The House on Haunted Hill*, 1999 remake).

I'll let one stand in for the lot. *Hellbound: Hellraiser II* (1988), the sequel to Clive Barker's horror classic *Hellraiser*, takes place largely at the Channard Institute. In the previous film, heroic Kristy solves a special puzzle box that sends Pinhead, a black-leathered "cenobite" whose bald dome is covered with geometrically placed needles, back to Hell. In the sequel, we find Kristy at the asylum. The trauma of fighting Pinhead was apparently too much for her psyche.

The Channard Institute has everything one might expect in a film asylum, from the protagonist's confusion as to where she is to the establishing shot on a stormy night. The superintendent is Dr. Phillip Channard, a perfect villain with his aristocratic British accent and French-sounding name (reminiscent of the pejorative "canard"). To access the subbasement, Channard steps into a rather plain-looking elevator. We watch as he looks at the button panel: "1" illuminates, then "Ground," then "Basement," and finally, "Maintenance." The doors open to screams. This subbasement is damp, dark, steamy, and industrial. We watch an attendant drag a patient along a wide hallway. On the sides are small padded cells fitted with peep windows. Channard pauses to watch the helpless deranged rant away in their tiny prisons. These unfortunates are clearly psychotic and unmedicated. Their purpose seems to be of the guinea pig variety. Channard watches with scientific interest.

Channard eventually ruins himself through hubris after he uses Kristy's knowledge to resurrect her evil stepmother. Using the blood of a subbasement patient, he accesses a labyrinth of Hell, where he tries to take over in order to become the ultimate superintendent. He succeeds in transforming himself into a cenobite thanks to a grotesque drill-lobotomy, after which he re-enters the Channard Institute crying out, "The doctor is in!" He proceeds to tear apart his patients, who have not been getting well but rather have been busily working as unpaid laborers to open demon puzzle boxes for him. Channard gets his comeuppance when a surviving waif patient opens the puzzle box that destroys him.

The Channard Institute's subbasement is a metaphor for the superintendent's own dark character. It also reaffirms the malign nature of the celluloid asylum and the gothic history of psychiatric horror. By summoning this history, Channard's psychiatric underworld taps the base from which the superstructure of pop culture institutional medicine springs. It is the gravest foundation.

THE TREATMENTS

Inside the movie asylum, we can expect to find torture. Pulling the protagonist into the darker reaches of the plotline via institutional medical punishment is a common trope. ECT is a leading method. In the bizarre 1985 Disney sequel to *The Wizard of Oz*, *Return to Oz*, Dorothy goes back to the Land of Oz to discover that it is suffering under the rule of the evil Nome King. Dorothy gets there not by tornado but by way of an asylum breakout. Aunt Em and Uncle Henry have sent her to Dr. Worley's gothic sanitarium to cure her of her post-Oz depression, where she is to be hooked up to a terrifying Victorian ECT machine. Dorothy gets shuffled down a dark hallway in a gurney by a Ratched-type named Nurse Wilson but is saved at the last minute by an electrical storm that knocks out the power.[33]

Hollywood really outdid itself threatening Dorothy with ECT. By trying to cure her "delusions" with electricity, Dr. Worley is essentially trying to destroy her. The filmmakers felt no need to tell us how ECT works, what it's supposed to do, or even that it had not yet been invented. Like the asylum, movie ECT is timeless. In their article "The Portrayal of ECT in American Movies," Andrew McDonald and Gerry Walter cite a study from the early 1950s in which a patient refused ECT treatment based on just having watched *The Snake Pit*. Another study, unsurprisingly, found that people who had seen *One Flew Over the Cuckoo's Nest* were "put off" by the treatment. Reviewing movies from the 1940s through the 1990s, McDonald and Walter find that ECT depictions had become standardized. "Although unmodified ECT has obvious dramatic potential," they explain, "one begins to suspect that much of the medical research in these films involved watching how ECT was performed in earlier movies." We typically get this routine: "the swabbing of the temples, the obligatory shoving-in of the mouth guard, the porters with white bow ties, and the unconscious patient rolled out of the ECT suite after treatment." McDonald and Walter describe *Return to Oz* as "a trenchant antipsychiatry metaphor." It is a reasonable argument.[34]

In some movies, ECT machines are literal killing devices. In *Death Wish II* (1982), the bad guy gets slain by one; evil doll Chucky kills a no-good psychiatrist with an ECT headband in *Child's Play* (1988); and, in *The House on Haunted Hill* (1999), a woman is electrified while the lights flash and sparks fly. The use of ECT as agent of destruction really hits the mark in *Requiem for a Dream* (2000). This disturbing film includes a scene in which a mother broken by diet pills gets subject to unanesthetized ECT. Ellen Burstyn plays Sara Goldfarb, who signs a release form in a hospital from hell. We watch as Burstyn is transported by gurney down a long hallway, then has electrodes stuck to her forehead and two metal rods placed at her temples. We see the panic in her eyes as the mouthpiece gets rammed in. With each blast, her eyes squeeze shut in agony, and she convulses. Then she opens her eyes, fully conscious, before being blasted yet again. This is bad, but the fact that the horror is intercut with fast-cuts of her son getting his arm amputated, her son's girlfriend demeaning herself in a public sex act, and her son's friend scrubbing a prison floor while vomiting, makes for a truly spectacular if grotesque scene. Afterward, we see the effect of ECT when her friends stop by the hospital for a visit. Burstyn has become a zombie. ECT has literally burned away her personality and appearance. She was nominated for an Academy Award for her performance.[35]

Requiem for a Dream puts an exclamation point on the Hollywood ECT narrative. Though anesthetics have been in use since as early as the 1940s, they are almost never depicted in film. Whereas in real life ECT involves "a short, controlled set of electrical pulses for a few seconds," in movies it's more like Dr. Frankenstein pulling the switch. The surging volts go on and on, often accompanied by blaring horns or sharp violins. Or there might be no soundtrack, emphasizing the electric crackle, as in *One Flew Over the Cuckoo's Nest* and *Changeling*. *Shock Corridor* superimposes wild imagery over the suffering character as the music blares. In *Shock Treatment* and *Brain Dead*, the camera sharply pulls back, as if recoiling. In *Insanitarium* (2008), the doctor holds shock handles while foam pours from the patient's mouth and the lights elsewhere in the building flicker. History need not get in the way of a good blast, as *Changeling* and *Return to Oz* show us. In the 1999 remake of *The House on Haunted Hill*, a woman is electrocuted in an ECT blast straight out of a Universal Pictures monster rally, despite the fact that the asylum was closed in 1931, seven years before the treatment was invented.[36]

While ECT is the most common movie asylum torture, insulin therapy gets a few nods, such as in *Frances* (1982) and *A Beautiful Mind* (2001). In the latter film, John Nash is taken into a bleach-white room with a single bed covered in leather straps. Masked nurses stand at attention and attendants tie him in. A close-up shows the needle penetrating skin, the nurse announcing, "administering insulin." The scene cuts between Nash and his wife, who is helplessly watching from an observation window. Then come the convulsions. His wife looks away as Nash thrashes violently, a thick tube up his nose. According to the director, "This sequence was very well researched . . . Patients don't always have the grand mal seizure, but they're not uncommon . . . We presented an intense version." With the foreboding music, the uniformed staff, the blanched look on Nash's face, the white room, and the surveillance apparatus, there is no other way to read this scene than as horror.[37]

Then there is lobotomy. Made notorious in *Cuckoo's Nest*, lobotomies have featured as punishment in a number of films before and since. In Kesey's novel, it is the method used to shut down McMurphy's rebellion. Others have similarly emphasized it as the endgame of the psychiatric threat. Lobotomies figure prominently in *Suddenly, Last Summer*, *A Fine Madness*, *Planet of the Apes*, *Asylum* (1972), and *Frances*, among other films. A panicky kid in *E.T.* does not want to alert the authorities to the little alien because "they'll give it a lobotomy or do experiments or something." In *Session 9* (2001), a movie about a crew cleaning up an abandoned asylum, we are treated to a graphic lobotomy description (complete with chopstick prop) as well several leukotomy attacks. In *Insanitarium*, a mad doctor tells the transorbital history while simultaneously jabbing a pick into the eye socket of his victim. The lobotomy is horror prop in period asylum fantasies like *Sucker Punch* (2011) and *American Horror Story: Asylum* (2012–2013). In *Cheech and Chong's Nice Dreams* (1981), it's a punchline, with a friendly, female psychiatrist leading Pee Wee Herman off, sweetly saying, "It's time for your lobotomy." Even an episode of the classic TV show *The Hulk* has a lobotomizing asylum doctor.[38]

Though the historical moment of the transorbital lobotomy was a brief one, filmmakers have not felt so constrained. In *From Hell* (2001), a conspiracy movie about Jack the Ripper, a modified icepick procedure makes its way back to fin de siècle London. At the Royal London Hospital, we see a screaming woman tied to a gurney, sedated with chloroform, and brought into an operating theater. Surrounded by male observers, a doctor uses a hammer and knife-like tool to tap into her lobes through the skull. The procedure speaks to writer Rafael Yglesias's intention to make a film about "sexual hypocrisy." In *From Hell*, lobotomy is a tool for erasing the minds of the inconvenient, first the woman who carried the crown prince's baby, and then the Ripper himself, who is no longer needed by the royals. The result of the operation is as might be expected—victims become vegetables.[39]

Perhaps the most innovative celluloid asylum torture is in *The Jacket* (2005), in which the patient is drugged and straitjacketed and then locked into a mortuary drawer. In the film, Adrien Brody is Jack Starks, a Gulf War vet who suffers from amnesia. After a series of misadventures, he lands in Alpine Grove Psychiatric Hospital, wrongly convicted of murder and declared insane thanks to his PTSD. Alpine Grove offers the usual collage: screams, long corridors, sparse rooms, paper cups full of pills, and rough attendants. The novelty happens when Jack gets gagged, injected with a mysterious green substance, and taken down into the subbasement. Here he's strapped into a ghastly looking canvas straitjacket and placed on a steel bed before being slammed into a mortuary drawer. The purpose is therapeutic. Explains Dr. Becker (Kris Kristofferson), the technique is designed to "adjust, maybe even reset his violent proclivities, peel away some layers of hate." The rationale: "You can't break something that's already broken." Someone notes that this procedure was "banned in the Seventies," making it part of the mythical *Cuckoo's Nest* era. What the treatment actually does is transport Jack into the future, where he learns how he dies. The torture has created the plot.[40]

PRÉCIS—*GIRL, INTERRUPTED*

Girl, Interrupted (1999) is a master class in the celluloid asylum. The girl in question, Susanna Kaysen (Winona Ryder), is a sensitive soul who winds up in an asylum called Claymoore after a condescending family psychiatrist remands her there for "rest." Though Kaysen signs herself in, it is a classic railroading; we feel the massive patriarchal pressure on her to do so. She is not crazy.[41]

Claymoore is based on McLean Hospital, which is where the real Susanna Kaysen spent time. In the movie, it's a big, gothic, brick structure with long corridors, white rooms, a padded seclusion cell, a tiled hydrotherapy chamber, a glassed-in nurse's station, and a big, bright dayroom. Director James Mangold shot at the Harrisburg State Hospital, using extant lighting. He wanted the film to feel "naked and true."[42]

Girl, Interrupted has a colorful cast of patients. In the dayroom (called the "TV room"), we meet a girl who reads the *Wizard of Oz* and is a "pathological liar;" an obese woman who behaves like a small child; a loud blond who sings plantation songs and refuses to eat; and Lisa, the resident McMurphy. Played by Angelina Jolie, Lisa is a scrapper who always tries to escape, like the titular hero in *Hogan's Heroes*. Her perennial flight attempts to remind us of her purpose, which is to undermine the system. She sees Claymoore for what it is—a prison for nonconformists. Mangold calls Lisa "a total rebel." Eventually, she gets Susanna to escape with her in the film's final act.[43]

The treatments draw from *Cuckoo's Nest*, beginning with scenes of patients lining up to receive their pills from the nurse. In this case, the nurse has a loud Irish brogue. She bellows out names and then waits for the patients to obediently swallow their meds. There are references to ECT as well, and it's clearly viewed as barbaric. The only person who receives it is Lisa. We see her dragged off to the ECT room while a nurse shoots her in the arm with a needle. Afterward, she tells Susanna, "They gave me shocks again. Jamie I have to get out of here." Kaysen recognizes the signs of brain damage, answering softly, "I'm Susanna."

Interestingly, James Mangold explicitly said that he did not want to make "a *Cuckoo's Nest* with women." This just happened "to be a period piece and it happens to involve mental health and a mental institution." His references to *The Wizard of Oz*, for instance, are intended to showcase the bizarre unreality of asylum life, rather than following Kesey's insight that asylums symbolize the real world. Mangold also did not want to suggest that mental illness is not real or simply a label used for social oppression. As he explains in the DVD commentary, mental illness is related to "genetic predispositions and chemical imbalances. There's millions of mysteries in the human mind that can explain how we fall astray." Clearly, Mangold protests too much. Without Forman, this film would have looked much different. The atmosphere, the mythical 1960s moment, the cast, the set, the rebel, the treatments, and even the lighting inexorably evoke this referent. It is better to say that this movie riffs on Forman while adding other themes.[44]

In the July 2000 issue of *Boston Review*, a doctor who served as director of the psychiatric training program at McLean while Kaysen was there commented on the accuracy of the film and compared it to the novel. The movie, he wrote, is "flawed and banal," while the book is an "elliptical meditation on the experience, with layers of irony, humor, and compassion for the keepers as well as for the kept." Sadly, the movie is just another case of Hollywoodization. McLean has become "The Land of Oz," Lisa "Jack Nicholson's McMurphy," and Kaysen's relationship with her "Thelma and Louise." Others had different quarrels. A *Cineaste* contributor asked why the women in the film showed "no solidarity." Regardless, *Girl, Interrupted* was a box office hit and it garnered numerous awards, including a Best Supporting Actress Oscar for Angelina Jolie. And despite Mangold's wishes, it did become a female *Cuckoo's Nest*. Even the critical praise for its avoiding "snake-pit clichés'" mirrored past reviews of Forman's movie. Just as people connected with Forman's film, late 1990s audiences loved the boldness of Jolie (who was also nominated for "Best Hissy Fit" at the 2000 Teen Choice Awards) and empathized with Ryder's efforts to defeat stifling social expectations. The movie worked because it was a believable allegory for problems the audience could identify with.[45]

Girl, Interrupted demonstrates the power of standardization. Claymoore is built along cinematic lines, fabricated out of identifiable stereotypes and stuffed with recognizable figures. It lets Mangold play with the tropes and manipulate them to suit his narrative goals of adolescent rebellion and growth. Standardization creates the stage upon which his drama is set.

CHAPTER 11

RETURN OF THE GOTHIC

> If you're anywhere remote—the woods, an old house, an abandoned mental institution in the middle of a blackout—then yes, your chances of being in a horror movie are much higher.
> —Seth Grahame-Smith, *How to Survive a Horror Movie*

Movies have depicted Hogarthian "period" bedlams since 1946's *Bedlam*, a movie that configures the historical asylum as a gloomy exemplar of a pre-Enlightenment past, when medicine meant pain and abuse. Postwar, Freudian, hero narratives checked this, giving us asylums that might be crowded but at least had heroic doctors and human attendants. In the era following deinstitutionalization, however, the dark, historical frame returned with a vengeance. As the century closed, Americans reveled in a new gothic sensibility. Notes Mark Edmundson, we became fixated on the shadow selves of celebrities, leered at superstar murderers, pored through vampire horrors, experimented with S&M, discovered terrible "recovered memories," tracked right-wing militia conspiracies, and intoxicated ourselves with self-help and Prozac. Back of this fin de siècle gothicism, I'd emphasize, were deepening structural traumas: a service economy replacing an industrial one; finance and technology revolutionizing capital accumulation; and deindustrialization and deinstitutionalization leaving us with big, empty, rotting structures to explore.[1]

As state hospitals shuttered, filmmakers saw fit to adjoin the *Cuckoo's Nest* era (1950s–1970s) to an abhorrent past. In Forman's film, shot in a real place while the institutional model still shakily stood, the horrors of the asylum are mainly metaphorical. A serene Nurse

Ratched and a clean, hospital environment stand-in for modern control and bureaucracy. The ECT scene is carried out in a bright space, with McMurphy surrounded by competent nurses and physicians. By the turn of the twenty-first century, this era would be imaginatively overhauled, unencumbered by the niceties of adept medical practice. Moving the dark past into the recent past and recent treatments into the dark past, filmmakers flattened out the history of the asylum, making it into one continuous, seamless nightmare.

POE MEETS CALIGARI

In *Shutter Island* (2010), Leonardo DiCaprio plays Teddy, a US Marshal sent to an isolated island asylum to investigate a missing patient named Rachel Solando. Though Shutter Island sits off the coast of Boston, it might as well be on another planet. It is a gray, authoritarian environment covered with walls, guards, and barbed wire. The dark, loud music tells us we are entering a perilous landscape, the jeep Teddy and his partner Chuck ride in evoking a military context. Through a series of gates they go, each manned by guards. Inside the main building the Marshals meet the superintendent, Dr. Cawley (Ben Kingsley). Cawley is an aristocratic man of mystery, equipped with the hint of a British accent, a pipe, and a goatee. We immediately do not trust him. On his office walls, we see classics of asylum horror, including an illustration of Benjamin Rush's Tranquilizing Chair. Dr. Cawley tries to educate his visitors. Unlike in the bad old days, we "try to heal, try to cure. And if that fails at least we provide them with a measure of comfort in their lives, calm."[2]

As we might expect, Teddy will find evidence of exactly the opposite. He learns of a secret building, a lighthouse "tower" in which dark experiments are performed. According to a strange woman he meets in a cave, in the tower doctors conduct mind-altering procedures including the transorbital lobotomy. Such operations are designed to render patients "obedient" and "tractable." She compares these with recent Nazi and Soviet efforts. The film's director Martin Scorsese ratchets the tension by progressively stripping Teddy of his authority and independence. First, he surrenders his gun. Then he changes out of his wet, G-Man suit and into hospital whites. Finally, he becomes a patient himself.

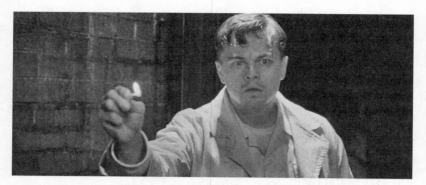

Teddy Daniels (Leonardo DiCaprio) uncovers dark secrets in the asylum in *Shutter Island* (2010)

Ironically, Teddy thinks he's playing a double game. Ostensibly only looking for Rachel Solando, he is also secretly hunting Andrew Laeddis, an inmate who had set the fire that killed Teddy's wife. When he learns about the tower, he fantasizes about "blow[ing] the lid off" the place. The more Teddy explores, the darker the landscape gets. He breaks into the "dangerous" ward and finds a dripping dungeon replete with flickering lights, shadows, stone walls, and bars. Patients lurk in dank cells, some naked and reduced to animal states. Finally, Teddy makes it to the lighthouse. Up the tower he climbs, where he finds the evil superintendent in his lair. But everything Teddy thinks is wrong.

Teddy is not a Marshal. He's not even Teddy. He's a patient, incarcerated at Shutter Island for killing his wife in response to her murdering their three children. Dr. Cawley and Chuck (who turns out to be Dr. Lester Sheehan) tell him that they've been conducting the "most radical cutting-edge roleplay ever attempted in psychiatry." They have allowed him to live the delusion that he's a Marshal (he only formerly was one) named Teddy, in order for him to cathartically realize his illusion through deduction. Teddy is Andrew Laeddis—an anagram for Edward (Teddy) Daniels; Rachel Solando is an anagram for his dead wife, Dolores Chanal. The purpose of the experiment is to save him from a lobotomy. Sadly, the next day, he's back to being Teddy again. We see Dr. Sheehan nod to Dr. Cawley, and then attendants escort him away. The tip of an icepick protrudes from towels carried by one of them.

Like many other asylum films, Scorsese's makes use of tradition. It re-creates "Tarr and Fether," with Dr. Cawley playing the Monsieur Maillard role. Cawley has "taken over" the asylum by convincing the board to allow him to carry out his radical, therapeutic technique. Just as Maillard's patients believe they are teapots and chickens, Cawley lets Andrew Laeddis believe he is a Marshal. Teddy, in turn, plays the young adventurer. He enters the strange asylum and ultimately uncovers its secrets. Just like in Poe's tale, the protagonist is the last to figure out what is happening, and he remains willfully in the dark even at the end.

If *Shutter Island* evokes Poe in its characterizations, its structure conjures *Caligari*. As Walter C. Metz explains, in both movies "a narrator tells a story of a mad killer and we come to learn that the 'killer' is the director of a mental institution housing the insane narrator." Both films want us to think one thing, and then topple our assumptions with a flourish. Both configure the asylum as a dark and twisted place, and both force the viewer into an uncomfortable alliance with the mad. We are aware of the nightmare, but unsure as to the content of its ultimate reality.[3]

Shutter Island's gothic film noir rests on a certain historical claim. Postwar psychiatric treatments have become gothic horrors. These horrors, as other filmmakers have implied, carry up to present in an unbroken chain of despair. For instance, in *The Silence of the Lambs*, Clarice literally descends into a subterranean dungeon with dripping stone walls located under a modern mental hospital, giving lie to the pretense of modern treatments. Here she finds a vampire. This return of the gothic is a recent trend. Only five years earlier, director Michael Mann had put Lecter in a bright, white space.

Movies like *Shutter Island* and *Silence of the Lambs* use gothic themes to address modern dilemmas while misrepresenting psychiatric history. Few do this with more flair than 2003's *Gothika*. Starting with the title, the movie presents the modern mental hospital as a nightmare prison space, haunted by ghosts and having no redeeming therapeutic value. The Woodward Penitentiary Psychiatric and Correctional Facility for Women has classically gothic features, including a dark, shadowy interior; long, concrete corridors with pipes along the ceilings; and a looming, castle-like, stone edifice (initially shown in a lightning storm). Note that the word "Penitentiary" comes first, summoning the old dream of rehabilitation through penitence. The combination "Psychiatric" and "Correctional Facility" tells us that this institution is part of a prison complex. Combining places of psychiatric and criminal control with gender, Woodward frames the protagonist's dilemma. Like the film's title, Dr. Miranda Grey's name loudly communicates the gothic theme. She begins the film as a doctor but will become a patient.

At the start of the film we see Dr. Grey (Halle Berry) attempt to analyze a violent, sexual patient named Chloe (Penelope Cruz). Grey is unhappy with Chloe's progress, thinking that she is overmedicated. The condescending superintendent calms her, joking that only he can see the big picture, since he's "God . . . or just an overworked hospital bureaucrat." Within the first seven minutes, the dynamics are all in place. This is a gothic institution of control for women. A female doctor is trying to save patients with talk and understanding. She's hampered by ineffective drugs and a masterly superintendent, who, it turns out, also happens to be her husband.

Suitably, the trigger for events is a Woman in White encountered along a lonely highway at night. Swerving to avoid her, Grey gets out of her car and approaches. The young lady spontaneously combusts and grabs Grey, and the screen goes black. Grey awakens in a cell. She has been thrust into her own asylum, accused of murdering her husband. She has no memory of this. She gets agitated and has to be restrained and sedated. The camera focuses on the needle entering her arm, intercut with her crying and thrashing, followed by a slow distortion of her perspective as the drug takes effect. Ultimately, we learn that the female on the highway is the ghost of a woman raped and murdered by the evil superintendent. The ghost possesses Grey to avenge herself, using Grey's body to kill the villain. The local sheriff is the superintendent's partner in crime, and he has also been raping Chloe in her cell. The truth is finally outed when Grey breaks out of the asylum and discovers the torture barn set up by her husband and the sheriff. She kills the sheriff in an act of self-defense, earning her own freedom.

Gothika makes explicit connections between incarceration and institutionalization. The massive, panopticon-style dayroom announces the nightmare. It is a big, concrete space with a massive, tall window gridded with steel, a barred entranceway, a glassed-in observation booth, and televisions bolted up high. Tinny classical music pumps in from somewhere. The inmates wear hospital gowns and rock themselves or stare off into space. In the dayroom, Grey gets a sisterly pep talk from Chloe: "Even if you tell the truth, no one will listen," because "you're crazy. And the more you try to prove them wrong, the crazier you'll appear."[4]

Grey has stereotypical experiences: cups of pills administered by a Ratched-type nurse, injections from big needles while pinned, a concentration-camp style group shower in a poorly lit room, horrific flashbacks and nightmares, and a psychiatric reframing of her legitimate experiences as craziness. Even her professional credentials are turned against her. As her attorney explains, "The fact that you're a brilliant psychiatrist is gonna have the juries thinking, 'Hey if she wanted to kill somebody, she could probably fake insanity and get away with it.' "[5]

Gothika not only makes a modern institution "look" gothic and has it perform the gothic function of dragging dark truths to light, but it also updates old themes. For instance, the imperiled waif is an African American psychiatrist, and the Woman in White is a literal ghost. The evil superintendent is also African American, and he winks ironically at the God-like power typically assigned to his archetype. More to the point, as in *The Silence of the Lambs*, this asylum thrusts modern treatments and technologies into a dismal, gothic space, purposely blurring past and present. It is an alchemy that, if not always convincing, is representative of the post-deinstitutionalized landscape.[6]

HISTORY LESSONS

On November 4, 2004, a small group of state legislators and reporters opened the storage room at the Oregon State Hospital where the cremated remains, or "cremains," of some 3,500 people sat on the shelves. Over the next several years, news articles, books, and a new memorial would bring attention to these forgotten souls. Explained the superintendent, "The story of the cremains is in large part a metaphor of what has happened here in terms of the mental health system . . . It is, of course, ironic that people, in essence, seem more concerned about the dead than the living." This irony is what drives the new

gothic narrative. Conjuring horrors in order to historicize and quarantine our fears, we ignore the living. As if to parody this sentiment,
there is 2014's *House of Dust*, its title echoing *Library of Dust*, the book
which told of the cremains discovery. In this micro-budget shocker,
a group of college kids breaks into an abandoned asylum and discovers urns of cremains. After they accidentally inhale the dust, they are
possessed by the malevolent spirits of dead inmates, some of whom
perished via power-drill lobotomies. We are told that this story is "Inspired by True Events." The "True Events" are apparently the discovery
of the urns.[7]

House of Dust and other films endeavor to perform an educative
function. They want to teach us about the history of psychiatry. In
Shutter Island, for example, though Dr. Cawley might look like a classic, evil superintendent, from his lips we learn the trajectory of institutional medicine. He tells Teddy that there is a "war" afoot. The "old
school . . . believes in shock therapy, partial lobotomies, spa treatments for the most docile patients. Psychosurgery is what we call it.
The new school is enamored of psychopharmacology. It's the future,
they say. Maybe it is. I don't know." For Cawley, the answer is neither
school. He proffers instead the "radical idea that if you treat a patient
with respect and listen to what he's trying to tell you, you just might
reach him." Cawley neatly summarizes the dark past and knits it to
the dark present, while opening up a therapeutic escape hatch, however small. For we know that psychopharmacology will win out, and
that the mentally ill will remain stigmatized and mistreated. The im-
plication is that we must do better, though the going will be tough.
Psychopharmacology is powerful, as it has "money behind it." The historical take away is the classic American tragedy of reform derailed
by the Almighty Dollar.[8]

Other movies also aim to enlighten. *Session 9* (2001), as previously
discussed, tells of a cleanup crew working an abandoned institution
in New England and has a character teach us about the transorbital
lobotomy over a Chinese takeout lunch. Holding a chopstick to a
young crewman's eye, he explains, "Insert a thin metal pipette into
the orbital frontal cortex and enter the soft tissue of the frontal lobe.
A few simple smooth up and down jerks to sever the lateral hypothal-
amus, all resulting in a rapid reduction of stress for our little patient
here. Total time elapsed two minutes. Only side effect—black eye.

Recommended treatment? Sunglasses." The movie culminates with the killer fatally lobotomizing a team member with a leukotome.[9]

John Carpenter's *The Ward* (2010) fully engages the educative impulse. Set in a mental hospital in 1966, the opening credit sequence is a slide show of psychiatry's greatest nightmares, including Hogarth paintings, Rush's Tranquilizer Chair, ECT, lobotomy, restraints, and victimized patients. Over the course of the film, Carpenter heroically manages to pack in: forced showers, death by ECT, death by icepick lobotomy, pills in paper cups, a naturally lit dayroom, thunderstorms, straitjackets, hypnotherapy, scary corridors, damp tunnels, subbasements, burly attendants, a Nurse Ratched character, a mysterious, British-accented superintendent carrying out experimental treatments, off-the-wall fellow inmates, a McMurphy rebel, and a ghost named Alice. One patient actually says, "*Nobody* gets out." To ice the cake, Carpenter sets the film in Oregon.[10]

Carpenter shot *The Ward* in a vacant building on the campus of the Eastern State Hospital. A working institution in Washington State enduring the effects of deinstitutionalization, Eastern has gone from a high of over two thousand patients in the 1950s to just 317 beds today. Setting the movie in the 1960s lets Carpenter put us right into the mythic *Cuckoo's Nest* era. In an interview, Carpenter explained, "In the Sixties, you could be forcibly kept against your will . . . so you could be thrown in, like you are in the movie, and no matter what you want they keep you there, and do what they want to do with you."[11]

We get a similar history lesson in *Stonehearst Asylum* (2014). An update of "Tarr and Fether," *Stonehearst Asylum* concerns a newly minted physician who arrives at a desolate sanitarium to pursue a career in mind medicine in 1899. The inmates have already taken over, led by the mad Dr. Silas Lamb (Ben Kingsley in another superintendent role). Dr. Lamb is an R. D. Laing type, who tells the newcomer, we don't "sedate our patients into a stupor with bromides and the like" but rather "celebrate them in their natural unadulterated state." Unlike Maillard, however, Lamb is not trying to effect any cure. He claims that he's more enlightened than the previous doctor, whom we see in flashback torturing patients with spinning chairs, tube feedings, straitjackets, hosings, heat boxes, and the famous tranquilizer chair. But Lamb himself, for some reason, is personally shown to pioneer ECT. His device, cranked by hand, kills the previous doctor and sets a brutal attendant's head on fire.[12]

Stonehearst Asylum communicates the gothic idea of the horrible past bridging into the present. On the cusp of the twentieth century, Lamb banishes the old tortures while introducing a new one—ECT— continuing the timeline of institutional barbarity into modern times. In a final twist, we learn that the visiting doctor is actually an escaped mental patient here to woo a waif (Kate Beckinsale). Poe's critique of disastrous democratic reform is transmogrified into a historical morality tale about the irony of psychiatric "progress."

Fiction offered plenty of new gothic asylums apace with film. In Lisa Carey's 2004 novel *Love in the Asylum*, two young people, Alba and Oscar, build a relationship in a fancy New England sanitarium. Theirs is not a gothic tale, but the second story woven within *Love in the Asylum* is. Alba discovers the unsent letters of a former patient named Mary. Mary is the daughter of an Abenaki Indian mother and is tormented by epileptic fits that her Native American uncle calls her "gift." He is right; when Mary succumbs, she travels to the Land of the Dead. But instead of becoming a Shaman she is sent off to Saint Dyphna's (the former name of the hospital) by her brutal, white husband. At Dyphna's, the nuns rule with an iron fist. "I have seen women hit across the face," Mary writes, "dragged across the cafeteria floor by their arms; sometimes the nuns force porridge into patients' mouths." Thanks to her ability to enter the Land of the Dead, Mary discovers that she can provide succor to her fellow unfortunates. When Dyphna's gets modernized and sold off by the Catholic Church, Mary's life takes a turn for the worse. In the new hospital setting, she's administered the "sleep cure" along with insulin therapy. After a blast of ECT destroys her ability to enter the Land of the Dead, she kills herself.[13]

Carey's book juxtaposes Alba and Oscar's comfortable modern sanitarium with a brutal, historical place where Mary is unjustly imprisoned and ultimately destroyed for her difference. The very ground of Abenaki Hospital portends doom. It was bought by a white doctor from the tribe after its men died fighting in the American Revolution and its women were killed in a massacre. The land is said to be cursed by "spells left behind by grudge-hungry Indians." The unfortunate Mary (real name: Mesatawe) is similarly annihilated by the white man. Like in *Shadowland*, here is a hospital tainted by an im-perial past. In a timeline of evil, we learn the history of institutional psychiatry and how "modern" somatic treatments proved to be more destructive than mere physical violence.[14]

Young adult readers could learn the gothic psychiatric history plot as well, in books like *Asylum* by Madeleine Roux, which provides a tour of a haunted asylum taken by adventurous youngsters. Youthful angst, love, and friendship get tested by ghosts once subjected to psy-chiatric torture. The book includes artistically rendered, abandoned asylum pictures.[15]

MONSTERS

In 2007, director Rob Zombie remade *Halloween*. The gothic dis-tance traveled since 1979 is evident. In Carpenter's original film, My-ers's evil is something inborn and unknowable. In the remake, Rob Zombie shifts the perspective and the critique. He makes Myers, not Lori Strode, the hero. The opposite of Carpenter's average joe, blank slate creation, this Myers is huge, with long, ropy hair over his face à la Samara. He wears a variety of masks until he finally dons the classic one—though this version looks distinctly weathered and dead-looking. Much of Zombie's film involves Myers's origin story, appropriate for the new perspective. We learn that Michael is the product of a dysfunctional and impoverished household. His mom is a stripper, and his dad is an abusive alcoholic who ridicules his mas-culinity. Myers is thus the result of working-class desperation, a boy who abuses small animals just as he himself is abused. He begins his murderous rampage by killing a bully, and his later murders follow the moral economy of retaliation. He slaughters his dad, then his sister's crude boyfriend, and then his cruel sister. He's thrown into Smith's Grove Sanitarium, which we are told happens after "one of the lengthiest and most expensive trials in the state's history." The social cost of Michael's neglect, in blood and in dollars, is staggering.

Whereas Carpenter's Smith's Grove is a nondescript office building suitable to the monster's anonymity, in the remake it's a big, gloomy structure, filled with aging tile walls, bilious yellow hallways, and metal bars. Michael appears to be the only patient. For that matter, nobody seems to be in charge. In this horrible storage depot for the forgotten, the best advice comes from a Latino, ex-con attendant, who tells him not to "let those walls get you down. Believe me, I know. I spent a little time behind walls. I know they can drive you crazy. You gotta look beyond the walls, you know, learn to live inside your head." Taking the advice literally, Michael does not speak to anyone for fifteen years. More than merely failing Michael as it did in the first film, this bleak asylum transforms him into a true monster. The new, guiltier Dr. Loomis suits the new narrative. He admits to Michael that he has failed him. Keeping in line with the hero archetype, Myers escapes while in the act of saving a female inmate from the sexual predations of two attendants. A classic slasher rampage commences, a flock of sexy teens and clueless adults going down one by one, until Loomis and Lori Strode kill Michael with a handgun.

This *Halloween* is a gothic parable of modern social undeath. Whereas in the original the asylum is merely ineffective, here it is a penitentiary that ruins a soul already injured by his impoverished environment. The lesson of past sins haunting the present is never clearer than in an abysmal institution that takes in a troubled child and vomits him out fifteen years later as an unrecognizable, enormous killing machine. Like Frankenstein's monster, Michael is the product of a botched experiment. The cynicism runs deep; it is hard to like any of Zombie's characters. Lori is reduced to mere plot cypher and Dr. Loomis is a hypocritical pop-psychologist who cashes in on his failure to heal by writing a book about Michael. As intended, we sympathize with the abused giant. We are pleased when he murders those who seem to "have it coming," while we tragically understand that he must ultimately be destroyed, because he is a monster, after all. In his sacrifice, we purge ourselves of any guilty feelings.

Perhaps the most popular modern gothic asylum is Arkham Asylum. The home of Batman's most deranged foes, Arkham is featured in numerous contemporary films, stories, video games, comics, and graphic novels. It has a surprisingly long historical lineage, starting in the writings of a weird fiction author whose work in the 1920s and 1930s proved foundational in the shaping of modern horror. H. P. Lovecraft created "Arkham Sanitarium" along with other institutions and populated them with monsters and the supernaturally afflicted. In 1974, Jack C. Harris, a future DC Comics editor, proposed the idea of an "Arkham Asylum" in the world of Batman to writer Denny O'Neil.

Harris recalled, "What better asylum could there be for such maniacs than Arkham, the dark dwelling of tormented souls from Lovecraft's horrific tales?" Lately, Arkham has seen a vibrant resurgence as gothic repository for monstrous villains.[16]

Howard Phillips Lovecraft grew up in Providence, Rhode Island, about a mile and a half away from the Butler Hospital for the Insane. Though he never entered its buildings, he knew Butler well. Both of his parents died there. His father perished after five years of "paralysis" (likely neurosyphilis), and his mother, committed for "traumatic psychosis" due to "an awareness of approaching bankruptcy," died from a botched gall bladder surgery at the hospital. Lovecraft's view of the asylum as a place of horrors was undoubtedly colored by his family history, as well as by his absorption of the worst of his era's virulent xenophobic, jingoistic, social-Darwinist thinking. His fiction, which often includes references to asylums or even takes place in them, explicitly makes connections between incarcerated insanity and monstrosity, degeneracy, and racial degradation.[17]

In "The Thing on the Doorstep" (1937), Edward Derby is possessed by his wife's dead father. He rants and raves until his "frenzy" subsides into catatonia. Because he is a man of wealth, his personal "doctor, banker, and lawyer" are all consulted, as well as two "specialist colleagues" of his family physician. They collectively find him to be insane and have him committed to the "Arkham Sanitarium." The story's narrator and Derby's best friend, Daniel Upton, eventually goes in and kills Derby, knowing that he is possessed. Some four decades later, Arkham Sanitarium re-entered the popular culture's bloodstream as "Arkham Hospital," and later still as Arkham Asylum. But it wouldn't be until the success of Frank Miller's 1986 *Batman: The Dark Knight Returns* that Arkham fully came into its own.[18]

Originating as a four-part comic miniseries and then reprinted as a graphic novel, *Batman: The Dark Knight Returns* finds the retired caped crusader coping with grief over the death of Robin. When an old foe, Two Face, returns, Batman relaunches his career. Noting the reappearance of his nemesis, the Joker, hitherto catatonic at the Arkham Asylum, returns to consciousness and escapes, thanks to the poison gas he unleashes while on a talk show. In Miller's modern noir, Arkham is literally a warehouse for the storage of an old enemy who can reactivate and escape once his heroic adversary comes back. Three years later, DC released the innovative and well-received graphic novel *Arkham Asylum: A Serious House on Serious Earth*. In this work, Batman learns that the criminal patients have taken over Arkham and are holding hostages. Entering to find the Joker and friends, the Dark Knight discovers that institutional treatment is worthless and has even made some (like Two Face) worse. The incarcerated are deformed and deranged, yet also manically celebratory. Combining Poe's cynical social commentary with Lovecraft's ideas of biological degeneracy, this tale cements Arkham as a gothic hell. Eventually, Batman must face his own demons, which he manages with the help of some heavy-handed Jungian symbolism. Other Arkham Asylum adventures follow, including the 1992 graphic novel *Batman: The Last Arkham*, in which the cowled crusader fakes insanity in order to get inside and solve a crime à la *Shock Corridor*.[19]

Arkham Asylum made it to the big screen in *Batman Forever* (1995), the third film in the revamped film series started by Tim Burton in 1989. Here Edward Nygma, a.k.a. The Riddler, loses his mind after getting blasted by his own mind control device. We see him at the end of the movie ranting in a striped, untied straitjacket in a dark padded cell at the end of a long corridor. Arkham Asylum looks like a mansion, introduced on a rainy night, looming behind an ornate iron gate. In *Batman & Robin* (1997), the asylum is reimagined as a castle, tall and geometrical, sitting on an isolated rock across a bridged chasm. Again, we see it on a rainy night. Inside lives Mr. Freeze. A guard tells him, "Get used to it. You're going to be here a very long, long time." Freeze is freed by Poison Ivy and Bane, but when he's defeated, back to Arkham he goes, now with Poison Ivy as his cellmate. When the series received a reboot under director Christopher Nolan, Arkham Asylum became a true nightmare factory. In *Batman Begins* (2005), within Arkham's bleak walls, an evil psychiatrist called The Scarecrow experiments on his patients, using a terrifying hallucinatory drug to torment them. He will pump the drug out into the water supply from beneath the asylum, infecting the city. Nolan has reconfigured Arkham as a malefic site of contamination, ground zero in a plot to destroy Gotham. Lovecraft's asylum has thus become the ultimate, post-deinstitutionalized, gothic location, a horror house for monstrous villainy. Inside, evil can be stored or even exported—but never treated.[20]

HAUNTED WRECKS

The closest relative to the new gothic asylum is the haunted house, appropriate given that so many have become haunted "attractions" for tourists. The haunted house evokes past sins and contemporary shortcomings. Shirley Jackson's *Haunting of Hill House* sets out some parameters. She writes, "No live organism can continue for long to exist sanely under conditions of absolute reality; even larks and ka-tydids are supposed, by some, to dream. Hill House, not sane, stood by itself against its hills, holding darkness within." This is a "place of despair," with "maniac" architectural angles and long halls of "un-lovely exactness," inlaid with "a series of doors, all closed." Bad things happen here.[21]

Like Hill House, abandoned institutions personify insane and stored-up evil. Living second lives as zones of horror, they are perfect for filmmakers looking for scary, ready-made sets. In this section, I'd like to suggest that the guiding metaphor for abandoned asylums in film is the battery. Silent yet alive with stored energy, these mon-strosities crackle with the carnage of "evil" medicine. The first film to capitalize on this seems to be *Doom Asylum*, a 1987 direct-to-video schlockfest, mainly remembered for the small part played by Kristin Davis, a woman later famous for her role in *Sex and the City*. In *Doom Asylum*, she spends much of her time wandering around the ruins of a real New Jersey mental hospital in a swimsuit, until she gets butch-ered by the maniac. The plot is that, ten years ago, a man and his fian-cée were in a car wreck nearby. The fiancée died, but the man sprang to life on the autopsy table. He killed the coroner and then decided to stay, even after the institution shut down. Now he haunts the place, going under the name The Coroner. Enter an all-girl punk band and a group of teens. Though cheaply shot, *Doom Asylum* makes good use of an abandoned asylum and at just the right time—this was when the state hospitals closed by deinstitutionalization began to rot and look scary.[22]

In the late 1980s, the haunted asylum came into its own. Compare *A Nightmare on Elm Street 3: Dream Warriors* (1987) with *A Nightmare on Elm Street 5: The Dream Child* (1989). In *Dream Warriors*, Freddy Krueger attacks kids in a working institution where it is revealed that he's the product of the gang rape of his mother, who was trapped over

Christmas in the violent ward. In *The Dream Child*, we relive the episode of conception. But this asylum looks much different from the one in *Dream Warriors*. No longer a dorm, *Dream Child*'s institution might be called Cartoon Hogarth, with its stylized shadows, dingy yellow lights, and a writhing throng in dirty white uniforms. After the attendants leave, a heavy iron door slams shut and the camera pans down on the helpless nun as she disappears beneath a mass of groping hands. The heroes later re-enter the now-abandoned asylum, and it resembles an ancient factory, complete with gothic clock towers protruding into a cloudy night sky. The movie culminates in a scene inspired by Escher, with staircases going every direction. Freddy is here, powered by the place that created him.[23]

The battery imagery is also apparent in post-deinstitutionalized fiction. In John Saul's six-part serial novel *The Blackstone Chronicles* (1997), an abandoned mental institution leaks evil into a small town, infecting it with despair and death. The tale revolves around a mysterious figure who haunts the defunct asylum, sending different items to various townsfolk. Each part of the novel concerns a different item, each bringing destruction with it. A doll, for example, convinces a woman to leap from her roof. A cigarette lighter ignites a house along with its occupant. And so on. Eventually, we learn that these items come from the asylum, and their "targets" are relatives of people who suffered within. The sender is the town's newspaperman, Oliver Metcalf, although he doesn't realize what he is doing. His father, the now-deceased superintendent, twisted his son's mind so badly that he enters a delusional state when he sends the gifts.

The Blackstone Chronicles is situated in a big, abandoned institution as a depot of malevolent energy, powered by its psychiatric past and carrying evil into the present. Though long closed, the asylum is merely "sleeping." In flashbacks, we learn about the source of the charge, with scenes of punitive and unanesthetized ECT, icepick lobotomies, patient suicide, forced tube-feeding, restraints, and vivisection. One patient was committed for refusing to conform to her gender: "Little boys don't wear dresses, do they?" the matron scolds. We ominously read how no one "beyond the Asylum's walls [would] ever see the child again." Ruminating on the hydrotherapy room, a man touring the wrecked hospital asks his companion, "What the hell kind of place was this?" to which she responds, "No different from hundreds of others, I suspect." In other words, such evil batteries might be anywhere. The book closes with the main character climbing into a demolition machine and destroying the building's edifice, battering away at the "evil that cloaked itself in the guise of medical science."[24]

By the dawn of the twenty-first century, there were enough abandoned asylums to make for plenty of hair-raising celluloid experiences. *Session 9* (2001) is a smashing example. It concerns the asbestos abatement crew working the deserted Danvers asylum in Massachusetts. This is a real place, and the movie was actually filmed there. There was also real asbestos, mold, and toxic substances, which quarantined filming to certain sections. *Session 9* follows the abatement crew as the madness stored in the place infects them.

Session 9 owes much to *The Shining*, with its long, creeping hallway shots, wide angles, big slow aerials, opening tour at the facility, jarring day-titles, and growing derangement of the lead character. In a history lesson early on, a guard explains, "Nearly all these places got closed down in the eighties ya know, the budget cuts. It's called deinstitutionalization." The youngest crewmember is shocked: "So they just dumped the people on the street?" Responds the guard, "Some. Some went to like, home care type programs." We also learn that some of the ex-patients chose to come back and squat in the wreckage. The guard concludes, "God knows why . . . I'd rather sleep in the street personally, but then, I'm not nuts." A local official gives us some more information, leading a tour and talking about the Kirkbride architecture. It makes the place resemble a "giant flying bat" with a "bat body" and "giant crooked bat wings." He laments that history itself has entombed the horror; because Danvers is on the historical registry, they can't tear it down and replace it with "a Walmart, maybe." He also boasts how the "prefrontal lobotomy was perfected here at Danvers." To drive it home, he informs the crew that they called the ward for violent patients "the Snake Pit."[25]

Session 9 wants to enlighten as it terrifies. It wants us to know that the psychiatric horrors were real. We get the detailed explanation of lobotomy, along with lingering shots of cracked paint, newspaper and magazine pictures pasted to cell walls, broken toilets, bizarre murals, barred windows, hydrotherapy tubs, and a leukotome icepick. One of the characters discovers a book and reads aloud the various

diagnostic categories for asylum commitment used in the past. Another plays dusty recordings of therapy sessions with a multiple personality case.

Session 9 makes the institution into a gothic metaphor for contemporary concerns. In this case, the institution represents the death of
upward mobility. The crew is white, working class, and they all dream
of something better, an "exit strategy," as one of them says. Cleaning the wreckage, they fantasize about improving their lot and escaping the dreary confines of their lives. The commotion they make
out of the $10,000 bonus for finishing early punctuates this theme.
The director confirms that the movie is really "about the American
Dream gone awry." Deinstitutionalization went apace of deindustrialization. Dreams of a bright future turned into nightmares for both
mental patients and the industrial working class at the same time.
Whether by globalization or by deinstitutionalization, ruins slowly
replaced physical symbols of progress. But the ruins could still produce something—nightmares.

AMERICAN HORROR STORIES

As educational passports to a dismal psychiatric past, the redux
gothic asylum is a gift to the horror film industry. Whether abandoned[26] or occupied, they offered an open invitation to the wildest fantasies of the creative filmmaker. Jack Snyder's *Sucker Punch*
(2011) answers the question, "Just how wild are we talking about?" In
Lennox House for the Mentally Insane, we find robots, giant samu-
rai, dragons, and machine guns, along with leukotomes and group
drama therapy. The protagonist is a girl named Babydoll, committed
after a violent confrontation with her evil stepfather in which she
gets blamed for her sister's death. Since her recently deceased mother
has left everything to her daughters, we find ourselves in the classic
narrative of the inconvenient woman locked away so that the greedy
relation can get their money. To add a layer of menace, the stepfather
pays a corrupt attendant to forge a doctor's signature so Babydoll
can receive a lobotomy. Elaborates the attendant, "She won't even remember her name when I'm done with her." Babydoll is strapped into
what looks like a dentist's chair, a large diagram of a transorbital procedure in the background for reference. In comes the doctor, icepick

and hammer in hand. We get a shot of the leukotome taking position, and the hammer beginning its descent.

Without detailing the complex layering techniques that Snyder employs, the gist is that the asylum transforms into a prison-dancehall-brothel where, Oz-like, the patients and staff play completely new characters. Babydoll instigates an escape plot which takes us into another layer of fantasy, in which the prostitute/patients become mini-skirted action heroes battling a variety of bizarre enemies (such as undead, steampunk, Kaiser soldiers). The asylum drops away, not returning until the very end of the film, when Babydoll gets shot while helping a fellow prostitute escape. The bullet that strikes her down syncs to the hammering of the lobotomist's icepick. Now zombified, the helpless Babydoll gets attacked by the evil attendant but saved by a sympathetic psychiatrist and some police officers. Of course, she is still ruined, her mind ravaged by the procedure.

Sucker Punch uses a gothic asylum as shorthand for the subjection of strong but "inconvenient" females, resurrecting the moral message of Elizabeth Packard. Set in the pre-Friedan early 1960s, *Sucker Punch* creates a mythical environment of unopposed male control and sexual violence. With no other recourse available, heroic women must employ brute force to save themselves. Critics were not impressed, most going along with the *New York Times*'s caustic assessment that *Sucker Punch* represented a "fantasia of misogyny," with scantily clad sex objects feigning empowerment but really just sating the male gaze.[27]

What is most pertinent here is Snyder's casual use of the asylum as stand-in for violence against women. Tapping a deep and tortuous history of patriarchal medicine and female resistance, Snyder assembles a bricolage of imagery and ideas to create a new myth of anti-psychiatry. Even with all the CGI and the kicking industrial beat, Snyder's film is no fresh expression; it's rather an homage dressed in techno-gothic, a traditional reading incorporating Wollstonecraft and Chesler and Piercy, with historical accumulations of fascism, surveillance technology, and deinstitutionalization in evidence.

The new gothic asylum received its fullest realization in the second season of the cable TV show *American Horror Story*. Airing over the winter of 2012–2013, *American Horror Story: Asylum* (*AHS: Asylum*) is set in the Briarcliff Mental Institution in Massachusetts. Linking post-deinstitutionalized decay to an equivalently scary past, the first episode summarizes the agenda. Two lovebirds are romping through a big, abandoned asylum, the last stop in their "haunted honeymoon tour." The woman reviews the institution's history for us on her cell phone. They then find a room with a reclining table and straps. The man ties the woman in, and, taking ancient and rotting ECT headphones, performs a fake electroshock on her. Suddenly, they hear something. The woman wonders if it is Bloody Face, the legendary serial killer who was once locked inside these walls. Mayhem follows. The two prove the Hollywood logic that no asylum can be entered without consequences.

The bulk of *AHS: Asylum* takes place in 1964, prime *Cuckoo's Nest* territory. In heroic fashion, the filmmakers display an impressive collection of asylum horrors: sedative-free ECT, icepick lobotomy, Sodium Pentothal, pills in paper cups, forced showers, injections, hydrotherapy, aversion therapy, psychoanalysis, oedipal complexes, straitjackets, human experimentation, burly attendants, a mysterious, foreign asylum doctor, concentration camp allusions, a Nurse Ratched–type, a serial killer who breaks out, a creepy dayroom with unnervingly happy music (always the same song), subterranean chambers, dripping tunnels, a maniac in a Santa costume, raving patients, zombified patients, a female inmate with a fake baby, and asylum-created, subhuman monsters. One innovative turn is the reimagining of the old, evil nun story. The vicious Mother Superior

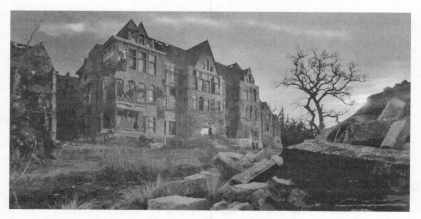

Briarcliff Mental Institution, *American Horror Story: Asylum* (2012–2013)

Sister Jude lords over her patients, especially Lana. Lana has been institutionalized for being gay and escapes to return with a camera crew, thus reenacting Geraldo Rivera's Willowbrook exposé. To complete the historical cycle, the now-abandoned asylum ends up a haunted tourist site. *AHS: Asylum* manages to compress two hundred years of the pop culture asylum into thirteen gothic episodes. It is an achievement.

The viewer obviously recognizes that this not "Inspired by a True Story." With a cast that includes the Angel of Death, space aliens, and a woman who claims, and might actually be, Anne Frank, we know we have entered fantasyland. Yet it is also strongly implied that there is a history lesson for us here. As the show's co-creator Ryan Murphy explained, "All those abuses that you see, we studied pictures of and recreated all that stuff. We did a lot of research."[28]

EPILOGUE

REAL HORRORS

> Marge Simpson: C'mon, grandpa, you're not staying on skid row.
> Chief Wiggum: Yeah, that's shameful, shoving poor old people out
> on the street. This place is for the mentally ill.
> —*The Simpsons* (TV show)

W e still live in the shadow of the asylum. America's historic and ongoing failure to treat and accept those suffering from mental illness is part of the reason. So is the unresolved paradox of freedom restored through total control. Edgar Allan Poe brilliantly captured the dilemma, and entertainment value, in "The System of Dr. Tarr and Prof. Fether." He showed us a dark setting for lies and twisted dreams. He also blueprinted a collection of themes used ever since—the lunatics running the asylum, the insane superintendent, the gothic manor-prison, the torturous "cures," the beautiful waif, and the madhouse rebellion. In Poe's day, the asylum could allegorize a panoply of topics and concerns: utopian reforms, slavery, democracy, and the chaotic market. In later years, women's rights, consumerism, civil rights, fascism, and psychiatry came into play.

Yet the asylum is also a real place. Actual people suffered here, and true stories have always elbowed alongside the fantastical ones. Conjunctures of the real and the imaginary provided creative tensions that birthed the most enduring asylum narratives. Kesey's experiences on the ward and growing up as a Cold War kid combined in *Cuckoo's Nest*. His hospital resonates on tandem levels of reality and myth. It is hard to separate them. Perhaps Kesey's ultimate lesson is this: we must all wrestle with those things troubling our society, and what we cannot overcome, we transmute into metaphor.

Today, many of the old state hospitals have become shipwrecks, attracting legions of "ruin porn" aficionados. A whole industry is building up around them. Private investors repurpose them, banking on the horror. One of the biggest haunted sites in America is the Trans-Alleghany Lunatic Asylum, a massive Kirkbride structure located in the town of Weston, West Virginia. It has hosted a variety of ghost-hunting TV shows and houses a museum along with a variety of tours and entertainments. In the fall of 2016, I spent a night there.

I began with a tour of the place. Led by a docent dressed in an old-time nurse's uniform, I traveled through a few empty, rotting wards. In the yard, I learned that at Halloween, thrill-seekers can pay to ride in the back of open-bed trucks and shoot paint balls at "zombie" actors. I couldn't help but snicker at this reimagining of *Night of the Living Dead*–style asylum breakouts. Later in the evening I returned with a thermos of hot coffee, a notepad, a headband-mounted flashlight, and an electronic ghost-detector (purchased online for $29.95). I spent the night with a tour guide and a group of fellow investigators, creeping about in the pitch-black. At night, you really get a sense of the history, smelling ancient tobacco and dust kicked up with each step. My guide and I spent some time trying to talk to a spirit named Big Jim, who allegedly killed another patient by driving a bedpost through his head. Alas, I did not find any spirits. Perhaps they sensed my skepticism.

Recently, mental health-care advocates have begun challenging the use of asylums and the institutionalized as horrors. Recent Halloween attractions at theme parks that depict wild patients in straitjackets and demented doctors have come under fire. For instance, after an online petition in 2016, the Six Flags New England attraction, "Psycho-Path Haunted Asylum," was shut down. Research shows that popular attractions, movies, and language all have an ongoing and stigmatizing impact. One 2014 study found that

> MHCEs [Mental Health Care Environments] are often depicted as unhygienic, dilapidated buildings where restraints, seclusion rooms, ECT, and psychosurgery are frequently used . . . Often, people will refuse to seek treatment due to the perception of mental ill health . . . this may be related to the fact that the general public gets a great deal of information from the media and film,

and in the case of modern horror, MHCEs and mental health practitioners are presented in a negative and stigmatizing light.

Similarly, the Hogg Foundation for Mental Health makes the case that words can have deleterious, stigmatizing effects in its "Language Matters in Mental Health" program.[1]

But there is more than horror happening. The pop culture asylum has historically played a vital role in helping the public uncover injustices and initiate dialogues for meaningful reforms. Elizabeth Packard's writings helped improve the lives of women shuttled off without recourse on the whims of abusive husbands. Clifford Whittingham Beers's *A Mind That Found Itself* awakened a Progressive middle class to the shortcomings of the state hospitals. *The Snake Pit* and *Shame of the States* provided frameworks for a critique of the massive, underfunded institutions that held naked, filth-covered patients. *One Flew Over the Cuckoo's Nest* energized a generation frustrated with stifling Cold War conformity. Yet narratives and films can obscure too. *David and Lisa* presents a sympathetic portrait of treatment, yet it paints schizophrenia as a quirk of teenage angst brought about by bad mothers. *Girl, Interrupted* (1999) takes us into a believable place, yet shoehorns patients into stereotypical foils for the protagonist's voyage to adulthood. More deeply, as Hayden White notes, the form *itself* has a content. Narrative conventions employ their own logic. For instance, Packard's tale of incarceration is crafted as melodrama, replete with a master villain, a setting of gothic terror, and a trapped female's flight to freedom. The form worked toward the betterment of mental health—like *Uncle Tom's Cabin*—Packard produced a sense of moral outrage that was successfully channeled along legislative lines. Yet her characterizations also repeated clichés of captivity and flight, reinforcing gendered and racial hierarchies, converting trauma into a commodity. Packard's depiction of Lizzie Bonner, the brutal Irish attendant, fortified Anglo whiteness while selling lasciviousness. The reader comes away with a hostile view of immigrants and a heart-wrenching pity for the fate of imperiled, white women.

More problematically, popular culture often deals in disastrously inaccurate images of mental illness and treatments. Much research indicates that negative portrayals have real-world effects, be they a disinclination to receive help or a stigmatizing view of those who suffer mental health issues. As Carrie Fisher reports in one of her memoirs, she did not want ECT because, "I, too, of course believed what pretty much the entire Western world believes, thanks in large part to Hollywood's portrayal of it—I believed that this treatment was an extreme measure primarily administered as punishment to mental patients for being crazily uncooperative." More academically, one might consult a 2006 study: "Viewers of fictional films and television programs frequently are confronted with negative images of mental illness, and these images have a cumulative effect on the public's perception of people with mental illness. In turn, this has consequences for people with mental illness, who experience stigma and may be less likely to seek help as a result of this collective impression of what mental illness means."[2]

Yet storytelling and metaphors are irreducible components of human communication. Making asylums and their denizens stand-ins for social concerns permit critiques of difficult, social problems. Reviewers of Forman's *Cuckoo's Nest* often remarked that the film was unoriginal in its asylum portrayal, yet nonetheless praised its message about social control. Nicholson's fictional martyrdom inspired real demands for patient rights and institutional reform. Art can inform change, even when we know it's just art. The problem is that pop culture formations can elide truth even as they access it. Patients should have rights; but Ratcheds are not the issue, nor is ECT routinely used to punish individualism.

Much has changed since Poe, but change is often lost in the enduring metaplot of despair and tyranny. Patient management regimes, medical presuppositions, psychological frameworks, biological understandings, technologies, and diagnoses have improved, yet these are largely left out of the main story. Further, we seem to have traded old horrors for new ones. According to João Biehl, society quarantines the unproductive and "unsound," using medical categories and punitive laws, into places where the public doesn't have to see them. Many sufferers of mental illness experience this "negative" citizenship and become, in Biehl's words, "ex-humans." Though Biehl writes of Brazil, one finds resonance in today's America. Our mentally ill have extremely high unemployment rates, high incarceration rates, high homelessness rates, and, notes Andrew Scull, a life expectancy that has actually decreased in the wake of deinstitutionalization. The term "trans-institutionalization" describes the process in which those who might have been lifetime mental patients become denizens of prisons, jails, and squalid federally-funded SROs. These are the new institutions, which are hardly a step up from the snake pits. The largest psychiatric care facility in America is the Los Angeles County Jail, where an estimated 20 percent of the inmate population suffer serious mental illness. Then there is the street, where dangers include sexual abuse, physical violence, and exposure to the elements. There is not much safety in prison or jail either. Sufferers of schizophrenia and bipolar disorders often find themselves beaten by guards and fellow inmates or locked into solitary confinement, which has a demonstrably deleterious effect on one's mental health. As one inmate told a documentary film crew, "Ask yourself, can you live in a bathroom for ten years?"[3]

The socially abandoned are silent. Asylum narratives have long relegated certain groups invisible, including the poor, the immigrant, the racial minority, and the illiterate. These people are not the protagonists of asylum stories. If they enter the picture, it is as monstrous Others. Visible victims are almost invariably white and middle class. African Americans have long been asylum residents, yet my survey of one hundred thirty-odd years of popular narratives and representations finds them typically absent, comedic, or villainous. Their historically segregated facilities simply do not enter the public radar. This is despite the fact that, as Jonathan M. Metzl argues, African Americans since the 1960s have been *more* likely to be labeled schizophrenic than their white counterparts. Rare is the film like *Pressure Point* (1962) that features a helpful African American psychiatrist. The same historical amnesia goes for institutionalized, non-English–speaking immigrants and Native Americans.[4]

Today's horror asylum is not like anything we would recognize from most mental hospital narratives. Our tradition utterly fails to help us conceptualize the mechanisms by which society quarantines people in penitentiaries and halfway houses. One reason for this is that the tools that dismantled the state institutions have not been incorporated into pop culture. Rather than descriptions of the demise of state welfare and the rise of pharmaceuticals, we are likely to see psychiatric tortures or miracle drugs in our movie-made history. Dismissing structure for simplistic "history lessons" suits the new gothic frame—the cause of decline is *moral*, suitable to metanarratives of good versus evil, democracy versus tyranny. Entering alternative frames of interpretation neither sells tickets nor lures advertisers.

The "asylum" evokes stigma, terror, and abandonment. It always has. A long, dark history weighs it down with an unmanageable burden. All agree that more is needed for those who suffer from the waking nightmare of mental illness. Perhaps it is time to write a new story.

ACKNOWLEDGMENTS

I appreciate the patience shown to me by friends, family, and colleagues. Special thanks to the staffs and volunteers at the Connecticut Valley Hospital at Middletown, Fairfield Hills Hospital, the Trans-Alleghany Lunatic Asylum, and the Oregon State Hospital and Museum. Thanks to the librarians and staffs of Buley Library at Southern Connecticut State University, Blackstone Library, Yale Sterling Memorial Library, the Disability History Museum, and the Library of Congress. In particular, thanks to Beth Paris at Buley and Rosemary Hanes at the Library of Congress Moving Image Section. Thanks as well to Dennie Brooks, Dr. Ulista Brooks, Kathleen Wilson, Kathryn Dysart, Sarah Profit, Heather Vrana, and Dan Cruson. I appreciate Troy Paddock and the International Association for the Study of Environment, Space, and Place for providing me an early opportunity to present my thesis. Special thanks to Laura Davulis at Johns Hopkins University Press and to Michael E. Staub.

Thanks to my colleagues in the History Department of Southern Connecticut State University, and to my friends—Luis Rodriguez, Xochitl Mercado, Mike Carter, Ericka Carter, Jon Purmont, Byron Nakamura, Lisa Nakamura, Brien Porter, Cara Porter, Josh Zeitz, Dr. Bruce Caldarone, Jen Klein, James Berger, Steve Amerman, Leah Glaser, Ginger Sullivan, and Marilyn Miller. Thanks to Brenda Sullivan Miller for sending on all of those interesting articles.

Thanks to my wonderful family, David Quinn, Jeff, and Rochelle, and to my amazing kids, Rowan and Catalina. Thanks especially to my life partner, Kath, without whose love, support, and ear, none of this would have been remotely possible. Finally, I'd like to dedicate this book to the memory of my late father-in-law, Dr. Alan Miller, a kind and caring model of the psychiatric profession.

NOTES

INTRODUCTION

1. Author interview with Dennie Brooks, March 11, 2017; Kathleen Wilson, "Echoes from the Set (1967–2017): Fifty Years of Filming Hollywood and Oregon's Cinematic Literary Voices" (unpublished manuscript). Special thanks to Kathleen Wilson for sharing this with me.

2. Rick Dodgson, *It's All a Kind of Magic: The Young Ken Kesey* (Madison: University of Wisconsin Press, 2013), 158; "Laff With, Not At, Mental Patients," *Variety*, April 17, 1974. Dean Brooks quoted in Ray Loynd, "'Cuckoo's Nest' Aloft and Well," *Los Angeles Herald-Examiner*, March 9, 1975. On Brooks's assistance, see Ted Mahar, "'Cuckoo's' Cast Praises Oregon Doctor for Help," *Oregonian*, December 19, 1975.

3. "Roughing It Back toward Sanity," *Life* (October 27, 1972), 61; Diane L. Goeres-Gardner, *Inside Oregon State Hospital: A History of Tragedy and Triumph* (Charleston, SC: History Press, 2013), 211, 216, 219, 220.

4. Author interview with Dennie Brooks, March 11, 2017; Dean Brooks, "'Cuckoo's Nest': Inside and Out," address to the American Psychiatric Association, Institute on Hospital and Community Psychiatry (September 1976).

5. Larry Sturhan, "Interview with Milos Forman," *Filmmakers Newsletter* 9, no. 2 (December 1975), 26; "Michael Douglas: Streets to 'Nest,'" *Los Angeles Times*, August 26, 1974; Marc Eliot, *Michael Douglas: A Biography* (New York, NY: Crown, 2012), 42, 45; "Laff With, Not At, Mental Patients," *Variety*, April 17, 1974.

6. According to my research, between 1901 and 2018, there were at least 500 mainstream movies and TV episodes featuring asylums. *Off to Bloomingdale Asylum* (orig. *L'omnibus des toqués blancs et noirs*), directed by Georges Méliès (1901). See also David Coleman, *The Bipolar Express: Manic Depression and the Movies* (Lanham, MD: Rowman and Littlefield, 2014), 20–21.

7. Author interview with Dennie Brooks, March 11, 2017; Saul Zaentz in *Completely Cuckoo*, directed by Charles Kiselyak (1997); Kesey quoted in Peter O. Whitmer and Bruce Van Wyngarden, *Aquarius Revisited: Seven Who Created the Sixties Counterculture That Changed America; William Burroughs, Allen Ginsberg, Ken Kesey, Timothy Leary, Norman Mailer, Tom Robbins, Hunter S. Thompson* (New York, NY: Macmillan, 1987), 209; Rupert Hawksley, "'One Flew Over the Cuckoo's Nest': 10 Things You Didn't Know about the Film," *The Telegraph* (UK), http://www.telegraph.co.uk/culture/film/10665661/, accessed May 26, 2017.

8. Author interview with Dennie Brooks, March 11, 2017; *Completely Cuckoo*, directed by Charles Kiselyak (1997); Wilson, "Echoes from the Set."

9. C. P. L. Freeman and K. E. Cheshire, "Review: Attitude Studies on Electroconvulsive Therapy," *Convulsive Therapy* 2, no. 1 (1986), 38.

10. Robert Fuller, *An Account of the Imprisonment and Sufferings of Robert Fuller of Cambridge* (Boston, MA: printed for the author, 1833), 19, 20; Isaac H. Hunt, *Astounding Disclosures! Three Years in a Mad-House* (published by author, 1851), 4; Mary Wollstonecraft, *Maria, or, The Wrongs of Woman* (Mineola, NY: Dover Publications, 2005), 10.

11. Jonathan Sadowsky makes an excellent argument for this in *Electroconvulsive Therapy in America: The Anatomy of a Medical Controversy* (New York, NY: Routledge, 2017).

CHAPTER 1. THE ENCHANTER'S CASTLE

1. Edgar A. Poe, "The System of Dr. Tarr and Prof. Fether," *Graham's Magazine* 28, no. 5 (November 1845), 193.

2. Poe, "The System of Dr. Tarr and Prof. Fether," 194.

3. Poe, "The System of Dr. Tarr and Prof. Fether," 196.

4. Poe, "The System of Dr. Tarr and Prof. Fether," 198–99.

5. Poe, "The System of Dr. Tarr and Prof. Fether," 199–200.

6. Jonathan Elmer, *Reading at the Social Limit: Affect, Mass Culture, and Edgar Allan Poe* (Stanford, CA: Stanford University Press, 1995), 142–48; Joan Dayan, "Poe, Persons, and Property," *American Literary History* 11, no. 3 (Autumn 1999), 405–25; Bernard A. Drabeck, "'Tarr and Fether': Poe and Abolition," *American Transcendental Quarterly* 14 (1972), 177–84; J. Gerald Kennedy, "A Mania for Composition: Poe's Annus Mirabilis and the Violence of Nation Building," *American Literary History* 17, no. 1 (Spring 2005), 1–35; Benjamin Reiss, *Theaters of Madness: Insane Asylums and Nineteenth-Century American Culture* (Chicago, IL: University of Chicago Press, 2008), chap. 5.

7. Lady Emmeline Stuart-Wortley, *Travels in the United States, etc.: During 1849 and 1850* (Paris: A. and W. Galignani, 1851), 142–43; Seth Rockman, *Scraping By: Wage Labor, Slavery, and Survival in Early Baltimore* (Baltimore, MD: Johns Hopkins University Press, 2010), 244–25; Arthur Hobson Quinn, *Edgar Allan Poe: A Critical Biography* (New York, NY: D. Appleton-Century, 1941), 186–87.

8. Charles Dickens, *American Notes for General Circulation*, vol. 1 (London: Chapman and Hall, 1842), 60, 185.

9. Alexis de Tocqueville, *Democracy in America*, vol. 2, trans. Henry Reve (New York, NY: D. Appleton, 1904), 624; Brown quoted in Gordon S. Wood, *The Idea of America: Reflections on the Birth of the United States* (New York, NY: Penguin Press, 2011), 117.

10. David S. Reynolds, *Waking Giant: America in the Age of Jackson* (New York, NY: HarperCollins, 2008), 3.

11. Benjamin Rush, "Influence of the American Revolution," in *The Selected Writings of Benjamin Rush*, ed. Dagobert D. Runes (New York, NY: Philosophical Library, 1947), 333; Norman Dain, *Concepts of Insanity in the United States, 1789–1865* (New Brunswick, NJ: Rutgers University Press, 1964), 88; Constance M. McGovern, *Masters of Madness: Social Origins of the American Psychiatric Profession* (Hanover, NH: University Press of New England, 1985), 26; Edward Jarvis, "On the Supposed Increase in Insanity," *American Journal of Insanity* 8, no. 4 (April 1852): 333–64;

and Amariah Brigham, "Insanity and Insane Hospitals," *North American Review* 44 (1837), 91–121; Nancy J. Tomes, "Devils in the Heart: Historical Perspectives on Women and Depression in the Nineteenth Century," *Transactions and Studies of the College of Physicians of Philadelphia* 5 (1991), 370–71; Dain, *Concepts of Insanity in the United States, 1789–1865.*

12. Joan Burbick, *Healing the Republic: The Language of Health and the Culture of Nationalism in Nineteenth-Century America* (Cambridge, UK: Cambridge University Press, 1994), 28; Benjamin Rush, *Medical Inquiries and Observations upon Diseases of the Mind*, 5th ed. (Philadelphia, PA: Grigg and Elliot, 1835), 209. Shryock, "The Beginnings: From Colonial Days to the Foundation of the American Psychiatric Association," and William Malamud, "Psychiatric Therapies," in *One Hundred Years of American Psychiatry*, 11–12, 275–76; Nancy Tomes, "Notes and Documents: The Domesticated Madman: Changing Concepts of Insanity at the Pennsylvania Hospital, 1780–1830," *Pennsylvania Magazine of History and Biography* 106, no. 2 (April 1982), 276; Andrew Scull, *Social Order, Mental Disorder: Anglo-American Psychiatry in Social Perspective* (Berkeley: University of California Press, 1989), 100; Samuel Thomson, "Receipt to Cure a Crazy Man," in *Madness: An American History of Mental Illness and Its Treatment*, ed. Mary de Young (Jefferson, NC: McFarland, 2010), 72.

13. Erika Janik, *Marketplace of the Marvelous: The Strange Origins of Modern Medicine* (Boston, MA: Beacon Press, 2014); Reynolds, *Waking Giant*; Reiss, *Theaters of Madness*, chap. 3; Paul Starr, *The Social Transformation of American Medicine* (New York, NY: Basic Books, 1995), 30–31; Dain, *Concepts of Insanity in the United States, 1789–1865*, 57–58; Amariah Brigham, *Remarks on the Influence of Mental Cultivation upon Health* (Hartford, CT: F. J. Huntington, 1832), 70; Brigham, "Insanity and Insane Hospitals"; Rush, *Medical Inquiries*, 60; Carla Yanni, *The Architecture of Madness: Insane Asylums in the United States* (Minneapolis: University of Minnesota Press, 2007), 26; Samuel Cartwright, "Report on the Diseases and Physical Peculiarities of the Negro Race," *New Orleans Medical and Surgical Journal* (1851); Gerald N. Grob, "Psychiatry's Holy Grail: The Search for the Mechanism of Mental Disease," *Bulletin of the History of Medicine* 72 (1998), 189–219. Madness was "the price," noted premier alienist Isaac Ray, which "we pay for civilization." Ray quoted in David J. Rothman, *The Discovery of the Asylum: Social Order and Disorder in the New Republic* (Boston, MA: Little, Brown, 1990), 112. For a discussion of drapetomania, see Jonathan M. Metzl, *The Protest Psychosis: How Schizophrenia Became a Black Disease* (Boston, MA: Beacon Press, 2009), ix; "Startling Facts from the Census," *American Journal of Insanity* 8 (October 1851), 153–55.

14. Lawrence B. Goodheart, *Mad Yankees: The Hartford Retreat for the Insane and Nineteenth-Century Psychiatry* (Amherst: University of Massachusetts Press, 2003), 93; Ian Dowbiggin, *The Quest for Mental Health: A Tale of Science, Medicine, Scandal, Sorrow, and Mass Society* (New York, NY: Cambridge University Press, 2011), 34, 36; Lynn Gamwell and Nancy Tomes, *Madness in America: Cultural and Medical Perceptions of Mental Illness before 1914* (New York, NY: Cornell University Press, 1995), 90; Mary Ann Jimenez, *Changing Faces of Madness: Early Attitudes and Treatment of the Insane* (Hanover, NH: published for Brandeis University Press by University Press of New England, 1987), 168; Kenneth J. Weiss, "Isaac Ray's Affair with Phrenology,"

Journal of Psychiatry and Law 34, no. 4 (Winter 2006): 455–94. Phrenologists like F. Coombs argued that we might better understand and treat people in "hospitals for the insane" via understanding their brain organs. See *Coombs's Popular Phrenology* (Boston, 1841), 100–101.

15. Mariana Valverde, *Diseases of the Will: Alcohol and the Dilemmas of Freedom* (Cambridge, MA: Cambridge University Press, 1998), 45.

16. David Brion Davis, *Homicide in American Fiction, 1798–1860: A Study in Social Values* (Ithaca, NY: Cornell University Press, 1957), 108; Poe defines monomania: "Then came the full fury of my monomania, and I struggled in vain against its strange and irresistible influence. In the multiplied objects of the external world I had no thoughts but for the teeth. All other matters and all different interests became absorbed in their single contemplation." Edgar Allan Poe, "Berenice: A Tale," in *The Annotated Poe*, ed. Kevin J. Hayes (Cambridge, MA: Harvard University Press, 2015), 55. See Phillips, "Mere Household Events"; C. T. Pridgeon, Jr., "Insanity in American Fiction from Charles Brockden Brown to Oliver Wendell Holmes" (PhD diss., Duke University, 1969), 234.

17. Janet Miron, *Prisons, Asylums, and the Public: Institutional Visiting in the Nineteenth Century* (Toronto, ON: University of Toronto Press, 2011), 22; "Peter McCandless, "Curative Asylum, Custodial Hospital: The South Carolina Lunatic Asylum and State Hospital, 1828–1920," in *The Confinement of the Insane: International Perspectives, 1800–1965*, ed. Roy Porter and David Wright (Cambridge, UK: Cambridge University Press, 2003), 173; Fuller and Torrey, *The Invisible Plague*, 223; Samuel W. Hamilton, "American Mental Hospitals," in *One Hundred Years of American Psychiatry*, 73–166; Brigham, "Insanity and Insane Hospitals," 114–15; Gerald N. Grob, *Mental Institutions in America: Social Policy to 1875* (New York, NY: Free Press, 1973), 166, 168; Goodheart, *Mad Yankees*, 111; Linda V. Carlisle, *Elizabeth Packard: A Noble Fight* (Urbana, IL: University of Illinois, 2010), 17; John Duffy, "Masturbation and Clitoridectomy: A Nineteenth-Century View," *JAMA* 186 (October 19, 1963), 166–68; Burbick, *Healing the Republic*, 4, 285; Ellen Dwyer, *Homes for the Mad: Life Inside Two Nineteenth-Century Asylums* (New Brunswick, NJ: Rutgers University Press, 1987), 134.

18. Benjamin Rush, "An Enquiry into the Effects of Public Punishments upon Criminals and upon Society. Read in the Society for Promoting Political Enquiries, convened at the house of His Excellency Benjamin Franklin, Esquire, in Philadelphia, March 9th, 1787" (Philadelphia, PA: Joseph James, 1787), 10–11; Robert R. Sullivan, "The Birth of the Prison: The Case of Benjamin Rush," *Eighteenth-Century Studies* 31, no. 3 (Spring, 1998), 333–44; Thomas L. Dumm, *Democracy and Punishment: Disciplinary Origins of the United States* (Madison: University of Wisconsin Press, 1987), 89–96.

19. Mark E. Kann, *Punishment, Prisons, and Patriarchy: Liberty and Power in the Early American Republic* (New York, NY: New York University Press, 2005), 61, chap. 4; Peter McCandless, *Moonlight, Magnolias, and Madness: Insanity in South Carolina from the Colonial Period to the Progressive Era* (Chapel Hill: University of North Carolina Press, 1996), 38; David J. Rothman, "Perfecting the Prison: United States, 1789–1865," in *The Oxford History of the Prison: The Practice of Punishment in Western Society*, ed. Norval Morris and David J. Rothman (Oxford, UK: Oxford

University Press, 1998), 104; Simone Browne, *Dark Matters: On the Surveillance of Blackness* (Durham, NC: Duke University Press, 2015); Toni Morrison, *Playing in the Dark: Whiteness and the American Literary Imagination* (Cambridge, MA: Harvard University Press, 1992), 7.

20. Dickens, *American Notes for General Circulation*, 1:105, 1:109.

21. John F. Sears, *Sacred Places: American Tourist Attractions in the Nineteenth Century* (New York, NY: Oxford University Press, 1989), 89–91.

22. Quoted in Gamwell and Tomes, *Madness in America*, 59.

23. Dickens, *American Notes for General Circulation*, 1:221–23.

24. Alex Beam, *Gracefully Insane: The Rise and Fall of America's Premier Mental Hospital* (New York, NY: Public Affairs, 2001), 20–23.

25. Robert Fuller, *An Account of the Imprisonment and Sufferings of Robert Fuller of Cambridge* (Boston, MA: printed for the author, 1833), 12, 22–23.

26. Fuller, *An Account of the Imprisonment and Sufferings of Robert Fuller*, 13, 15, 16, 19, 25.

27. Fuller, *An Account of the Imprisonment and Sufferings of Robert Fuller*, 28–29.

28. Fuller, *An Account of the Imprisonment and Sufferings of Robert Fuller*, 30.

29. Elizabeth T. Stone, *A Sketch of the Life of Elizabeth T. Stone, and of her Persecutions, with an Appendix of her Treatment and Sufferings While in the Charlestown McLean Assylum Where She was Confined under the Pretense of Insanity* (printed for the author, 1842), 19–20.

30. Stone, *A Sketch of the Life of Elizabeth T. Stone*, 20–21, 24–27, 31.

31. Stone, *A Sketch of the Life of Elizabeth T. Stone*, 35, 36.

32. Quoted in Jeffrey L. Geller and Maxine Harris, *Women of the Asylum: Voices from Behind the Walls, 1840–1945* (New York, NY: Doubleday, 1994), 56–57.

33. Gerald N. Grob, *Mental Institutions in America*, 134–36; Nancy Tomes, *A Generous Confidence: Thomas Story Kirkbride and the Art of Asylum Keeping, 1840–1883*.

34. Edmund Wilson, *Patriotic Gore: Studies in the Literature of the American Civil War* (New York, NY: W. W. Norton, 1994), 10; Leslie Aaron Fiedler, *Love and Death in the American Novel* (New York, NY: Criterion Books, 1960), 127.

35. Robert H. Wiebe, *The Opening of American Society: From the Adoption of the Constitution to the Eve of Disunion* (New York, NY: Knopf, 1984), 367; Mark Edmunson, *Nightmare on Main Street: Angels, Sadomasochism, and the Culture of Gothic* (Cambridge, MA: Harvard University Press, 1997), 17; Karen Halttunen, *Murder Most Foul: The Killer and the American Gothic Imagination* (Cambridge, MA: Harvard University Press, 1998), chap. 3.

36. On the importance of architecture, see Mike Davis, *Reading the Text That Isn't There: Paranoia in the Nineteenth-Century American Novel* (New York, NY: Routledge, 2005), 10–14. Herman Melville, "The Paradise of Bachelors and the Tartarus of the Maids," in *The Oxford Book of American Short Stories*, ed. Joyce Carol Oates (Oxford, UK: Oxford University Press, 1992), 82.

37. Orpheus Everts, "The American Style of Public Provision for the Insane, and Despotism in Lunatic Asylums," *American Journal of Insanity* 37 (1881), 113–39. Utica also put out a journal, the *Opal*. See Maryrose Eannace, "Lunatic Literature: New York State's *The Opal, 1850–1860*" (PhD diss., University of Albany, SUNY, 2001).

38. Isaac H. Hunt, *Astounding Disclosures! Three Years in a Mad-House* (published by author, 1851), 216; Hiram Chase, *Two Years and Four Months in a Lunatic Asylum* (Saratoga Springs, 1868), 9.

39. Halttunen, *Murder Most Foul*, 5.

40. David S. Reynolds, introduction to *Quaker City; or, the Monks of Monk Hall: A Romance of Philadelphia Life, Mystery, and Crime*, by George Lippard, ed. David S. Reynolds (Amherst: University of Massachusetts Press, 1995), vii.

41. Lippard, *Quaker City*, 3.

42. Lippard, *Quaker City*, 105, 106; Cynthia Hall, "'Colossal Vices' and 'Terrible Deformities' in George Lippard's Gothic Nightmare," in *Demons of the Body and Mind: Essays on Disability in Gothic Literature*, ed. Ruth Beinstock Anolik (Jefferson, NC: McFarland Publishing, 2010), 35–46.

43. Lippard, *Quaker City*, 435, 527.

44. Lippard, *Quaker City*, 356–57, 399, 431; also see Edmundson, *Nightmare on Main Street*, 7–8.

45. Lippard, *Quaker City*, 532–37.

46. Lippard, *Quaker City*, 527.

47. Also, the fact that many of the large public institutions were based on private asylum designs didn't help clear things up.

48. Greenhorn [Thompson], *Dashington*, 42, 6.

49. Greenhorn [Thompson], *Dashington*, 49.

50. Lippard, *Quaker City*, 41.

51. Greenhorn [Thompson], *Dashington*, 49, 50, 82.

52. A. J. H. Duganne's *Knights of the Seal* is another story featuring a Philadelphia asylum. See Lisa M. Hermsen, "*Knights of the Seal*: Mad Doctors and Maniacs in A. J. H. Duganne's Romance of Reform," in *Demons of the Body and Mind*, ed. Ruth Beinstock Anolik, 157–69; Greenhorn [Thompson], *Dashington*, 75.

53. Richard Henry Dana, *Two Years Before the Mast and Twenty-Four Years After* (New York, NY: P. F. Collier, 1909), 16, 19, 105, 382.

54. Philip F. Gura, *Truth's Ragged Edge: The Rise of the American Novel* (New York, NY: Farrar, Straus and Giroux, 2014), 209. Also in *White-Jacket*, Melville uses terms like "state prison afloat" and "a large manufactory" to describe the *Neversink*. See Herman Melville, *White-Jacket, or, The World in a Man-of-War* (New York, NY: Grove Press, 1850), 46, 172. Mary Elene Wood, *The Writing on the Wall: Women's Autobiography and the Asylum* (Urbana: University of Illinois Press, 1994), 35. Herman Melville, *Moby-Dick; or, The Whale* (New York, NY: Charles Scribner's Sons, 1902), 60.

55. Melville, *Moby-Dick*, 409.

56. Melville, *Moby-Dick*, 145, 158–60. Also see Burbick, *Healing the Republic*, 165–75. Note Melville's play on phrenology at numerous points.

57. Critic quoted in Ruland and Bradbury, *From Puritanism to Postmodernism: A History of American Literature*, 161. On Melville and madness, see Paul McCarthy, "*The Twisted Mind*": *Madness in Herman Melville's Fiction* (Iowa City, IA: University of Iowa Press, 1990); Pridgeon, "Insanity in American Fiction," 372; Henry Nash Smith, "The Madness of Ahab," in *Democracy and the Novel: Popular Resistance to Classic American Writers* (New York, NY: Oxford University Press, 1978): 35–55; Torrey and Miller, *The Invisible Plague*, 232–35.

58. Melville, *Moby-Dick*, 200.

59. Melville, *Moby-Dick*, 141.

CHAPTER 2. WOMAN IN WHITE, ANGEL IN BLACK

1. T. J. Jackson Lears, *Fables of Abundance: A Cultural History of Advertising in America* (New York, NY: Basic Books, 1994), 78; Kari J. Winter, *Subjects of Slavery, Agents of Change: Women and Power in Gothic Novels and Slave Narratives, 1790–1865* (Athens, GA: University of Georgia Press, 1992), 21–22.

2. Sandra M. Gilbert and Susan Gubar, *The Madwoman in the Attic: The Woman Writer and the Nineteenth-Century Literary Imagination* (New Haven, CT: Yale University Press, 2000), 617.

3. Barbara Welter, "The Cult of True Womanhood: 1820–1860," *American Quarterly* 18, no. 2 (Summer 1966), 151–74; Thomas Cooley, *The Ivory Leg and the Ebony Cabinet: Madness, Race, and Gender in Victorian America* (Amherst, MA: University of Massachusetts, 2001), 117; Nancy F. Cott, *The Bonds of Womanhood: "Woman's Sphere" in New England, 1780–1835* (New Haven, CT: Yale University Press, 1997).

4. Wilkie Collins, *The Woman in White*, 2nd ed. (New York, NY: New American Library, 1985), 32–41.

5. Collins, *The Woman in White*, 6.

6. Elaine Showalter, *The Female Malady: Women, Madness, and English Culture, 1830–1980* (New York, NY: Penguin, 1987); Introduction, Edgar Allan Poe, "The Fall of the House of Usher," in *The Fall of the House of Usher and Other Tales* (New York, NY: Penguin, 2006), 116, 128; Gilbert and Gubar, *The Madwoman in the Attic*, 620.

7. Carla Yanni, *The Architecture of Madness: Insane Asylums in the United States* (Minneapolis: University of Minnesota Press, 2007), 6; Ian Robert Dowbiggin, *The Quest for Mental Health: A Tale of Science, Medicine, Scandal, Sorrow, and Mass Society* (New York, NY: Cambridge University Press, 2011), 72; Darby Penney and Peter Stastny, *The Lives They Left Behind: Suitcases from a State Hospital Attic* (New York, NY: Bellevue Literary Press, 2008), 40; Gerald N. Grob, *The Mad among Us: A History of the Care of America's Mentally Ill* (Cambridge, MA: Harvard University Press, 1994), 80; Fanny Fern, *Ruth Hall and Other Writings* (New Brunswick, NJ: Rutgers University Press, 1986), 109; Charles Reade, *Hard Cash*, vol. 1 (New York, NY: George D. Sproul, n.d.).

8. Louisa May Alcott, "A Whisper in the Dark," in *Louisa May Alcott Unmasked: Collected Thrillers*, ed. Madeleine Stern (Boston, MA: Northeastern University Press, 1995), 53, 55.

9. Alcott, "A Whisper in the Dark," 46, 53; Lynette Carpenter, "'Did They Never See Anyone Angry Before?': The Sexual Politics of Self-Control in Alcott's 'A Whisper in the Dark,'" *Legacy* 3, no. 2 (Fall 1986), 31–41.

10. Gregg D. Crane, *The Cambridge Introduction to the Nineteenth-Century American Novel* (New York, NY: Cambridge University Press, 2013), 137.

11. Gilbert and Gubar, *The Madwoman in the Attic*, 78; Marta Caminero-Santangelo, *The Madwoman Can't Speak: Or Why Insanity Is Not Subversive* (Ithaca, NY: Cornell University Press, 1998), 12–17; Sally Shuttleworth, introduction to *Jane Eyre*, by Charlotte Brontë, ed. Margaret Smith (Oxford, UK: Oxford University Press,

2000), xix. Brontë also made sure to note that "she came of a mad family:—idiots and maniacs through three generations!" 292. On the Creole (racialized) aspects of Bertha's madness, see Sue Thomas, "The Tropical Extravagance of Bertha Mason," *Victorian Literature and Culture* 27, no. 1 (1999), 1–17.

12. Brontë, *Jane Eyre*, 283–84.

13. Brontë, *Jane Eyre*, 300, 309, 427.

14. S. Weir Mitchell, *Fat and Blood: And How to Make Them*, ed. Michael S. Kimmel (Walnut Creek, CA: Rowman and Littlefield, 2004), 37; G. M. Goshgarian, *To Kiss the Chastening Rod: Domestic Fiction and Sexual Ideology in the American Renaissance* (Ithaca, NY: Cornell University Press, 1992), 59; Karen Halttunen, *Murder Most Foul: The Killer and the American Gothic Imagination* (Cambridge, MA: Harvard University Press), 188–89.

15. Denise Russell, *Women, Madness, and Medicine* (Cambridge, MA: Polity Press, 1995), 13. Gynecologist William Goodell quoted in Andrew Scull, *Madhouse: A Tragic Tale of Megalomania and Modern Medicine* (New Haven, CT: Yale University Press, 2005), 334n17. Mitchell, *Fat and Blood*, 37, 44, 79; Elaine Showalter, "Hysteria, Feminism, and Gender," in *Hysteria Beyond Freud*, ed. Sander L. Gilman (Berkeley, CA: University of California Press, 1993), 286–344.

16. Mary Wollstonecraft, *The Wrongs of Woman* in *Mary; and The Wrongs of Woman*, ed. Gary Kelly (New York, NY: Oxford University Press, 2007), 69. Also see Kari J. Winter, *Subjects of Slavery, Agents of Change: Women and Power in Gothic Novels and Slave Narratives, 1790–1865* (Athens, GA: University of Georgia Press, 1992), 21–22.

17. Wollstonecraft, *The Wrongs of Woman*, 69, 70, 77, 168; Phyllis Chesler, *Women and Madness*, rev. and updated ed. (New York, NY: Palgrave Macmillan, 2005), 62; Lydia A. Smith, *Behind the Scenes; or, Life in an Insane Asylum*, quoted in Geller and Harris, *Women of the Asylum*, 135–36.

18. Andrew Mangham, "What Could I Do? Nineteenth-Century Psychology and the Horrors of Masculinity in *The Woman in White*," in *Victorian Sensations: Essays on a Scandalous Genre*, ed. Kimberly Harrison and Richard Fantina (Columbus, OH: The Ohio State Press, 2006), 119.

19. Harriet Prescott Spofford, "Her Story," reprinted in *The Other Woman: Stories of Two Women and a Man*, ed. Susan Koppelman (Old Westbury, NY: Feminist Press, 1984), 71–72, 77–79, 84.

20. Spofford, "Her Story," 73, 87.

21. Lillie Devereux Blake, *Southwold: A Novel* (New York, NY: Rudd and Carleton, 1859), 226. For an analysis, see Grace Farrell, *Lillie Devereux Blake: Living a Life Erased* (Amherst: University of Massachusetts Press, 2002), chap. 3; Edward Hammond Clarke, *Sex in Education; or, A Fair Chance for the Girls* (Boston, MA: James R. Osgood, 1873), 87.

22. In Geller and Harris, *Women of the Asylum*, 51. On the realities of the asylum for women in this period, see Ellen Dwyer, "A Historical Perspective," in *Sex Roles and Psychopathology*, ed. Cathy Spatz Widom (New York, NY: Plenum Press, 1984), 19–48; Constance McGovern, "The Myths of Social Control and Custodial Oppression: Patterns of Psychiatric Medicine in Late Nineteenth-Century Institutions," *Journal of Social History* 20 (1986), 3–23.

23. Charlotte Perkins Stetson (Gilman), *The Yellow Wallpaper* (Boston, MA: Small, Maynard, 1892), 20, 25.

24. Gilman, *The Yellow Wallpaper*, 35; Charlotte Perkins Gilman, *The Living of Charlotte Perkins Gilman: An Autobiography* (Madison: University of Wisconsin Press, 1990), 96–97; Gilman, "Why I Wrote the Yellow Wallpaper," reprinted in *The Heath Anthology of American Literature*, 6th ed., ed. Paul Lauter, vol. C, *Late Nineteenth Century: 1865–1910* (Boston, MA: Wadsworth, 2010), 692. Compared to her 1913 essay, in her posthumously published autobiography she is a bit more circumspect. See *The Living of Charlotte Perkins Gilman*, 121.

25. Gilman, *The Yellow Wallpaper*, 42–44, 55.

26. David Gollaher, *Voice for the Mad: The Life of Dorothea Dix* (New York, NY: Free Press, 1995), 3; Dorothea Dix, *Memorial to the Legislature of Massachusetts* (1843), 16, http://www.disabilitymuseum.org/dhm/lib/detail.html?id=737&page=all.

27. Gollaher, *Voice for the Mad*, 20.

28. Dix, *Memorial to the Legislature of Massachusetts*.

29. Gollaher, *Voice for the Mad*, 150; Dix, *Memorial to the Legislature of Massachusetts*.

30. Gollaher, *Voice for the Mad*, 166, 213.

31. Gollaher, *Voice for the Mad*, 158, 171, 181–87, 325–33; Marie Hamilton, Judith A. Cook, and Jessica A. Jonikas, "Dorothea Dix," in *Encyclopedia of Disability* 1, ed. Gary L. Albrecht (Thousand Oaks, CA: Sage Publications, 2006), 513; Seaton W. Manning, "The Tragedy of the Ten-Million-Acre Bill," *Social Service Review* 36, no. 1 (March 1962), 47.

32. Elizabeth Packard quoted in Linda V. Carlisle, *Elizabeth Packard: A Noble Fight* (Urbana: University of Illinois Press, 2010), 86.

33. Packard, *The Prisoners' Hidden Life, or, Insane Asylums Unveiled* (Chicago, IL: J. N. Clarke, 1871), 81.

34. Carlisle, *Elizabeth Packard*, 60; Packard, *The Prisoners' Hidden Life*, 37; Garrison quoted in Benjamin Reiss, *Theaters of Madness: Insane Asylums and Nineteenth-Century American Culture* (Chicago, IL: University of Chicago Press, 2008), 175.

35. Carlisle, *Elizabeth Packard*, 168.

36. Packard, *The Prisoners' Hidden Life*, 23, 102.

37. Elizabeth Packard, *Modern Persecution, or Insane Asylums Unveiled* (New York, NY: Pelletreau and Raynor, 1873), 51.

38. Packard, *Modern Persecution*, 62, 120.

39. Packard, *Modern Persecution*, 235–37, 281.

40. Elizabeth Packard, *Modern Persecution, or Married Woman's Liabilities* (New York, NY: Case, Lockwood and Brainard, 1874), 115; Mary Elene Wood, *The Writing on the Wall: Women's Autobiography and the Asylum* (Urbana: University of Illinois Press, 1994), 31.

41. Nancy Tomes, "Historical Perspectives on Women and Mental Illness," in *Women, Health, and Medicine in America: A Historical Handbook*, ed. Rima D. Apple (New York, NY: Garland, 1990), 155. On Packard's "domestic feminism," see Hendrik Hartog, "Mrs. Packard on Dependency," *Yale Journal of Law and the Humanities* 1, no. 1 (1989), 79–103.

42. "Who Is This Insane Girl?," *New York Sun*, September 25, 1887; "In and About the City," *New York Times*, September 26, 1887.

43. "A Day with Lunatics: Inside View of the Asylum on Blackwell's Island," *New York Times*, December 27, 1870; Nellie Bly, *Ten Days in a Mad-House* (New York, NY: Ian L. Munro, 1887), 56.

44. Bly, *Ten Days in a Mad-House*, 5, 16–17.

45. Bly, *Ten Days in a Mad-House*, 21, 29–30, 57.

46. Brooke Kroeger, *Nellie Bly: Daredevil, Reporter, Feminist* (New York, NY: Random House, 1994), 85–99.

CHAPTER 3. MONSTERS OF THE ASYLUM

1. David J. Rothman, *Conscience and Convenience: The Asylum and Its Alternatives in Progressive America* (Boston, MA: Little, Brown, 1980), 320, 335; George W. Dowdall, *The Eclipse of the State Mental Hospital: Policy, Stigma, and Organization* (Albany, NY: State University of New York Press, 1996), 49; Kim Jacks, "Weston State Hospital" (master's thesis, West Virginia University, 2008), 38; Andrew Scull, *Madness in Civilization: A Cultural History of Insanity from the Bible to Freud, from the Madhouse to Modern Medicine* (Princeton, NJ: Princeton University Press, 2015), 419n77. An 1854 meeting of asylum superintendents saw one member decrying the negative association of "asylum" with "poor house." See *American Journal of Insanity* 11 (July 1854), 44–45. Discussed in Constance McGovern, *Masters of Madness: Social Origins of the American Psychiatric Profession* (Hanover, NJ: University Press of New England, 1985), 130. Another word coined in this era, "sanitarium," would also eventually grow into a monstrous reference. See Andrew Scull, *Madhouse: A Tragic Tale of Megalomania and Modern Medicine* (New Haven, CT: Yale University Press, 2005), 35. Thomas Paine, *Common Sense* (London, UK: Penguin Books, 1986), 84.

2. Karl Marx, *Capital: A Critique of Political Economy*, vol. 1, trans. Samuel Moore and Edward Aveling (Mineola, NY: Dover Publications, 2011), 834. For a useful discussion of the above quotes, see Mark Neocleous, "The Political Economy of the Dead: Marx's Vampires," *History of Political Thought* 24, no. 4 (Winter 2003). Steve Fraser, *The Age of Acquiescence: The Life and Death of American Resistance to Organized Wealth and Power* (New York, NY: Little, Brown, 2015), 57–58.

3. Rothman, *Conscience and Convenience*; Jeffrey A. Lieberman and Ogi Ogas, *Shrinks: The Untold Story of Psychiatry* (New York, NY: Little, Brown, 2015), 34; Norman Dain, *Clifford W. Beers: Advocate for the Insane* (Pittsburgh, PA: University of Pittsburgh Press, 1980), xxiv, 20. Writes Richard Noll, compared to their European counterparts, in this period "American alienists tended to rely heavily on sedative drugs as a form of chemical restraint to keep order in overcrowded institutions." In *American Madness: The Rise and Fall of Dementia Praecox* (Cambridge, MA: Harvard University Press, 2011), 194. Gerald N. Grob, *From Asylum to Community: Mental Health Policy in Modern America* (Princeton, NJ: Princeton University Press, 1991), 5–6; Tom Burns, *Psychiatry: A Very Short Introduction* (London: Oxford University Press, 2006), 38; Grob, *The Mad among Us: A History of the Care of America's Mentally Ill* (Cambridge, MA: Harvard University Press, 1994), 125–26; Edward Shorter, *A History of Psychiatry: From the Era of the Asylum to the Age of Prozac* (New

York, NY: John Wiley and Sons, 1997), 53–59; Susan Burch and Hannah Joyner, *Unspeakable: The Story of Junius Wilson* (Chapel Hill, NC: University of North Carolina Press, 2007), 44. For a contemporary and highly critical report, see John Maurice Grimes, *Institutional Care of Mental Patients in the United States* (Published by author, 1934).

4. Edgar Allan Poe, "The Premature Burial," in *The Portable Edgar Allan Poe*, ed. J. Gerald Kennedy (New York, NY: Penguin Books, 2006), 57; Sigmund Freud, "The Uncanny," in *The Standard Edition of the Complete Psychological Works of Sigmund Freud*, vol. 27, trans. James Strachey (London, UK: Hogarth Press, 1971), 244; Noel Carroll, *The Philosophy of Horror, or, Paradoxes of the Heart* (New York, NY: Routledge, 1990), 32; Ellen Dwyer, *Homes for the Mad: Life inside Two Nineteenth-Century Asylums* (New Brunswick, NJ: Rutgers University Press), 1.

5. Frederick Douglass, *The Life and Times of Frederick Douglass* (Mineola, NY: Dover Publications, 2003), 121; David Walker, *Appeal to the Coloured Citizens of the World*, ed. Sean Wilentz (New York, NY: Hill and Wang, 1995), 72; Harriet Jacobs, *Incidents in the Life of a Slave Girl, Written by Herself* (Boston, MA, 1861), 220. On slavery as social death, see Orlando Patterson, *Slavery and Social Death: A Comparative Study* (Cambridge, MA: Harvard University Press, 1982). Elizabeth Stone, *A Sketch in the Life of Elizabeth T. Stone, and of Her Persecutions* (printed for the author, 1842), 40; Packard, *Modern Persecution*, 2:188. Even earlier, "The Declaration of Sentiments" argued that man "has made her, if married, in the eyes of the law, civilly dead." In *One Half the People: The Fight for Woman Suffrage*, ed. Anne Firor Scott and Andrew MacKay Scott (Urbana: University of Illinois Press, 1982), 57. Lucy Stone would also argue that "marriage is to woman a state of slavery." See Nancy F. Cott, *Public Vows: A History of Marriage and the Nation* (Cambridge, MA: Harvard University Press, 2002), 64. Susan B. Anthony spoke of the "living death!" of "ill-assorted marriage homes." See Debra Bernardi, "Domestic Horrors: Disfiguring the American Home, 1860–1903" (PhD diss., University of Madison Wisconsin, 1996), 246. Anne Bingham Russell excerpted in *Women of the Asylum: Voices from Behind the Walls, 1840–1945*, ed. Jeffrey L. Geller and Maxine Harris (New York, NY: Anchor Books, 1994), 194. An Inmate [William Hotchkiss], *Five Months in the New-York State Lunatic Asylum* (Buffalo, NY: L. Danforth, 1849), 9. The prison was also a place of living death. See Caleb Smith, *The Prison and the American Imagination* (New Haven, CT: Yale University Press, 2009).

6. Daniel J. Kevles, *In the Name of Eugenics: Genetics and the Use of Human Heredity* (New York, NY: Knopf, 1985), 3, 21; R. L. Dugdale, *The Jukes: A Study in Crime, Pauperism, Disease and Heredity*, 5th ed. (New York, NY: J. P. Putman, 1895). Also see R. C. Scheerenberger, *A History of Mental Retardation* (Baltimore, MD: Paul H. Brookes, 1983). Madison Grant quoted in Ron Powers, *No One Cares about Crazy People: The Chaos and Heartbreak of Mental Health in America* (New York, NY: Hachette Books, 2017), 94. Hitler apparently wrote a letter to Grant claiming "the book is my Bible." See Powers, *No One Cares about Crazy People*, 97. For eugenics in its context of New Disability History, see Douglas C. Baynton, "Disability and the Justification of Inequality in American History," in *The New Disability History: American Perspectives*, ed. Paul K. Longmore and Lauri Umansky (New York: New York University Press, 2001), 33–57.

7. Janet Miron, *Prisons, Asylums, and the Public: Institutional Visiting in the Nineteenth Century* (Toronto, ON: University of Toronto Press, 2011), 41. In Horatio Alger's *Adrift in the City*, a crazed old "monomaniac" doctor tries to vivisect the hero after paying for a nice dinner. In *Adrift in the City; or, Oliver Conrad's Plucky Fight* (Philadelphia, PA: Henry T. Coates and Company, 1895), 163.

8. Kate Lee, *A Year at Elgin Insane Asylum*, excerpted in *Women of the Asylum: Voices from Behind the Walls, 1840–1945*, ed. Jeffrey L. Geller and Maxine Harris (New York, NY: Doubleday, 1994), 204. Florence Seyler Thompson and George W. Galvin, M.D., *A Thousand Faces* (Boston, MA: Four Seas, 1920), 285–86.

9. George du Maurier, *Trilby*, in *Novels of George Du Maurier* (London, UK: Pilot Press, 1947), 44, 47, 255, 286. On "reverse colonization," see Stephen D. Arata, "The Occidental Tourist: 'Dracula' and the Anxiety of Reverse Colonization," *Victorian Studies* 33, no. 4 (Summer 1990), 629. On Svengali and Shylock references in Dracula, see David J. Skal, *Hollywood Gothic: The Tangled Web of Dracula from Novel to Stage to Screen* (New York, NY: Norton, 1990), 45, 48; Judith Halberstam, "The Technologies of Monstrosity: Bram Stoker's *Dracula*," *Victorian Studies* 36, no. 3 (Spring 1993): 333–52.

10. Bram Stoker, *The New Annotated Dracula*, ed. Leslie S. Kinger (New York, NY: W. W. Norton, 2008), 78.

11. Stoker, *The New Annotated Dracula*, 130, 170, 259–60, 388.

12. David J. Skal refers to Dracula as a "sanguinary capitalist" who "relocates from Transylvania after draining the local peasants." In *The Monster Show: A Cultural History of Horror*, rev. ed. (New York, NY: Faber and Faber, 2001), 159. Also see Franco Moretti, "The Dialectic of Fear," in *Signs Taken for Wonders*, trans. Susan Fischer, David Forgacs, and David Miller (London, UK: Verso, 1983), 83–108.

13. Hamilton Deane and John L. Balderston, *Dracula: A Stage Play in Three Acts* (New York, NY: Samuel French, 1960), 7, 8. Raymond Huntley's contemporaneous stage depiction would also be clean shaven and debonaire.

14. Scull, *Madhouse*, 121. Burdette G. Lewis, "The Winning Fight against Mental Disease," *Review of Reviews* 65 (April 1922), quoted in Scull, *Madhouse*, 71.

15. John R. Sutton, "The Political Economy of Madness: The Expansion of the Asylum in Progressive America," *American Sociological Review* 56 (October 1991): 665–78; Ian Dowbiggin, *Keeping America Sane*, 85; Harry Bruinius, *Better for All the World: Forced Sterilization and America's Quest for Racial Purity* (New York, NY: Vintage Books, 2007); Nancy Ordover, *American Eugenics: Race, Queer Anatomy, and the Science of Nationalism* (Minneapolis: University of Minnesota Press, 2003); Stefan Kuhl, *For the Betterment of the Race: The Rise and Fall of the International Movement for Eugenics and Racial Hygiene* (New York, NY: Palgrave Macmillan, 2015).

16. As the *Detroit Free Press* noted in its review of his work, "A great many men have entered asylums for the purpose of making investigations. Mr. Beers began at the other end." In "Tells in Book of Asylum Life," *Detroit Free Press*, May 31, 1908. Albert Deutsch, "History of Mental Hygiene," in the American Psychiatric Association, *One Hundred Years of American Psychiatry* (New York, NY: Columbia University Press, 1944), 357–58.

17. Clifford Beers, *The Mind That Found Itself* (New York, NY: Longmans, Green, 1908), 19, 39, 82.

18. Beers, *The Mind That Found Itself*, 117–18, 151–52, 256.

19. Noel Carroll, *The Philosophy of Horror*, 32–34; Dwyer, *Homes for the Mad: Life inside Two Nineteenth-Century Asylums*, 140; Grob, *The Mad among Us*, 153.

20. The *Washington Post* compared his book to Reade's *Hard Cash* and hoped it would "eventually bring about as great reform in these institutions here as Charles Reade" had done in England. "Experiences of a Man Who Suddenly Recovered His Sanity but Feigned Madness in Order to expose Brutal Keepers," *Washington Post*, March 22, 1908. Thompson and Galvin, *A Thousand Faces*, 5.

21. Thompson and Galvin, *A Thousand Faces*, 85–86, 14, 11.

22. Thompson and Galvin, *A Thousand Faces*, 289–91, 176, 173, 177, 178.

23. Thompson and Galvin, *A Thousand Faces*, 92, 93, 95.

24. Thompson and Galvin, *A Thousand Faces*, 196, 197.

25. Thompson and Galvin, *A Thousand Faces*, 208, 212, 260. Also see Julius Chambers, *A Mad World and Its Inhabitants* (New York, NY: D. Appleton, 1877), 84n1.

26. Thompson and Galvin, *A Thousand Faces*, 262–63, 265.

27. *The Escaped Lunatic*, directed by Wallace McCutcheon (1904); *Maniac Chase*, directed by Edwin S. Porter (1904); *Dr. Dippy's Sanitarium*, Biograph Company (1906); *House of Darkness*, directed by D. W. Griffith (1913); *The Unfortunate Marriage*, directed by Ernest C. Warde (1917, 1920). Other pioneering asylum efforts include *Dr. Goudron's System (The Lunatics)*, a.k.a. *Le Systeme du Docteur Goudron et du Professeur Plume*, directed by Maurice Tourneur (1913).

28. *The Cabinet of Dr. Caligari*, directed by Robert Wiene (1920).

29. "The Screen," *New York Times*, April 4, 1921; "Psychopathic Film, 'The Cabinet of Dr. Caligari,' At the Capitol Theater," *New York Tribune*, April 3, 1921; "Weirdly New: 'The Cabinet of Dr. Caligari' at Miller's Theater," *Los Angeles Times*, May 8, 1921; Mae Tinee, "Whoops, My Dear! Do Bring on the Strait Jacket: 'The Cabinet of Dr. Caligari,'" *Chicago Daily Tribune*, May 15, 1921.

30. *The Monster*, directed by Roland West (1925).

31. On the history of "Igor," see Steve Biodrowski, "Antecedents of Igor: The History and Etymology of Mad Scientists' Assistants," http://cinefantastiqueonline.com /2008/09/antecedents-of-igor/, accessed May 10, 2017. As David J. Skal explains, "While a truly ridiculous film, *The Monster* is significant in formalizing certain mad science plot conventions." In *Screams of Reason: Mad Science and Modern Culture* (New York, NY: Norton, 1998), 104.

32. Melvin E. Matthews, *Fear Itself: Horror on Screen and in Reality during the Depression and World War II* (Jefferson, NC: McFarland Publishing, 2009). *Dracula*, directed by Tod Browning (1931); *The Mummy*, directed by Karl Freund (1932); *The Invisible Man*, directed by James Whale (1933); H. G. Wells quoted in Skal, *Screams of Reason*, 146.

33. Susan Tyler Hitchcock, *Frankenstein: A Cultural History* (New York, NY: W. W. Norton, 2007); Elizabeth Young, *Black Frankenstein: The Making of an American Metaphor* (New York, NY: New York University Press, 2008). Skal, *The Monster Show*, 132.

34. *Frankenstein*, directed by James Whale (1931).

35. *The Ghost of Frankenstein*, directed by Erle C. Kenton (1942).

36. *House of Frankenstein*, directed by Erle C. Kenton (1944).

37. *House of Frankenstein*, directed by Erle C. Kenton (1944); *Arsenic and Old Lace*, directed by Frank Capra (1944). In *Bedlam*, directed by Mark Robson (1946), Karloff finally plays an asylum superintendent himself.

CHAPTER 4. FREUDIAN RESCUES

1. Howard L. Kaye, "Why Freud Hated America," *Wilson Quarterly* 17, no. 2 (Spring 1993), 118–25; Ernst Falzeder, "'A Fat Wad of Dirty Paper': Freud on America, Freud in America, Freud and America," in *After Freud Left: A Century of Psychoanalysis in America*, ed. John Burnham (Chicago, IL: University of Chicago Press, 2012), 85–110. Freud called America "Dollaria" (92).

2. Eva Illouz, *Saving the Modern Soul: Therapy, Emotions, and the Culture of Self-Help* (Berkeley, CA: University of California Press, 2008), 36. The American press also tended to use Freud as a stand-in for *all* psychiatric innovations. See Nathan G. Hale, *The Rise and Crisis of Psychoanalysis in the United States: Freud and the Americans, 1917–1985* (New York, NY: Oxford University Press, 1995), 276.

3. See Lawrence R. Samuel, *Freud on Madison Avenue: Motivation Research and Subliminal Advertising in America* (Philadelphia, PA: University of Pennsylvania Press, 2010); Enoch Callaway, *Asylum: A Mid-Century Madhouse and Its Lessons about Our Mentally Ill Today* (Westport, CT: Praeger, 2007), xv.

4. Van Wyck Brooks, *Days of the Phoenix: The Nineteen-Twenties I Remember* (New York, NY: E. P. Dutton, 1957), 184, 185, 189. Also see James Hoopes, *Van Wyck Brooks: In Search of American Culture* (Amherst, MA: University of Massachusetts Press, 1977), 185–88. Anonymous, *Snake Pit Attendant*, ed. Jesse Walter Dees, Jr. (New York, NY: Exposition Press, 1950), 22.

5. Andrew Scull, *Madness in Civilization: A Cultural History of Insanity from the Bible to Freud, from the Madhouse to Modern Medicine* (Princeton, NJ: Princeton University Press, 2015), 391; Gail A. Hornstein, *To Redeem One Person Is to Redeem the World: The Life of Frieda Fromm-Reichmann* (New York, NY: Free Press, 2000), 97.

6. Gerald N. Grob, *The Mad Among Us: A History of the Care of America's Mentally Ill* (Cambridge, MA: Harvard University Press, 1994), 170; Paul Starr, *The Social Transformation of American Medicine* (New York, NY: Basic Books, 1995), 345; Jeffrey A. Lieberman and Ogi Ogas, *Shrinks: The Untold Story of Psychiatry* (London, UK: Wiedenfeld and Nicolson, 2016), 71–72; Susan Burch and Hannah Joyner, *Unspeakable: The Story of Junius Wilson* (Chapel Hill, NC: The University of North Carolina Press, 2007), 55. A report by John Grimes told of the poor conditions and was basically submerged by the APA. For this story, see Robert Whitaker, *Mad in America: Bad Science, Bad Medicine, and the Enduring Mistreatment of the Mentally Ill* (Cambridge, MA: Perseus Publishing, 2002), 70–71.

7. Mary de Young, *Encyclopedia of Asylum Therapeutics, 1750-1950s* (Jefferson, NC: McFarland Publishing, 2015), 125; Edward Shorter, *A History of Psychiatry: From the Era of the Asylum to the Age of Prozac* (New York, NY: John Wiley and Sons, 1997), 208–24; Alex Beam, *Gracefully Insane: The Rise and Fall of America's Premier Mental Hospital* (New York, NY: Public Affairs, 2001), 81. On insulin, Metrazol, and ECT, see Edward Shorter and David Healy, *Shock Therapy: A History of Electroconvulsive Treatment in Mental Illness* (New Brunswick, NJ: Rutgers University Press, 2007);

Whitaker, *Mad in America*, 98–99. Notably, as Jonathan Sadowsky points out, the relationship was more complex than simple opposition. See *Electroconvulsive Therapy in America: The Anatomy of a Medical Controversy* (New York, NY: Routledge, 2017), chap. 4.

8. *The Man from Beyond*, directed by Burton L. King (1922).

9. Anne Austin, *One Drop of Blood: A Mystery Novel* (New York, NY: Macmillan, 1932), 270, 313.

10. Austin, *One Drop of Blood*, 4, 144; Mary Jo Buhle, *Feminism and Its Discontents: A Century of Struggle with Psychoanalysis* (Cambridge, MA: Harvard University Press, 1998), 55; Eli Zaretsky, *Secrets of the Soul: A Social and Cultural History of Psychoanalysis* (New York, NY: Alfred A. Knopf, 2004), 55, 201–2.

11. Inmate Ward 8 [Marle Woodson], *Behind the Door of Delusion* (New York, NY: Macmillan, 1932), 8–9.

12. Woodson, *Behind the Door of Delusion*, 99, 106, 114.

13. Woodson, *Behind the Door of Delusion*, 158–59, 224.

14. William Seabrook, *Asylum* (New York, NY: Harcourt, Brace, 1935), vii, 71, 207–8, 212.

15. Seabrook, *Asylum*, 54, 148–49.

16. Seabrook, *Asylum*, 54, 44, 186, 184n1.

17. Seabrook, *Asylum*, 71, 209.

18. Michel Foucault, *Madness and Civilization: A History of Insanity in the Age of Reason*, trans. Richard Howard (New York, NY: Vintage Books, 1988), 278.

19. Henry Bellamann, *Kings Row* (New York, NY: Simon and Schuster, 1940), 4. For instance, there is a poor part of town, "nigger-town," that is racially segregated and little spoken of.

20. Bellamann, *Kings Row*, 35, 249, 340–42.

21. Bellamann, *Kings Row*, 463.

22. Bellamann, *Kings Row*, 93, 94, 502–3, 576, 577, 589.

23. Bellamann, *Kings Row*, 507. See Sigmund Freud, *Civilization and Its Discontents* (London, UK: Penguin Classics, 2014); Gay, *Freud: A Life for Our Time*, 547. *Daily News*, June 7, 1940, quoted in Janet Walker, *Trauma Cinema: Documenting Incest and the Holocaust* (Berkeley: University of California Press, 2005), 33.

24. *Kings Row*, directed by Sam Wood (1942); Walker, *Trauma Cinema*, 36.

25. Bellamann, *Kings Row*, 597; Richard L. Lael, Barbara Brazos, and Margot Ford McMillen, *Evolution of a Missouri Asylum: Fulton State Hospital, 1851–2006* (Columbia: University of Missouri Press, 2007), 138.

26. Bellamann, *Kings Row*, 568, 632.

27. Olive Higgins Prouty, *Pencil Shavings* (Cambridge, MA: Riverside Press, 1961), 156; Jeanne Thomas Allen, "Introduction: *Now, Voyager* as Women's Film: Coming of Age Hollywood Style," in *Now, Voyager*, ed. Thomas Allen (Madison: University of Wisconsin Press, 1984), 27.

28. Olive Higgins Prouty, *Now, Voyager* (New York, NY: Feminist Press, 2004), 73.

29. Prouty, *Pencil Shavings*, 15; Prouty, *Now, Voyager*, 46.

30. Casey Robinson, "*Now, Voyager* Screenplay," in *Now, Voyager*, ed. Thomas Allen, 62–63. Interestingly, as a child Prouty used to travel to the nearby "insane asylum," describing it as a "big dreary rectangular building surrounded by bog

dreary grounds and an iron fence. Its windows also had bars. Once peering through the fence I saw a figure at one of the windows grasping the bars as if shaking them and I was torn by pity." In *Pencil Shavings*, 42.

31. Prouty, *Now, Voyager*, 141–42.

32. Prouty, *Pencil Shavings*, 115, 180–81, 194; Prouty, *Now, Voyager*, 198.

33. For instance, at one point Jaquith lectures Charlotte about the importance of "sublimation." Prouty, *Now, Voyager*, 195.

34. Janet Walker, *Couching Resistance: Women, Film, and Psychoanalytic Psychiatry* (Minneapolis: University of Minnesota Press, 1993), 4; Prouty, *Pencil Shavings*, 21, 56, 89, 205–6.

35. *Spellbound*, directed by Alfred Hitchcock (1945).

36. *Strange Illusion*, directed by Edgar Ulmer (1945).

37. A *New York Times* search finds the expression "snake pit" used ten times between 1925 and 1945 and 356 times between 1946 and 1966. Author keyword search May 17, 2017.

38. Leslie Fishbein, "*The Snake Pit* (1948): The Sexist Nature of Sanity," in *Hollywood as Historian: American Film in a Cultural Context, Revised Edition*, ed. Peter C. Rollins (Lexington: University Press of Kentucky, 2013), 138–39.

39. Mary Jane Ward, *The Snake Pit* (New York, NY: Random House, 1946), 87.

40. Ward, *The Snake Pit*, 74.

41. Though her experience in the wet pack, evoking a damsel in distress in an island prison cell, also makes for disturbing gothic reading. See Ward, *The Snake Pit*, 169–72.

42. Ward, *The Snake Pit*, 42–44.

43. On the development of ECT, see Timothy W. Kneeland and Carol A. B. Warren, *Pushbutton Psychiatry: A History of Electroshock in America* (Westport, CT: Praeger, 2002), chap. 3; Shorter and Healy, *Shock Therapy*; Richard Abrams, *Electroconvulsive Therapy*, 4th ed. (Oxford, UK: Oxford University Press, 2002), chap. 1; Sadowsky, *Electroconvulsive Therapy in America*, chap. 2.

44. Fishbein, "*The Snake Pit* (1948): The Sexist Nature of Sanity," 137.

45. Hedda Hopper, "Life with de Havilland: 'Snake Pit' and Snakes," *The Sun* (Baltimore), December 12, 1948.

46. *The Snake Pit*, directed by Anatole Litvak (1948; Beverly Hills, Twentieth Century Fox Entertainment, 2004), DVD; "Shocker," *Time*, December 20, 1948; "Sound and Fury" *Newsweek*, November 8, 1948.

47. Ward, *The Snake Pit*, 256–57, 274.

48. *The Snake Pit*, directed by Anatole Litvak (1948).

49. Glen O. Gabbard and Krin Gabbard, *Psychiatry and the Cinema*, 2nd ed. (Washington, DC: American Psychiatric Press, 1999), 60–63.

50. Gerald N. Grob, *From Asylum to Community: Mental Health Policy in Modern America* (Princeton, NJ: Princeton University Press, 1991), 77.

51. William Gibson, *The Cobweb* (New York, NY: Alfred A. Knopf, 1954); Robert W. Marks, *The Horizontal Hour* (New York, NY: David McKay Company, Inc., 1957); Millen Brand, *Savage Sleep* (Crown, 1967), 61.

52. The first *Diagnostic and Statistical Manual of Mental Disorders* (*DSM I*) in 1952 reified the turn toward early childhood psychological causes of mental illness.

See Jonathan M. Metzl, *The Protest Psychosis: How Schizophrenia Became a Black Disease* (Boston, MA: Beacon Press, 2009), 28–38; Foucault, *Madness and Civilization*, 277–78.

53. Burch and Joyner, *Unspeakable*, 1.

54. Burch and Joyner, *Unspeakable*, 44; "Insanity: Mental Illness among Negroes Exceeds Whites, Overcrowds Already Jammed 'Snake Pits,'" *Ebony*, April 1949, 19–23. Quoted in Metzl, *The Protest Psychosis*, 40.

CHAPTER 5. THE DAWNING AGE OF PARANOIA

1. Ginsberg quoted in Jonah Raskin, *American Scream: Allen Ginsberg's Howl and the Making of the Beat Generation* (Berkeley, CA: University of California Press, 2005), xiv; Ginsberg, "Howl for Carl Solomon" in *Howl: Original Transcript Facsimile, Transcript, and Variant Versions*, ed. Barry Miles (New York, NY: Harper Perennial Modern Classics, 2006), 7.

2. J. D. Salinger, *The Catcher in the Rye* (Boston, MA: Little, Brown, 2010), 3; Jack Salzman, ed., *New Essays on Catcher in the Rye* (Cambridge, UK: Cambridge University Press, 1991), 98. Salinger earlier published a short story about Holden Caulfield titled "I'm Crazy" in *Colliers*, December 22, 1945.

3. Erich Fromm, *The Sane Society* (New York, NY: Holt, 1955), 360; Paul Goodman, *Growing Up Absurd: Problems of Youth in the Organized System* (New York, NY: Random House, 1960), 72.

4. *Salinger*, directed by Shane Salerno (2013); David Shields and Shane Salerno, *Salinger* (New York, NY: Simon and Schuster, 2013), xvi, 116, 125, 158; J. D. Thomas Medicus, "Salinger's Psychological Catastrophe," *Boston Globe*, March 23, 2014; J. D. Salinger, "A Perfect Day for Bananafish," in *Nine Stories* (Boston, MA: Little, Brown, 1953), 8, 9, 13, 26.

5. Paul Fussell, *Wartime: The Experience of War, 1939–1945* (New York, NY: Oxford University Press, 1989); James Jones, *The Thin Red Line* (New York, NY: Scribner, 1962), 46, 101, 167, 111; Joseph Heller, *Catch-22* (New York, NY: Alfred A. Knopf, 1995), 56–57, 46–47.

6. Sloan Wilson, *The Man in the Gray Flannel Suit* (New York, NY: Simon and Schuster, 1955), 3, 98, 266.

7. There were also issues with confidentiality. Huston quoted in Lesley Brill, *John Huston's Filmmaking* (Cambridge, UK: Cambridge University Press, 1997), 112; also see John L. Michalczyk and Susan A. Michalczyk, "Troubled Silences: Trauma in John Huston's Film *Let There Be Light*," in *War and Film in America: Historical and Critical Essays*, ed. Marilyn J. Matelski and Nancy Lynch Street (Jefferson, NC: McFarland Publishing, 2003), 67–78.

8. Bosley Crowther, "The Screen: Bad Medicine," *New York Times*, March 9, 1946.

9. Michael Bronski, introduction to *Finistère*, by Fritz Peters (Vancouver, BC: Arsenal Pulp Press, 2006), xxii; "Arthur A. Peters, Writer of Psychological Novels," *New York Times*, December 29, 1979. The *Saturday Review* commented, it "with some reason might be called a male 'Snake Pit.'" September 17, 1949, 11. Fritz Peters (Arthur A. Peters), *The World Next Door* (New York, NY: Farrar, Straus, 1949), 34, 44, 117.

10. Lillian Faderman, *The Gay Revolution: The Story of the Struggle* (New York, NY: Simon and Schuster, 2015), 31; Peters, *The World Next Door*, 178, 260.

11. Peters, *The World Next Door*, 271, 298, 359.

12. Janet Walker, *Couching Resistance: Women, Film, and Psychoanalytic Psychiatry* (Minneapolis: University of Minnesota Press, 1993), 2; Gerald N. Grob, *From Asylum to Community: Mental Health Policy in Modern America* (Princeton, NJ: Princeton University Press, 1991), 13. Leo Rosten, *Captain Newman, M.D.* (New York, NY: Harper and Row, 1961), 38, 126; *Captain Newman, M.D.*, directed by David Miller (1963). A key report on psychic casualties of warfare is John W. Appel and Gilbert W. Beebe, "Preventative Psychiatry: An Epidemiologic Approach," *Journal of the American Medical Association* 131 (1946), 1469–75. On Freud and vets, see Robert Francis Wickware, "Psychoanalysis," *Life* 22 (February 3, 1947).

13. Joel T. Braslow, *Mental Ills and Bodily Cures: Psychiatric Treatment in the First Half of the Twentieth Century* (Berkeley, CA: University of California Press, 1997), 27; Steven J. Taylor, *Acts of Conscience: World War II, Mental Institutions, and Religious Objectors* (Syracuse, NY: Syracuse University Press, 2009), 1–2. Albert Deutsch, *The Shame of the States* (New York, NY: Harcourt, Brace, 1948), chap. 14.

14. Frank L. Wright, Jr., *Out of Sight, Out of Mind* (Philadelphia, PA: National Mental Health Foundation, 1947), 13–15, 35, 49–51, 52, 55, 62–63, 106–8. Eleanor Roosevelt quoted in Taylor, *Acts of Conscience*, 139.

15. Jeanne L. Brand, "Albert Deutsch: Historian as Social Reformer," *Journal of the History of Medicine and Allied Sciences* 18, no. 2 (1963), 149–57; Deutsch, *The Shame of the States*, 41, 49, 112.

16. Deutsch, *The Shame of the States*, 135, 161.

17. He writes America's asylums have become "little more than concentration camps on the Belsen pattern." Albert Q. Maisel, "Bedlam 1946," *Life*, May 6, 1946.

18. Wright, *Out of Sight, Out of Mind*, 42–43, 58; Ellen C. Philtine (Ellen Catt), *They Walked in Darkness* (New York, NY: Liveright Publishing, 1945), 241; Deutsch, *Shame of the States,* 96. Writes Deutsch, in asylums he witnessed "scenes that rivaled the horrors of the Nazi concentration camps" (28).

19. Benjamin L. Alpers, *Dictators, Democracy, and American Public Culture: Envisioning the Totalitarian Enemy, 1920s–1950s* (Chapel Hill: University of North Carolina Press, 2003), 285–86; David Seed, *Brainwashing: The Fictions of Mind Control: A Study of Novels and Films since World War II* (Kent, OH: Kent State University Press, 2004), 2.

20. This dating basically follows postwar noir analyses of Mark Osteen, Edward Dimendberg, John Belton, and others. See Osteen, *Nightmare Alley: Film Noir and the American Dream* (Baltimore, MD: Johns Hopkins University Press, 2013), 11; Dimendberg, *Film Noir and the Spaces of Modernity* (Cambridge, MA: Harvard University Press, 2001), 6; and Frank Krutnik, *In a Lonely Street: Film Noir, Genre, Masculinity* (London, UK: Routledge, 1991). An argument can be made that the genre originates in the Great Depression, and that it did not ever really "end." My own view is that noir is best viewed as an expression or coalescence of postwar anxieties building on modernist critiques, prewar pulp, and hard-boiled fiction, as well as innovations adopted from German Expressionism.

21. Jeffrey A. Lieberman and Ogi Ogas, *Shrinks: The Untold Story of Psychiatry*

(London, UK: Wiedenfeld and Nicolson, 2016), 73; Mary Jo Buhle, *Feminism and Its Discontents: A Century of Struggle with Psychoanalysis* (Cambridge, MA: Harvard University Press, 1998), 9; Andrew Scull, *Madness in Civilization: A Cultural History of Insanity from the Bible to Freud, from the Madhouse to Modern Medicine* (Princeton, NJ: Princeton University Press, 2015), 353.

22. *High Wall*, directed by Curtis Bernhardt (1947; Burbank, CA: Warner Home Video, 2010), DVD; "At the Capitol," *New York Times*, December 26, 1947.

23. Quoted in Michael T. Toole, "High Wall," Turner Classic Movies, http://www.tcm.com/this-month/article.html?isPreview=&id=191872%7C62536&name=High-Wall, accessed May 19, 2017.

24. Fredric Brown, *The Screaming Mimi* (New York, NY: E. P. Dutton, 1949), 8–19.

25. Writes Jack Seabrook, "*The Screaming Mimi* is a brilliant portrait of a world gone mad . . ." In *Martians and Misplaced Clues: The Life and Work of Fredric Brown* (Bowling Green, OH: Bowling Green State University Popular Press, 1993), 115.

26. Seabrook, *Martians and Misplaced Clues*, 116; *Screaming Mimi*, directed by Gerd Oswald (1958).

27. *Kiss Me Deadly*, directed by Robert Aldrich (1955; Santa Monica, CA: MGM Home Entertainment, 2001), DVD; Mickey Spillane, *Kiss Me, Deadly* (New York, NY: Simon and Schuster, 1952), 12; *Shock*, directed by Alfred Werker (1946; Beverly Hills, CA: Twentieth Century Fox Home Entertainment, 2006), DVD; *The Enforcer*, directed by Bretaigne Windust (1951; Santa Monica, CA: Artisan Home Entertainment, 2003), DVD; *Possessed*, directed by Curtis Bernhardt (1947; Burbank, CA: Warner Home Video, 2005), DVD; *Nightmare Alley*, directed by Edmund Goulding (1947; Beverly Hills, CA: Twentieth Century Fox Home Entertainment, 2005), DVD; *Ring of Fear*, directed by James Edward Grant (1954; Hollywood, CA: Paramount Home Video, 2005), DVD; *Shock Treatment*, directed by Denis Sanders (1964). Pulp novels such as *Shock Treatment* (1961) and *Nightmare in Pink* (1964) also dished out noir asylums.

28. Margot A. Henriksen, *Dr. Strangelove's America: Society and Culture in the Atomic Age* (Berkeley: University of California Press, 1997), 107; Michael E. Staub, *Madness Is Civilization: When Diagnosis Was Social, 1948–1980* (Chicago, IL: University of Chicago Press, 2011), 13, 35; Grob, *From Asylum to Community*, 44; Seed, *Brainwashing: The Fictions of Mind Control*, 45–49. Note that in *The Man in the Gray Flannel Suit*, Tom Rath's job is public relations aimed at promoting awareness of mental health.

29. Fromm, *The Sane Society*, 194, 169.

30. Nora Sayre, *Previous Convictions: A Journey through the 1950s* (New Brunswick, NJ: Rutgers University Press, 1995), 179; Sigmund Freud, "Formulations on the Two Principles of Mental Functioning," in *The Freud Reader*, ed. Peter Gay (New York, NY: W. W. Norton, 1989), 304; Menninger, *Psychiatry in a Troubled World*, 23, 45; Roy Porter, *Madness: A Brief History* (Oxford, UK: Oxford University Press, 2002), 199.

31. Corbett H. Thigpen and Hervey M. Cleckly, *The Three Faces of Eve* (New York, NY: McGraw-Hill, 1957), 5, 177. Kevin Young, *Bunk: The Rise of Hoaxes, Humbug, Plagiarists, Phonies, Post-Facts, and Fake News* (Minneapolis, MN: Graywolf Press, 2017), 211.

32. Thigpen and Cleckly, *The Three Faces of Eve*, 237, 235.

33. Thigpen and Cleckly, *The Three Faces of Eve*, 177.

34. Thigpen and Cleckley also critique simplistic Jungian explanations. See *The Three Faces of Eve*, 250–51, 259. Dr. Joost A. M. Meerloo was considered a multiple personality expert. See "Well, Then Who Am I," *New York Times*, March 24, 1957.

35. *The Three Faces of Eve*, directed by Nunnally Johnson (1957; Beverly Hills, CA: Twentieth Century Fox, 2013), DVD; Thigpen and Cleckley, *The Three Faces of Eve*, 274.

36. Robert Bloch, *Psycho* (New York, NY: Overlook Press, 2010), 170, 173. Bloch actually makes what seems to be a clever reference to the atomic age here. He writes, "The voices had exploded when triggered into fission, but now, almost miraculously, a fusion had taken place." The atom bomb was a fission bomb; the much bigger hydrogen bomb was a fusion weapon.

37. Judith Kruger, *My Fight for Sanity* (Philadelphia, PA: Chilton, 1959), 140. Noted Dorothy Thompson in October of 1945, the Bomb and arms race may lead "for a worldwide nervous breakdown." Quoted in Henriksen, *Dr. Strangelove's America*, 86. Psychiatrists could break down too—see Robert W. Marks, *The Horizontal Hour* (New York, NY: David McKay Company, Inc., 1957).

38. Kruger, *My Fight for Sanity*, 18, 21.

39. Kruger, *My Fight for Sanity*, 51.

40. Kruger, *My Fight for Sanity*, 31, 50–51.

41. Kruger, *My Fight for Sanity*, 197, 199, 211, 212, 244.

42. Robert Dahl, *Breakdown* (New York, NY: Ace Books, 1959), 8, 160, 161.

43. Yale Kramer, "Freud and the Culture Wars," *Public Interest* 124 (Summer 1996), 44.

44. Vladimir Nabokov, *The Annotated Lolita*, rev. and updated ed., ed. Alfred Appel, Jr. (New York, NY: Vintage Books, 1991), 14, 18, 308.

45. Jack Kerouac, "About the Beat Generation," in *The Portable Jack Kerouac*, ed. Ann Charters (New York, NY: Penguin Books, 1995), 560.

46. Kerouac, *On the Road* in *Jack Kerouac: Road Novels, 1957–1960* (New York, NY: Literary Classics, 2013), 7.

47. Nora Sayre, *Previous Convictions: A Journey through the 1950s* (New Brunswick, NJ: Rutgers University Press, 1995), 193; Jerome Neukirch, "The Janitor," in *The Beats: A Graphic History*, ed. Harvey Pekar, Ed Piskor, and Paul Buhle (New York, NY: Farrar, Straus and Giroux, 2009), 156; Paul Varner, *Historical Dictionary of the Beat Movement* (Lanham, MD: Scarecrow Press, 2012), 36.

48. Carl Solomon's asylum experience is treated in his *Mishaps, Perhaps* (San Francisco, CA: City Lights Books, 1969). Bill Morgan, *The Typewriter is Holy: The Complete, Uncensored History of the Beat Generation* (Berkeley, CA: Counterpoint, 2010), 5, 32, 46.

49. Christopher Gair, *The Beat Generation: A Beginner's Guide* (Oxford: Oneworld Publications, 2008), 74. Ginsberg, "Howl for Carl Solomon," 3–4.

50. Ginsberg, "Howl for Carl Solomon," 3, 5–7.

51. Morgan, *The Typewriter Is Holy*, 155; Ginsberg, "Howl for Carl Solomon," 6–8.

52. Raskin, *American Scream*, 93.

53. Kerouac, "About the Beat Generation," 561, and "The Vanishing American

Hobo," 764, in *The Portable Jack Kerouac*; Kerouac, *The Dharma Bums* (New York, NY: Penguin Books, 1976), 121.

CHAPTER 6. THEY'RE COMING TO TAKE YOU AWAY

1. Rick Dodgson, *It's All a Kind of Magic: The Young Ken Kesey* (Madison, WI: University of Wisconsin Press, 2013), 135–37; Terry Gross, "The Fresh Air Interview: Ken Kesey," in *Conversations with Ken Kesey*, ed. Scott F. Parker (Jackson: University of Mississippi Press, 2014), 113–14; Robert Cottrell, *Sex, Drugs, and Rock 'n' Roll: The Rise of America's 1960s Counterculture* (Lanham, MD: Rowman and Littlefield, 2015), 89–90.

2. Ken Kesey, *One Flew Over the Cuckoo's Nest: Text and Criticism*, ed. John C. Pratt (New York, NY: Viking Press, 1977). I use the critical edition, originally published in 1973, which differs slightly from the original 1962 version. One of the characters, "The Red Cross Lady" called "Gwen-doe-lin" is replaced by the "Public Relations Man" due to a lawsuit from Gwen Davis, who accused Kesey of defamation. This change, in my view, does not alter the substance of the book, though his portrayal of the Red Cross Lady does make the original book seem more anti-Semitic. See Dodgson, *It's All a Kind of Magic*, 157–58.

3. See Raymond M. Olderman, "The Grail Knight Arrives," in *Beyond the Waste Land: The American Novel in the Nineteen-Sixties* (New Haven, CT: Yale University Press, 1972), 35–51; Harold Bloom, ed. *Ken Kesey's "One Flew Over the Cuckoo's Nest,"* Bloom's Modern Critical Interpretations (New York, NY: Bloom's Literary Criticism, 2008). As *Life* magazine explained, Kesey "makes the tired old subject of life in a mental hospital into an absorbing Orwellian microcosm of all humanity." Quoted in Cottrell, *Sex, Drugs, and Rock 'n' Roll*, 93.

4. Kesey, *One Flew Over the Cuckoo's Nest*, 294. See Bloom, *Ken Kesey's "One Flew Over the Cuckoo's Nest"*; Kesey, "Criticism," in *One Flew Over the Cuckoo's Nest: Text and Criticism*; George J. Searles, ed., *A Casebook on Ken Kesey's One Flew Over the Cuckoo's Nest* (Albuquerque: University of New Mexico Press, 1992); Barbara T. Lupack, *Insanity as Redemption in Contemporary American Fiction* (Gainesville: University Press of Florida, 1996), chap. 3; M. Gilbert Porter, *The Art of Grit: Ken Kesey's Fiction* (Columbia: University of Missouri Press, 1982); Leslie Fiedler, *The Return of the Vanishing American* (New York, NY: Stein and Day, 1968).

5. Kesey, *One Flew Over the Cuckoo's Nest*, 68–69, 122. The book uses the acronym EST (electro-shock therapy), though I will use ECT for the sake of consistency with the rest of this book.

6. Kesey, *One Flew Over the Cuckoo's Nest*, 27–28.

7. Frederick Douglass, *Narrative of the Life of Frederick Douglass, An American Slave, Written by Himself* (Boston, MA: Antislavery Office, 1849), 84–85; Simone Browne, *Dark Matters: On the Surveillance of Blackness* (Durham, NC: Duke University Press, 2015), 10. Also see Christian Parenti, *The Soft Cage: Surveillance in America, from Slavery to the War on Terror* (New York, NY: Basic Books, 2007).

8. Kesey, *One Flew Over the Cuckoo's Nest*, 4–5.

9. Fanny Fern, *Ruth Hall and Other Writings* (New Brunswick, NJ: Rutgers University Press, 1986), 110; Elizabeth Packard, *The Prisoners' Hidden Life, Or, Insane*

Asylums Unveiled (Chicago, IL: J. N. Clarke, 1871), 206; Nellie Bly, *Ten Days in a Mad-House* (New York, NY: Ian L. Munro, 1887), 29; Florence Seyler Thompson and George W. Galvin, M.D., *A Thousand Faces* (Boston, MA: Four Seas, 1920), 255; Margaret Starr, *Sane or Insane? Or How I Regained Liberty* (Baltimore, MD: Fosnot, Williams, 1904), 31, 95; Olive Higgins Prouty, *Now, Voyager* (New York, NY: Feminist Press, 2004); Mary Jane Ward, *The Snake Pit* (New York, NY: Random House, 1946); Sylvia Plath, "Johnny Panic and the Bible of Dreams," in *Johnny Panic and the Bible of Dreams: Short Stories, Prose and Diary Excerpts* (New York, NY: Harper and Row, 1977), 291, 299. It should also be said that tyrannical women existed in many places in American literature. Even in *Now, Voyager*, the worst of the women is the protagonist's own mother, who personally hates asylums. On the archetypal, mid-century Viper Mother, see Barbara Ehrenreich and Deirdre English, *For Her Own Good: Two Centuries of Experts' Advice to Women*, rev. ed. (New York, NY: Anchor Books, 2005).

    10. Kesey, *One Flew Over the Cuckoo's Nest*, 58, 61.

    11. Kesey, *One Flew Over the Cuckoo's Nest*, 63, 288.

    12. Kesey, *One Flew Over the Cuckoo's Nest*, 15, 14.

    13. Kesey quoted in Peter O. Whitmer and Bruce VanWyngarden, *Aquarius Revisited: Seven Who Created the Sixties Counterculture That Changed America* (New York, NY: Citadel Press Books, 2007), 202; Ruth Sullivan, "Big Mama, Big Papa, and Little Sons in Ken Kesey's *One Flew Over the Cuckoo's Nest*," in *A Casebook on Ken Kesey's "One Flew Over the Cuckoo's Nest*," ed. George J. Searles, 49–66. Kesey, *One Flew Over the Cuckoo's Nest*, 281.

    14. Kesey, *One Flew Over the Cuckoo's Nest*, 58, 180, 55, 57.

    15. Kesey, *One Flew Over the Cuckoo's Nest*, 293, 268, 249, 291, 42, 242.

    16. Kesey, *One Flew Over the Cuckoo's Nest*, 292, 228.

    17. Dale Wasserman, *One Flew Over the Cuckoo's Nest: A Play in Two Acts* (New York, NY: Samuel French, 1974), 22; Michel Foucault, *Discipline and Punish: The Birth of the Prison*, trans. Alan Sheridan (New York, NY: Vintage Books, 1995), 217; Kesey, *One Flew Over the Cuckoo's Nest*, 47, 116, 183, 27, 190, 305.

    18. Erving Goffman, *Asylums: Essays on the Social Situation of Mental Patients and Other Inmates* (New Brunswick, NJ: Aldine Transaction, 2007), xx, 12, 16, 320. By way of historical comparison, Benjamin Rush praised asylums precisely because they were total, a "complete government over patients." See Rush, *Medical Inquiries and Observations upon Diseases of the Mind*, 5th ed. (Philadelphia, PA: Grigg and Elliot, 1835), 174. Staub, *Madness Is Civilization*, 69, 83; Rael Jean Isaac and Virginia C. Armat, *Madness in the Streets: How Psychiatry and the Law Abandoned the Mentally Ill* (New York, NY: Free Press, 1990), 46; David Seed, *Brainwashing: The Fictions of Mind Control, A Study of Novels and Films since World War II* (Kent, OH: Kent State University Press, 2004), 165; Olderman, "The Grail Knight Arrives," 36–37.

    19. Freeman was specifically inspired by an Uline Ice Company pick. See Jack El-Hai, *The Lobotomist: A Maverick Medical Genius and His Tragic Quest to Rid the World of Mental Illness* (Hoboken, NJ: Wiley, 2005), 183–86. Alternatively, according to Andrew Scull, Freeman got the idea for an out-patient lobotomy from an article "in the Italian medical literature." In Andrew Scull, *Madness in Civilization: A Cultural History of Insanity from the Bible to Freud, from the Madhouse to Modern*

Medicine (Princeton, NJ: Princeton University Press, 2015), 315. Also see Elliot Valenstein, *Great and Desperate Cures: The Rise and Decline of Psychosurgery and Other Radical Treatments for Mental Illness* (New York, NY: Basic Books, 1986); Jack D. Pressman, *Last Resort: Psychosurgery and the Limits of Medicine* (Cambridge, UK: Cambridge University Press, 1998); Joel T. Braslow, *Mental Ills and Bodily Cures: Psychiatric Treatment in the First Half of the Twentieth Century* (Berkeley, CA: University of California Press, 1997), 152, 167; Jenell Johnson, *American Lobotomy: A Rhetorical History* (Ann Arbor: University of Michigan Press, 2014). Walter Freeman, James W. Watts, and Thelma Hunt, *Psychosurgery: Intelligence, Emotion, and Social Behavior Following Prefrontal Lobotomy for Mental Disorders* (London, UK: Bailliere, Tindall, and Cox, 1942), 142.

20. E. B. White, "The Door," *New Yorker*, March 25, 1939; Robert Penn Warren, *All the King's Men* (Orlando, FL: Harcourt, 2006), 475–79.

21. Warren, *All the King's Men*, 478–79.

22. See William L. Laurence, "Surgery Is Tried on the Soul-Sick," *New York Times*, June 7, 1937; "Surgery Succeeds in Insanity Field," *Baltimore Sun*, June 13, 1941; H. A. Dannecker, "Psychosurgery Cured Me," *Coronet*, October 1942; "Medicine: Losing Nerves," *Time*, June 30, 1947; "Explorers of the Brain," *New York Times*, October 30, 1949. Kaempffert's article condensed and republished in *Hygeia* (AMA magazine) and further condensed into an article in *Reader's Digest* (October 1942).

23. Irving Wallace, "The Operation of Last Resort," *Saturday Evening Post*, October 20, 1951.

24. Bernard Wolfe, *Limbo* (New York, NY: Random House, 1952), 8, 22, 368. "Book Reviews," *Psychiatric Quarterly* 27 (January 1953), 338.

25. Tennessee Williams, *Suddenly Last Summer*, in *Tennessee Williams: Plays, 1957–1980* (New York, NY: Library of America, 2000), 112, 113, 147.

26. Williams, *Suddenly Last Summer*, 107; Albert J. Devlin and Nancy M. Tischler, *The Selected Letters of Tennessee Williams*, vol. 1, *1920–1945* (New York, NY: New Directions, 2000), 429.

27. Frank G. Slaughter, *Daybreak* (New York, NY: Pocket Books, 1958), 9–10, 13–14, 18. For an overview of Slaughter's life, see Paul Lewis, "Frank Slaughter, Novelist of Medicine, Is Dead at 93," *New York Times*, May 23, 2001.

28. Slaughter, *Daybreak*, 83–87.

29. Slaughter, *Daybreak*, 96, 140, 166.

30. Slaughter, *Daybreak*, 164. As a *New York Times* reviewer dramatically put it, Dr. Slaughter takes us "into the snake pit of a state mental hospital." Charles Lee, "A Miracle-Drug Called Reserpine," *New York Times*, May 18, 1958.

31. Slaughter, *Daybreak*, 126, 320. In the 1961 novel *Shock Treatment*, the evil Dr. Wolfgang Scheirwagen wants to lobotomize the hero before being overruled by a concerned superintendent who tells him he only lobotomizes as a "last resort." As a patient explains, "It would have left you a doddering idiot." Winfred Van Atta, *Shock Treatment* (New York, NY: Doubleday, 1961), 136, 146.

32. Elliott Baker, *A Fine Madness* (New York, NY: G. P. Putnam's Sons, 1964), 13, 14, 36.

33. Baker, *A Fine Madness*, 74–77.

34. Baker, *A Fine Madness*, 275–78, 293, 298, 319.

35. *A Fine Madness*, directed by Irvin Kershner (1966; Burbank, CA: Warner Home Video, 2006), DVD; Christopher Bray, *Sean Connery: A Biography* (New York, NY: Pegasus Books, 2011), 130.

36. Baker, *A Fine Madness*, 162. In the film, the female superintendent refers to lobotomy as "a form of castration."

37. Johnson, *American Lobotomy*, 91–96; *Planet of the Apes*, directed by Franklin J. Schaffner (1968). For a discussion, see Eric Greene, *"Planet of the Apes" as American Myth: Race and Politics in the Films and Television Series* (Jefferson, NC: McFarland Publishing, 1996), chap. 1.

38. According to Eric Greene, the lobotomized loss of "identity" "echoed the identity crisis of the West." In *"Planet of the Apes" as American Myth*, 47.

39. João Biehl, *Vita: Life in a Zone of Social Abandonment* (Berkeley, CA: University of California Press, 2013); Tennessee Williams, *A Streetcar Named Desire*, in *Best American Plays: Third Series, 1945–1951*, ed. John Gassner (New York, NY: Crown, 1952), 91–93; Ronald Hayman, *Tennessee Williams: Everyone Else Is an Audience* (New Haven, CT: Yale University Press, 1993), 42.

40. Dariel Telfer, *The Caretakers* (New York, NY: New American Library, 1959), 395.

41. Telfer, *The Caretakers*, 100. In his review, Frank G. Slaughter wrote that this "polemic attack upon society's handling of one of our greatest social problems" may not be well-written but could help wake society up. "Life in a Snake-Pit," *New York Times*, November 22, 1959. Slaughter suspected Telfer was familiar with the mental institution, and he was right. See Robert Gottlieb, *Avid Reader: A Life* (New York: Farrar, Straus and Giroux, 2016), 76.

42. *The Caretakers*, directed by Hall Bartlett (1963; Santa Monica, CA: MGM Home Video, 2010), DVD.

43. "WABC, WMCA Pull Napoleon from Playlists," *Billboard*, July 30, 1966. It was ranked no. 11 at the time. "Napoleon XIV" is obviously a reference to the ongoing, and quite old, trope in which patients imagine themselves to be the French Emperor.

44. Sigmund Freud, *Jokes and Their Relation to the Unconscious*, trans. James Strachey (New York, NY: W. W. Norton, 1989); *Dr. Strangelove, or How I Stopped Worrying and Learned to Love the Bomb*, directed by Stanley Kubrick (1964). See Charles Maland, *"Dr. Strangelove* (1964): Nightmare Comedy and the Ideology of Liberal Consensus," *American Quarterly* 31, no. 5 (Winter 1979): 697–717. *The Dirty Dozen*, directed by Robert Aldrich (1967; Burbank, CA: Warner Home Video, 2006), DVD.

45. Kesey, *One Flew Over the Cuckoo's Nest*, 138.

46. Ralph Ellison, *Invisible Man* (New York: Modern Library, 1994), 37–70. Dees, *Snake Pit Attendant*, 119–20.

47. *King of Hearts*, directed by Philippe de Broca (1966; New York, NY: Cohen Film Collection, 2018), DVD. Herbert Marcuse, *One-Dimensional Man* (Boston, MA: Beacon Press, 1964), 63–64.

48. Ralph Ellison, *Invisible Man* (New York, NY: Modern Library, 1994), 231–33, 236–37. This scene of white masters using electricity to make a black person "dance" echoes an earlier scene in the book, in which the protagonist as a youth has to pick

up coins on an electrified rug to the delight of observing whites. Also see Alexander Dunst, *Madness in Cold War America* (New York, NY: Routledge, 2017).

49. *Shock Corridor*, directed by Sam Fuller (1963; New York, NY: Criterion Collection, 2011), DVD; Richard Severo, "Sam Fuller, Director, Is Dead at 85," *New York Times*, November 1, 1997; in a 1980 interview, Fuller said, "As far as I am concerned, we are one big asylum." In *Sam Fuller: Interviews*, ed. Gerald Peary (Jackson: University Press of Mississippi, 2012), 74.

50. Susan Tyler Hitchcock, *Frankenstein: A Cultural History* (New York, NY: W. W. Norton, 2007), 230; "Nightmare at 20,000 Feet," in *Twilight Zone*, directed by Richard Donner (1963).

51. *The Disorderly Orderly*, directed by Frank Tashlin (1964; Hollywood, CA: Paramount, 2004), DVD; *One Froggy Evening*, directed by Chuck Jones (1955).

CHAPTER 7. THE ASYLUM NEXT DOOR

1. Jacqueline Susann, *Valley of the Dolls* (New York, NY: Grove Press, 2016), 19. For a typical snarky review, see Martin Levin, "Reader's Report," *New York Times*, April 10, 1966. See Arthur T. Vanderbilt II, *The Making of a Bestseller: From Author to Reader* (Jefferson, NC: McFarland Publishing, 1999), 66.

2. Betty Friedan, *The Feminine Mystique* (New York, NY: W. W. Norton, 1997), 425.

3. Susann, *Valley of the Dolls*, 42.

4. Friedan, *The Feminine Mystique*, 15, 17, 20–21, 29.

5. Friedan, *The Feminine Mystique*, 9, 268.

6. Friedan notes, for instance, that the most popular article run in *McCall's* was a 1956 piece, "The Mother Who Ran Away." In *The Feminine Mystique*, 50.

7. Friedan, *The Feminine Mystique*, 425.

8. Friedan, *The Feminine Mystique*, 447, 487.

9. "Their Sheltered Honeymoon," *Life*, August 10, 1959; Friedan, *The Feminine Mystique*, 182–83.

10. Friedan, *The Feminine Mystique*, 18–20, 34.

11. Friedan, *The Feminine Mystique*, 103, 118–21. Along similar lines, Kate Millett wrote, "All the forces of psychoanalysis came to be gathered to force woman to 'adjust' to her position." In *Sexual Politics*, 196. Also see Lawrence R. Samuel, *Shrink: A Cultural History of Psychoanalysis* (Lincoln: University of Nebraska Press, 2013), 152–53.

12. Friedan, *The Feminine Mystique*, 103, 117, 118, 123.

13. Paul Wilkes, "Mother Superior to Women's Lib," in *Interviews with Betty Friedan*, ed. Janann Sherman (Jackson: University Press of Mississippi, 2002), 15, 16. For a discussion of the psychological dimension of Friedan's work, see Ellen Herman, *The Romance of American Psychology: Political Culture in the Age of Experts* (Berkeley: University of California Press, 1995), 290–303. For her book in context, see Stephanie Coontz, *A Strange Stirring: "The Feminine Mystique" and American Women at the Dawn of the 1960s* (New York, NY: Basic Books, 2011), xv, 90; Ruth Rosen, *The World Split Open: How the Modern Women's Movement Changed America* (New York, NY: Penguin Books, 2000), chap. 1; and Joanne Meyerowitz, "Beyond the Feminine Mystique: A Reassessment of Postwar Mass Culture, 1946–1958," in *Not June Cleaver:*

Women and Gender in Postwar America, 1945–1960, ed. Meyerowitz (Philadelphia, PA: Temple University Press, 1994), 229–62.

14. Notes Gayle Greene, this book was part of a trend of "mad housewife" novels, including books by Faye Weldon, Margaret Laurence, and Margaret Drabble. See *Changing the Story: Feminist Fiction and the Tradition* (Bloomington: Indiana University Press, 1991), 54. Also see Imelda Whelehan, *The Feminist Bestseller: From Sex and the Single Girl to Sex and the City* (New York, NY: Palgrave Macmillan, 2005), chap. 3.

15. Sue Kaufman, *Diary of a Mad Housewife* (New York, NY: Random House, 1967), 5, 30, 44–45, 73, 81.

16. Elizabeth Winder, *Pain, Parties, Work: Sylvia Plath in New York, 1953* (New York, NY: HarperCollins, 2013), 247; Sylvia Plath, *The Bell Jar* (New York, NY: Harper and Row, 1971), 238.

17. Sylvia Plath, "Tongues of Stone" in *Johnny Panic and the Bible of Dreams: Short Stories, Prose and Diary Excerpts* (New York, NY: Harper and Row, 1979), 267–68. Also see N. B. Masal, "*The Bell Jar* and 'Tongues of Stone': A Comparative Study," in *Studies in American Literature,* ed. Mohit K. Ray (New Delhi, India: Atlantic Publishers and Distributors, 2002), 52–60. Luke Ferretter, *Sylvia Plath's Fiction: A Critical Study* (Edinburgh: Edinburgh University Press, 2010), 43–44.

18. Plath, *The Bell Jar,* 85, 114.

19. Plath, *The Bell Jar,* 93–94, 128–30, 83, 140. Plath's critique of patriarchy is implicit in the many destructive, male influences on Esther. On this, see Linda Wagner-Martin, "*The Bell Jar*": A Novel of the Fifties* (New York, NY: Twayne Publisher, 1992), chap. 7. Also see Plath's famous poem "Daddy," in which she imagines her father as a stifling, autocratic patriarch and pokes fun at Freudianism, in *Ariel* (New York, NY: HarperCollins, 1965), 50.

20. Plath, *The Bell Jar,* 142.

21. Plath, *The Bell Jar,* 143. Ken Kesey, *One Flew Over the Cuckoo's Nest: Text and Criticism,* ed. John C. Pratt (New York, NY: Viking Press, 1977), 270. Peter K. Steinberg, *Sylvia Plath* (Philadelphia, PA: Chelsea House, 2004), 41; Connie Ann Kirk, *Sylvia Plath: A Biography* (Westport, CT: Greenwood Press, 2004), 53; Alex Beam, *Gracefully Insane: The Rise and Fall of America's Premier Mental Hospital* (Cambridge, MA: Public Affairs, 2001), 154; Edward Shorter and David Healy, *Shock Therapy: A History of Electroconvulsive Treatment in Mental Illness* (New Brunswick, NJ: Rutgers University Press, 2007), 155. However, according to Andrew Scull, "as early as 1942 . . . ECT began to be administered with a muscle relaxant, first curare and then succinylcholine, which required the use of anaesthesia and oxygenation." This might mean that Plath suffered instead an "incomplete" seizure. On this, see Rael Jean Isaac and Virginia C. Armat, *Madness in the Streets: How Psychiatry and the Law Abandoned the Mentally Ill* (New York, NY: Free Press, 1990), 198.

22. Sylvia Plath, "Johnny Panic and the Bible of Dreams," in *Johnny Panic and the Bible of Dreams: Short Stories, Prose and Diary Excerpts* (New York, NY: Harper and Row, 1977), 166; Plath, "The Hanging Man," in *Ariel,* 69. Plath, *The Bell Jar,* 1. On Plath and the Rosenbergs, see Luke Ferretter, *Sylvia Plath's Fiction,* 101–7; also useful is Sally Bayley, "'I have your head on my wall': Sylvia Plath and the Rhetoric of Cold War America," in *Critical Insights: The Bell Jar by Sylvia Plath,* ed. Janet

McCann (Pasadena, CA: Salem Press, 2012), 129–52. For an insightful discussion of Plath and the electrocution theme, see Elaine Showalter, *The Female Malady: Women, Madness, and English Culture, 1830–1980* (New York, NY: Penguin Books, 1987), 217–18.

23. Plath, *The Bell Jar*, 159–60. Describing her first, painful round of ECT to a friend, Plath would similarly write, "Pretty soon, the only doubt in my mind was the precise time and method of committing suicide." Quoted in Beam, *Gracefully Insane*, 154.

24. Plath, *The Bell Jar*, 185–87, 189, 213–14.

25. Plath, *The Bell Jar*, 192–93.

26. In fact, Prouty wanted to send Plath to the same place *she* went, but her mother preferred McLean. See Kirk, *Sylvia Plath*, 56. Plath, *The Bell Jar*, 220; Sylvia Plath and Aurelia Schober Plath, *Letters Home: Selected Correspondence 1950–1963* (New York, NY: Harper and Row, 1975), 131–32.

27. Anne Sexton, "Sylvia's Death," in *The Complete Poems* (Boston, MA: Houghton Mifflin, 1981), 126; Diane Wood Middlebrook, *Anne Sexton: A Biography* (New York, NY: Vintage Books, 1992), 32, 40; Clare Pollard, "Her Kind: Anne Sexton, the Cold War, and the Idea of the Housewife," *Critical Quarterly* (October 1, 2006), 1.

28. Elizabeth Bishop, "The Second Chance," *Time*, June 2, 1967. In Bishop's 1950 asylum poem, "Visits to St. Elizabeths," she paints a disquieting picture of a madhouse, mimicking the meter of the child's rhyme "This Is the House that Jack Built." On confessional poetry, see Christopher Beach, *The Cambridge Introduction to Twentieth-Century American Poetry* (Cambridge, UK: Cambridge University Press, 2012), chap. 8.

29. Middlebrook, *Anne Sexton*, 40. Sexton even wrote a poem about Lowell in a manic state, "Elegy in the Classroom," in *To Bedlam and Part Way Back*. In Sexton, *The Complete Poems*, 32. Middlebrook adds as well Maxine Kumin, Denise Levertov, and Adrienne Rich.

30. Barbara Howes, "Voice of a New Poet," *New York Herald Tribune*, December 11, 1960; Sexton, "You, Dr. Martin," "Music Swims Back to Me," and "Noon Walk on the Asylum Lawn," in *The Complete Poems*, 3, 6–7, 27–28. For an analysis of mental institutions in Sexton's work, see "'To Bedlam and Almost All the Way Back': The Image and Function of the Institution in Confessional Poetry" in *Signifying Pain: Constructing and Healing the Self through Writing*, ed. Judith Harris (Albany: State University of New York Press, 2003), 219–37.

31. Sexton, "Flee on Your Donkey," in *The Complete Poems*, 97–105; Middlebrook, *Anne Sexton*, 177.

32. Or as Middlebrook explains, "Sexton's work offered the mental hospital as a metaphorical space in which to articulate the crazy-making pressures of middle-class life, particularly for women." In *Anne Sexton*, 98.

33. Gail A. Hornstein, *To Redeem One Person Is to Redeem the World: The Life of Frieda Fromm-Reichmann* (New York, NY: Free Press, 2000), xi, xiv.

34. Writes Andrew Scull, "While the median income in 1954 of their state hospital colleagues was a mere $9,000, among analysts the comparable figure was more than twice as much—$22,000." In *Madness in Civilization*, 341. See as well Hornstein, *To Redeem One Person Is to Redeem the World*. This did not mean other forms

of restraint were absent here. The hospital used some drugs and wet pack therapy. See Alfred H. Stanton and Morris S. Schwartz, *The Mental Hospital: A Study of Institutional Participation in Psychiatric Illness and Treatment* (New York, NY: Basic Books, 1954).

35. It was named for the enormous chestnut trees that inhabited the property. Hornstein, *To Redeem One Person Is to Redeem the World*; Stanton and Schwartz, *The Mental Hospital*, 44.

36. Frieda Fromm-Reichmann, *Principles of Intensive Psychology* (Chicago, IL: University of Chicago Press, 1950), 178; Hornstein, *To Redeem One Person Is to Redeem the World*, 281–96.

37. Joanne Greenberg, *I Never Promised You a Rose Garden* (New York, NY: Signet, 1964), 12, 11, 124.

38. See Winfred Van Atta, *Shock Treatment* (New York, NY: Doubleday, 1961). On the "tradition" of female therapists falling in love with patients, see Glen O. Gabbard and Krin Gabbard, *Psychiatry and the Cinema*, 2nd ed. (Washington, DC: American Psychiatric Press, 1999), chap. 5. A recent movie with this theme is *Suicide Squad* (2016) where asylum doctor Harley Quinn falls in love with the Joker.

39. Lisa Appignanesi, *Mad, Bad and Sad: Women and the Mind Doctors* (New York, NY: W. W. Norton, 2008), 315–19; Greenberg, *I Never Promised You a Rose Garden*, 106, 191.

40. Greenberg, *I Never Promised You a Rose Garden*, 140.

41. Stanton and Schwartz, *The Mental Hospital*, 33, 9, 73, 395; Nathan G. Hale, *The Rise and Crisis of Psychoanalysis in the United States: Freud and the Americans, 1917–1985* (New York, NY: Oxford University Press, 1995), 253; Beam, *Gracefully Insane*, 121–22; Hornstein, *To Redeem One Person Is to Redeem the World*.

42. J. R. Salamanca, *Lilith* (New York, NY: Simon and Schuster, 1961), 18, 97–98.

43. Salamanca, *Lilith*, 302.

44. Salamanca quoted in Suzanne Finstad, *Warren Beatty: A Private Man* (New York, NY: Three Rivers Press, 2005), 300.

45. Jurgen Muller, ed., *Movies of the 60s* (Los Angeles, CA: Taschen, 2004), 264–69; Suzanne Finstad, *Warren Beatty*, 301.

46. Greenberg, *I Never Promised You a Rose Garden*, 102–3, 350.

47. The phrase "schizophrenogenic mother" found in her 1948 paper, "Notes on the Development of Treatment of Schizophrenics by Psychoanalytic Psychotherapy," in Frieda Fromm-Reichmann, *Psychoanalysis and Psychotherapy: Selected Papers of F. Fromm-Reichmann*, ed. Dexter Bullard (Chicago, IL: University of Chicago Press, 1959), 164. For a discussion, see Hornstein, *To Redeem One Person Is to Redeem the World*, 133–35; Friedan, *The Feminine Mystique*, 189, 276, 279, 286–87. On the rise of the "pathological mother," see Barbara Ehrenreich and Deirdre English, *For Her Own Good: Two Centuries of Experts' Advice to Women*, rev. ed. (New York, NY: Anchor Books, 2005), chap. 7. Greer Williams, "Schizophrenics Can Recover," *Atlantic Monthly* 209 (January 1962), 28; Don D. Jackson, "Schizophrenia," *Scientific American* 207 (August 1962), 65–74; Martin B. Loeb, "Mental Health: New Frontiers," *The Nation*, May 18, 1963, 418–21; "Family Schizophrenia," *Time*, October 27, 1961. This is discussed in Michael E. Staub, *Madness Is Civilization: When Diagnosis Was Social* (Chicago, IL: University of Chicago Press, 2011), 53.

48. Joyce Rebeta-Burditt, *The Cracker Factory* (New York: Macmillan, 1977), 1, 174.

49. Susann, *Valley of the Dolls*, 322–24, 330, 338, 344.

50. Susann, *Valley of the Dolls*, 349, 369.

51. Susann, *Valley of the Dolls*, 249.

52. In the book, which is titled *Lisa and David*, the perspective is mainly the doctor's, with more direct psychoanalytical themes, including playing up David's "sexual confusion" as being the source of his madness. See Theodore Isaac Rubin, *Lisa and David* (New York, NY: Macmillan, 1961), 75. *Splendor in the Grass*, directed by Elia Kazan (1961; Burbank, CA: Warner Home Video, 2000), DVD; *David and Lisa*, directed by Frank Perry (1962; Chatsworth, CA: Image Entertainment, 2007), DVD.

53. *Inside Daisy Clover*, directed by Robert Mulligan (1965; Burbank, CA: Warner Home Video, 2009), DVD. Coincidentally, Wood herself was analyzed in the 1960s. See Samuel, *Shrink*, 139. International women's asylum fiction was also gaining popularity in America in this era. Works like Jennifer Dawson's *The Ha-Ha* (Kansas City, MO: Valancourt Books, 1961) and Janet Frame's *Faces in the Water* (George Braziller, 1961) deliver asylum episodes that resounded with feminist discontent.

54. Mary Jo Buhle, *Feminism and Its Discontents: A Century of Struggle with Psychoanalysis* (Cambridge, MA: Harvard University Press, 1998), 85, 209–10.

55. Benita Roth, "The Making of the Vanguard Center: Black Feminist Emergence in the 1960s and 1970s," in *Still Lifting, Still Climbing: Contemporary African American Woman's Activism*, ed. Kimberly Springer (New York: New York University Press, 1999), 70–90; Gayl Jones, "Asylum," in *White Rat* (New York, NY: Random House, 1977), 78, 79, 81; Wolfgang Karrer quoted in Casey Clabough, "Speaking the Grotesque: The Short Fiction of Gayl Jones," *Southern Literary Journal* 38, no. 2 (Spring 2006), 85.

56. Critics quoted in Clabough, "Speaking the Grotesque: The Short Fiction of Gayl Jones," 74; Gayl Jones, *Eva's Man* (New York, NY: Random House, 1976), 149, 153.

57. Frantz Fanon, *The Wretched of the Earth*, trans. Richard Philcox (New York, NY: Grove Press, 1963), 3.

CHAPTER 8. ASYLUMS DON'T WORK

1. Morton A. Meyers, *Happy Accidents: Serendipity in Major Medical Breakthroughs in the Twentieth Century* (New York, NY: Arcade, 2011), 34; Jeffrey A. Lieberman and Ogi Ogas, *Shrinks: The Untold Story of Psychiatry* (London, UK: Wiedenfeld and Nicolson, 2015), 176–80; Gerald N. Grob, *From Asylum to Community: Mental Health Policy in Modern America* (Princeton, NJ: Princeton University Press, 1991), 148; Gerald N. Grob, *The Mad among Us: A History of the Care of America's Mentally Ill* (New York, NY: Free Press, 2011), 229; Andrew Scull, ed., *Cultural Sociology of Mental Illness: An A-to-Z Guide* (Thousand Oaks, CA: Sage Publications, 2014), 885; Ann Braden Johnson, *Out of Bedlam: The Truth about Deinstitutionalization* (New York, NY: Basic Books, 1990), 48; Andrew Scull, *Madness in Civilization: A Cultural History of Insanity from the Bible to Freud, from the Madhouse to Modern Medicine* (Princeton, NJ: Princeton University Press, 2016), 367. Earlier, in 1958, the Council of State Governments had reported that "The new 'wonder' drugs" played a prominent role

in declining numbers. See William G. Staples, *Castles of Our Conscience: Social Control and the American State 1800–1985* (New York, NY: John Wiley and Sons, 2013), 109. For an even earlier contemporary discussion, see the June 14, 1954, *Time* magazine article, "Wonder Drug of 1954?"

2. As former Worcester State psychiatrist Enoch Callaway puts it, "The cart of deinstitutionalization had already started to move before the horse of psychopharmacology appeared on the scene." In *Asylum: A Mid-Century Madhouse and Its Lessons about Our Mental Illness Today* (Westport, CT: Praeger, 2007), 173. Maxwell Jones pioneered the idea of the "therapeutic community" in 1947 and codified it in 1953 in his *The Therapeutic Community: A New Treatment Method in Psychiatry* (New York, NY: Basic Books, 1953); Johnson, *Out of Bedlam*, 70, 73–75, 78, 89, 96; Murray Levine, *The History and Politics of Community Mental Health* (New York, NY: Oxford University Press, 1981), 40; John F. Kennedy, "Special Message to the Congress on Mental Illness and Mental Retardation," February 5, 1963. *The American Presidency Project*, http://www.presidency.ucsb.edu/ws/?pid=9546, accessed September 26, 2016; Richard G. Frank and Sherry A. Glied, *Better but Not Well: Mental Health Policy in the United States Since 1950* (Baltimore, MD: Johns Hopkins University Press, 2006), 54–55, 59–60; Rael Jean Isaac and Virginia C. Armat, *Madness in the Streets: How Psychiatry and the Law Abandoned the Mentally Ill* (New York, NY: The Free Press, 1990), chap. 4. Importantly, Mike Gorman already had the phrase, "We will provide greatly increased support for psychiatric research" put into the Democratic National Platform in July 1960. See E. Fuller Torrey, *American Psychosis: How the Federal Government Destroyed the Mental Illness Treatment System* (New York, NY: Oxford University Press, 2014), 39.

3. Gerald N. Grob, "Government and Mental Health Policy: A Structural Analysis," *Milbank Quarterly* 72, no. 3 (1994), 471–500. For a useful overview with links, see "Timeline: Deinstitutionalization and Its Consequences," *Mother Jones*, April 19, 2013, http://www.motherjones.com/politics/2013/04/timeline-mental-health -america, accessed June 7, 2018.

4. Hubert Selby, Jr., *Requiem for a Dream* (Cambridge, MA: Da Capo Press, 2000), 215, 224, 237–38, 263–64.

5. Seymour Krim, "The Insanity Bit," from *Views of a Nearsighted Cannoneer*, reprinted in *The Age of Madness: The History of Involuntary Mental Hospitalization Presented in Selected Texts*, ed. Thomas Szasz (New York, NY: Jason Aronson, 1974), 283, 285; D. Robinson, "Conspiracy USA: The Far Right Fights against Mental Health," *Look*, January 26, 1965, 30–32; Torrey, *American Psychosis*, 75. On the context of Cold War, see David Seed, *Brainwashing: The Fictions of Mind Control, A Study of Novels and Films since World War II* (Kent, OH: Kent State University Press, 2004), chap. 7. On the history of anti-psychiatry, see Norman Dain, "Psychiatry and Antipsychiatry in the United States," in *Discovering the History of Psychiatry*, ed. Mark S. Miscale and Roy Porter (Oxford, UK: Oxford University Press, 1994); Jonathan Sadowsky, *Electroconvulsive Therapy in America: The Anatomy of a Medical Controversy* (New York, NY: Routledge, 2017), chap. 5.

6. Alex Beam, *Gracefully Insane: The Rise and Fall of America's Premier Mental Hospital* (New York, NY: Public Affairs, 2001), 14; Marcuse quoted in Isaac and Virginia, *Madness in the Streets*, 26.

7. Thomas J. Scheff, *Being Mentally Ill: A Sociological Theory* (Chicago, IL: Aldine Publishing, 1966); Erving Goffman, *Asylums: Essays on the Social Situation of Mental Patients and Other Inmates* (Garden City, NY: Anchor Books, 1961); August B. Hollingshead and Frederick C. Redlich, *Social Class and Mental Illness: A Community Study* (New York, NY: Wiley, 1958); Robert Perrucci darkly argues: "In the mental hospital, as well as the prison, there is a conscious attempt at destruction of the patient's self that existed prior to institutionalization." In *Circle of Madness: On Being Insane and Institutionalized in America* (Englewood Cliffs, NJ: Prentice Hall, 1974), 53; J. K. Wing, "Institutionalism in Mental Hospitals," in *Mental Illness and Social Processes*, ed. Thomas J. Scheff (New York, NY: Harper and Row, 1967), 219–38; Kai T. Erikson, "Notes on the Sociology of Deviance," reprinted in *Mental Illness and Social Processes*, ed. Thomas J. Scheff, 300.

8. Thomas S. Szasz, "Some Observations on the Relationship between Psychiatry and the Law," *AMA Archives of Neurology and Psychiatry* 75 (March 1956), 297–315; Szasz, "Malingering: 'Diagnosis' or Social Condemnation?," *AMA Archives of Neurology and Psychiatry* 76 (October 1956), 432–43; Szasz, "The Problem of Psychiatric Nosology," *American Journal of Psychiatry* 114 (November 1957), 405–11; Szasz, "Politics and Mental Health: Some Remarks Apropos of the Case of Mr. Ezra Pound," *American Journal of Psychiatry* 115 (December 1958), 508–11; Szasz, "The Myth of Mental Illness," *The American Psychologist* 15, no. 2 (1960), 113–18; Szasz, *The Myth of Mental Illness: Foundations of a Theory of Personal Conduct* (New York, NY: Harper and Row, 1961); Szasz, *The Myth of Mental Illness: Foundations of a Theory of Personal Conduct*, rev. ed. (New York, NY: Harper and Row, 1974), 50; Szasz, *The Manufacture of Madness: A Comparative Study of the Inquisition and the Mental Health Movement* (New York, NY: Harper and Row, 1970), 138; Szasz, *Law, Liberty, and Psychiatry: An Inquiry into the Social Uses of Mental Health Practices* (New York, NY: Macmillan, 1963), 205; Szasz, *Liberation by Oppression: A Comparative Study of Psychiatry and Slavery* (New Brunswick, NJ: Transaction Publishers, 2009), xiii, 10. Szasz's early arguments are cogently discussed in Michael E. Staub, *Madness Is Civilization: When Diagnosis Was Social* (Chicago, IL: University of Chicago Press, 2011), 89–93.

9. Szasz, *The Manufacture of Madness*, chap. 10; Szasz, *The Myth of Mental Illness*, 267; Szasz, *Law, Liberty, and Psychiatry*, 218–19. On Szasz's varied appeal, see Staub, *Madness Is Civilization*, 106–7.

10. R. D. Laing, *The Politics of Experience* (New York, NY: Pantheon Books, 1967), 36, 83; R. D. Laing, "Massacre of the Innocents," *Peace News* 7 (January 22, 1965), quoted in Staub, *Madness Is Civilization*, 57. Scull notes "Laing was a self-proclaimed Marxist" in *Madness in Civilization*, 373. Thomas S. Szasz, *Schizophrenia: The Sacred Symbol of Psychiatry* (New York, NY: Basic Books, 1988), xii. These critics also all cited each other. Note Isaac and Armat, "Scheff draws liberally upon the writing of Szasz, Laing, Lemert, Foucault, Goffman, and Rosenhan; Laing draws on Szasz, Scheff, Goffman, Bateson, and Foucault; Goffman draws upon Szasz and Bateson; Leifer draws upon Szasz. (Szasz is the only one to move out of the magic circle.)" In *Madness in the Streets*, 57.

11. David L. Rosenhan, "On Being Sane in Insane Places," *Science* (January 1973), 250–58; Isaac and Armat, *Madness in the Streets*, 54–55; Scull, *Madness in Civilization*, 386.

12. Harry Solomon, "The American Psychiatric Association in Relation to American Psychiatry," in *New Directions in American Psychiatry 1944–1968: The Presidential Addresses of the American Psychiatric Association over the Past Twenty-Five Years* (Washington, DC: American Psychiatric Association, 1969), 185. On Rosemary Kennedy's lobotomy, see Torrey, *American Psychosis*, chap. 1. Isaac and Armat, *Madness in the Streets*, 117–18, 121–24; Buchenwald quote in Torrey, *American Psychosis*, 150.

13. William Peter Blatty, *The Exorcist* (New York, NY: Harpertorch, 1971), 337, 59, 60, 119, 148, 218. It is unclear whether Regan is possessed by the demon Pazuzu or the Devil himself, or perhaps legions of demons. Father Merrin seems to like the word "demon." On the idea that Blatty is giving us a tale about invasion from the Middle Eastern "Other," see Philip L. Simpson, "Fear of the Assimilation of the Foreign Other in *The Exorcist*" in *American Exorcist: Critical Essays on William Peter Blatty*, ed. Benjamin Szumskyj (Jefferson, NC: McFarland Publishing, 2008), 25–43.

14. *The Exorcist*, directed by William Friedkin (1973; Burbank, CA: Warner Home Video, 2010), DVD. Karras's brother implies the possibility of better care by mentioning that they can't afford a "private hospital." In the book, we get a near identical flashback: "*I'm not about to put her in a goddam asylum!*" Blatty, *The Exorcist*, 191. Barbara Creed, "Woman as Abject Monster," in *Studies in the Horror Film The Exorcist*, ed. Daniel Olson (Lakewood, CO: Centipede Press, 2011), 208.

15. Vincent Canby, "Why the Devil Do They Dig 'The Exorcist?,'" *New York Times*, January 13, 1974.

16. William Peter Blatty, *The Ninth Configuration* (New York, NY: Harper, 1978), 3; *The Ninth Configuration*, directed by William Peter Blatty (1980; Burbank, CA: Warner Home Video, 2002), DVD.

17. Mike White, *Cinema Detours* (Morrisville, NY: Lulu.com, 2013), 115–16; Blatty, *The Ninth Configuration*, 25, 85, 101.

18. Blatty, *The Ninth Configuration*, 26, 39. On Blatty's *Ninth Configuration* apologetics, see Geoffrey Reiter, "'Foot, You Are Wise!' The Apologetic Structure of *The Ninth Configuration*" in *American Exorcist*, ed. Benjamin Szumskyj, 99–111.

19. William Peter Blatty, *Legion* (New York, NY: Simon and Schuster, 1983), 113, 140, 186.

20. *The Exorcist III*, directed by William Peter Blatty (1990; Burbank, CA: Warner Home Video, 1999), DVD.

21. Kirk Douglas, *The Ragman's Son: An Autobiography* (New York, NY: Simon and Schuster, 1988), 364–69, 385; Howard Taubman, "Theater: 'Cuckoo's Nest,'" *New York Times*, November 14, 1963; Michael Douglas quoted in Marc Eliot, *Michael Douglas: A Biography* (New York, NY: Crown, 2012), 62. Also see Elaine B. Safer, "'It's the Truth Even If It Didn't Happen': Ken Kesey's *One Flew Over the Cuckoo's Nest*," *Literature/Film Quarterly* 5, no. 2 (Spring 1977), 132. Kesey was paid to write a script, which was rejected by the filmmakers, and was bought out. See Marc Eliot, *Nicholson: A Biography* (New York, NY: Crown, 2013), 143.

22. Eliot, *Michael Douglas*, 81; Douglas, *The Ragman's Son*, 390–91; *Completely Cuckoo*, directed by Charles Kiselyak (1997); Larry Sturhan, "Interview with Milos Forman," *Filmmakers Newsletter* 9, no. 2 (December 1975), 26. Quoted in Marsha McCreadie, "*One Flew Over the Cuckoo's Nest*: Some Reasons for One Happy Adaptation,"

Literature/Film Quarterly 5, no. 2 (Spring 1977), 131. Milos Forman and Jan Novak, *Turnaround: A Memoir* (New York, NY: Villard Books, 1994), 112, 273.

23. Commentary, *One Flew Over the Cuckoo's Nest*, directed by Milos Forman (2010; Burbank, CA: Warner Home Video, 2010), DVD; *"One Flew Over the Cuckoo's Nest* Trivia" Milosforman.com. https://milosforman.com/en/movies/one-flew -over-the-cuckoos-nest, accessed May 28, 2017; Forman and Novak, *Turnaround,* 125.

24. Commentary, *One Flew Over the Cuckoo's Nest*, directed by Milos Forman (2010), DVD.

25. Others were also supposedly considered ahead of Nicholson, including Burt Reynolds and James Caan. See Eliot, *Nicholson,* 145–46; *Completely Cuckoo*, directed by Charles Kiselyak (1997); Mark Christensen, *Acid Christ: Ken Kesey, LSD, and the Politics of Ecstasy* (Tucson, AZ: Schaffner Press, 2009), 359; Forman, "Commentary" in *One Flew Over the Cuckoo's Nest*; "Roles and Reality in the Nature of Nicholson," *Chicago Tribune*, March 16, 1975. And there is also, as Robin Wood has theorized, the "ultimate dread" of "women usurping the active, aggressive role that patri-archal ideology assigns to the male." In Wood, "An Introduction to the American Horror Film," in *Movies and Methods*, vol. 2, *An Anthology*, ed. Bill Nichols (Berkeley: University of California Press, 1985), 217.

26. *The Snake Pit*, directed by Anatole Litvak (1948; Beverly Hills, CA: Twentieth Century Fox Entertainment, 2004), DVD; *Fear Strikes Out*, directed by Robert Mulli-gan (1957; Hollywood, CA: Paramount, 2003), DVD; *Shock Corridor*, directed by Sam Fuller (1963; New York, NY: Criterion Collection, 2003), DVD.

27. Forman, "Commentary," *One Flew Over the Cuckoo's Nest*.

28. *Don't Look in the Basement* (orig. *The Forgotten*), directed by S. F. Brownrigg (1973; Narberth, PA: Alpha Video, 2003), DVD. There is no basement in the movie.

29. *One Flew Over the Cuckoo's Nest*, directed by Milos Forman (1975).

30. Eliot, *Nicholson,* 156; Eliot, *Michael Douglas,* 88. *One Flew Over the Cuckoo's Nest*, boxofficemojo.com; Charles Kiselyak, "Excerpts from *Notes from the Cuckoo's Nest*" (Warner Brothers Entertainment, 2001), 36.

31. Vincent Canby, "'Cuckoo's Nest'—A Sane Comedy about Psychotics," *New York Times*, November 23, 1975; Rex Reed, "Movies: One Flew Over the Cuckoo's Nest," *Vogue*, February 1, 1976; Ruth McCormick, review of *One Flew Over the Cuckoo's Nest*, directed by Milos Forman, *Cineaste* 7, no. 3 (Fall 1976), 42.

32. Pauline Kael, "The Bull Goose Loony," *New Yorker*, December 1, 1975; McCor-mick, review of *One Flew Over the Cuckoo's Nest*, 42; *Completely Cuckoo*, directed by Charles Kiselyak (1997); McCreadie, "*One Flew Over the Cuckoo's Nest*: Some Reasons for One Happy Adaptation," 131.

33. McCormick, review of *One Flew Over the Cuckoo's Nest*, 42.

34. H. Steven Moffic, "We Are Still Flying Over the Cuckoo's Nest," *Psychiatric Times* 31, no. 7 (July 1, 2014); Brian S. Everitt, *Health and Lifestyle: Separating the Truth from the Myth with Statistics* (Cham, Switzerland: Springer International Pub-lishing, 2016), 32; Sadowsky, *Electroconvulsive Therapy in America*, 41; Timothy W. Kneeland and Carol A. B. Warren, *Pushbutton Psychiatry: A History of Electroshock in America* (Westport, CT: Praeger, 2002), 78; Edward Shorter and David Healy, *Shock Therapy: A History of Electroconvulsive Treatment in Mental Illness* (New Brunswick,

NJ: Rutgers University Press, 2007), 153–63; Millen Brand, *Savage Sleep* (New York, NY: Crown, 1968), 270.

35. Carrie Fisher, *Wishful Drinking* (New York, NY: Simon and Schuster, 2008), 14, 13.

36. Michael Fleming and Roger Manvell, *Images of Madness: The Portrayal of Insanity in the Feature Film* (Rutherford, NJ: Farleigh Dickinson University Press, 1985), 179; Anthony Clare, review of *One Flew Over the Cuckoo's Nest*, Occasional Film, *The Lancet*, April 17, 1976.

37. As another added bonus, while inside they also discover an undercover "crusading girl reporter" played by Suzanne Somers. She does a Nelly Bly to Hutchinson's R. P. McMurphy. "Murder Ward," *Starsky and Hutch*, directed by Earl Bellamy (1977).

38. Frances Farmer, *Will There Really Be a Morning? An Autobiography of Frances Farmer* (New York, NY: G. P. Putnam's Sons, 1972), 11.

39. Farmer, *Will There Really Be a Morning?*, 13, 32–34, 168–71, 173.

40. Farmer, *Will There Really Be a Morning?*, 217–21.

41. Farmer, *Will There Really Be a Morning?*, 220–21, 212–13, 217, 220–23.

42. Review of *Will There Really Be a Tomorrow* [*sic*]?, by Frances Farmer, *New York Times*, August 20, 1972; Richard D. Lesen, review of *Will There Really Be a Morning?*, by Frances Farmer, *Women's Wear Daily*; Edward Wagenknecht, "A Phenomenal Number of Bad Breaks," *Chicago Tribune*, July 16, 1972; Clarence Petersen, "A Tale from Tinsel Town—with a Twist," *Chicago Tribune*, January 27, 1974; Kevin Kelly, "A Shirt of Flame," *Boston Globe*, September 9, 1973.

43. Phyllis Chesler, *Women and Madness* (Garden City, NY: Doubleday, 1972), 10, 25, 31; Jeffrey L. Geller and Maxine Harris, eds., *Women of the Asylum: Voices from Behind the Walls, 1840–1945* (New York: Anchor Books, 1994), xiii.

44. Marge Piercy, *Woman on the Edge of Time* (New York, NY: Knopf, 1976), 59–60, 68, 99. Also see Jane Donawerth, *Frankenstein's Daughters: Women Writing Science Fiction* (Syracuse, NY: Syracuse University Press, 1997), 82n40.

45. Piercy, *Woman on the Edge of Time*, 74, 362.

46. Barbara Gittings, "Preface: Show and Tell," in *American Psychiatry and Homosexuality: An Oral History*, ed. Jack Drescher and Joseph P. Merlino (Binghamton, NY: Harrington Park Press, 2007), xv; Piercy, *Woman on the Edge of Time*, 77, 255, 276–77.

47. Peter Shelley, *Frances Farmer: The Life and Times of a Troubled Star* (Jefferson, NC: McFarland Publishing, 2011), 60. The earliest version of Kenneth Anger's book was released in France in 1959. Anger, *Hollywood Babylon* (Phoenix, AZ: Associated Professional Services, 1965), 269; Anger, *Hollywood Babylon* (San Francisco, CA: Straight Arrow Books, 1975), 223–29.

48. William Arnold, *Frances Farmer: Shadowland* (New York, NY: McGraw-Hill, 1978), 7.

49. Arnold, *Frances Farmer: Shadowland*, 12, 95, 107, 108.

50. Arnold, *Frances Farmer: Shadowland*, 7–9.

51. Arnold, *Frances Farmer: Shadowland*, 28, 122–23, 124.

52. He seems to be taking his lead from Szasz here.

53. Arnold, *Frances Farmer: Shadowland*, 140–45.

54. Arnold, *Frances Farmer: Shadowland*, 150, 156–57.

55. Arnold, *Frances Farmer: Shadowland*, 161, 168.

56. Jeffrey Kauffman, *Frances Farmer: Shedding Light on Shadowland*, http://jeffreykauffman.net/francesfarmer/sheddinglight.html, accessed November 4, 2016; Jack El-Hai, *The Lobotomist*, 241; Margie Crow, *Off Our Backs* on July 31, 1978; William French, *The Globe and Mail* (Ontario, Canada), June 29, 1978.

57. Edith Herman, "Tempo: Frances Farmer: Did the Star Rebel of Hollywood Really Have a Cause?," *Chicago Tribune*, June 6, 1978.

58. Kauffman, *Frances Farmer: Shedding Light on Shadowland*.

59. Kauffman, *Frances Farmer: Shedding Light on Shadowland*.

60. Dale Pollack, "Film Clips: Screen Biography of Actress Frances Farmer Scheduled," *Los Angeles Times*, April 21, 1981; Richard Corliss and Martha Smilgis, "Morning Comes for Frances," *Time*, February 15, 1982; Aljean Harmetz, "Jessica Lange, Film Star Whose Future Is Here," *New York Times*, December 20, 1982, late East Coast edition.

61. On Harry York, see Kathleen J. Waites, "Graeme Clifford's Biopic, *Frances* (1982): Once a Failed Lady, Twice Indicted," *Literature/Film Quarterly* 33, no. 1 (2005), 12–19. Gary Storhoff, "Icon and History in 'Frances,'" *Literature/Film Quarterly* 23, no. 4 (1995), 271.

62. Stephen Hunter, "'Frances': Film Is Freak of Feminist Parable"; Gary Storhoff, "Icon and History in 'Frances,'" 267.

63. Freeman himself often bragged that "lobotomy got them home." For an overview, see Shelley, *Frances Farmer*, 64–65. Michael Azerrad, in *Come as You Are: The Story of Nirvana* (New York, NY: Broadway Books, 1993), 326–27.

CHAPTER 9. BREAKOUT

1. Ann Braden Johnson, *Out of Bedlam: The Truth about Deinstitutionalization* (New York, NY: Basic Books, 1990), 99; E. Fuller Torrey, *American Psychosis: How the Federal Government Destroyed the Mental Illness Treatment System* (New York, NY: Oxford University Press, 2014), 96; "Denying the Mentally Ill," *New York Times*, June 5, 1981.

2. *Halloween*, directed by John Carpenter (1978; Englewood, CO: Starz Home Entertainment, Restored Edition, 2007), DVD.

3. He later slows to a plod, stalking his victims with his blank mask and knife.

4. The filming location was a small hospital in Altadena, California.

5. Carpenter quoted in Jason Zinoman, *Shock Value: How a Few Eccentric Outsiders Gave Us Nightmares, Conquered Hollywood, and Invented Modern Horror* (New York, NY: The Penguin Press, 2011), 187.

6. Adam Rockoff, *Going to Pieces: The Rise and Fall of the Slasher Film, 1978–1986* (Jefferson, NC: McFarland Publishing, 2002), 51, 53–54; Director's commentary, *Halloween*, directed by John Carpenter (2007), DVD.

7. Phil Brown, *The Transfer of Care: Psychiatric Deinstitutionalization and Its Aftermath* (New York, NY: Routledge, 1988), 133–41. Ronald Sullivan, "Mental-Patient Releases Questioned," *New York Times*, March 13, 1978; Peter Koenig, "The Problem that Can't Be Tranquilized," *New York Times*, May 21, 1978; Gilles Boulenger, *John*

Carpenter: The Prince of Darkness (Los Angeles, CA: Silman-James Press, 2001), 97.

8. *When a Stranger Calls*, directed by Fred Walton (1979; Culver City, CA: Columbia Tristar Home, 2001), DVD.

9. Quoted in Joseph Maddrey, *Nightmares in Red, White, and Blue: The Evolution of the American Horror Film* (Jefferson, NC: McFarland Publishing, 2004), 133.

10. *Friday the 13th*, directed by Sean S. Cunningham (1980; Hollywood, CA: Paramount, 1999), DVD; *Friday the 13th Part III*, directed by Steve Miner (1982; Hollywood, CA: Paramount, 2011), DVD; *Friday the 13th: The Final Chapter*, directed by Joseph Zito (1984; Hollywood, CA: Paramount, 2011), DVD. And at the very, very end of this film, Tommy has a vision of Jason and then finds the mask in his dresser drawer in his hospital room. He "becomes" Jason.

11. *Jason Lives: Friday the 13th Part VI*, directed by Tom McLoughlin (1986; Hollywood, CA: Paramount, 2001) DVD; *Friday the 13th: A New Beginning*, directed by Danny Steinmann (1985; Hollywood, CA: Paramount, 2001), DVD; *Friday the 13th Part VII: The New Blood*, directed by John Carl Buechler (1988; Hollywood, CA: Paramount, 2009), DVD.

12. In Reagan-esque fashion, the blackout is caused by a nuclear reactor failure.

13. *Alone in the Dark*, directed by Jack Sholder (1982; Chatsworth, CA: Image Entertainment, 2005), DVD.

14. "Alone in the Dark," *New York Times*, November 19, 1982, late edition. One critic found this to be "a plausibility problem; to wit: one would think the system would fail with doors and windows locked rather than unlocked." Binn, "Alone in the Dark," *Variety*, July 28, 1982.

15. Mark Edmundson, *Nightmare on Main Street: Angels, Sadomasochism, and the Culture of Gothic* (Cambridge, MA: Harvard University Press, 1997), 55.

16. *Halloween II*, directed by Rick Rosenthal (1981).

17. *Halloween 4: The Return of Michael Myers*, directed by Dwight H. Little (1988; Beverly Hills, CA: Anchor Bay, 2009), DVD; *Halloween 5: The Revenge of Michael Myers*, directed by Dominique Othenin-Girard (1989; Beverly Hills, CA: Anchor Bay, 2009), DVD; *Halloween 6: The Curse of Michael Myers*, directed by Joe Chappelle (1995; Burbank, CA: Dimension Home Video, 2000), DVD.

18. *Halloween: Resurrection*, directed by Rick Rosenthal (2002; Burbank, CA: Miramax, 2011); *Halloween*, directed by David Gordon Green (2018; Universal City, CA).

19. *A Night to Dismember*, directed by Doris Wishman (1983; Scarborough, ME: Elite Entertainment, 2001), DVD; *Splatter University*, directed Richard W. Haines (1984; Scarborough, ME: Elite Entertainment, 2005), DVD; *Night Train to Terror*, directed by John Carr and Phillip Marshak (1985; Los Angeles, CA: Prism Entertainment, 1989), VHS; *Sorority House Massacre*, directed by Carol Frank (1986; Burbank, CA: Warner Home Video, 1989), VHS; *The Last Slumber Party*, directed by Stephen Tyler (1988; USA: United Home Video, 1998), VHS.

20. Robert Bloch, *Psycho II* (New York, NY: Warner Books, 1982), 84, 171. Though Bates, in a twist, turns out not to be the killer. It's his shrink.

21. Mark Seltzer, *Serial Killers: Death and Life in America's Wound Culture* (Hoboken, NJ: Taylor and Frances, 2013), 110; Robert Conrath, "Serial Heroes: A Sociocultural Probing into Excessive Consumption," in *European Readings of American Popular Culture*, ed. John Dean and Jean-Paul Gabilliet (Westport, CT: Greenwood

Press, 1996), 148; Leonard Cassuto, *Hard-Boiled Sentimentality: The Secret History of American Crime Stories* (New York, NY: Columbia University Press, 2008), 261. Italics mine. FBI special agent Robert Ressler would claim to have coined the term "serial killer" in the late '70s. See Seltzer, *Serial Killers*, 108; Philip Jenkins, *Using Murder: The Social Construction of Serial Homicide* (New York, NY: Aldine de Gruyter, 1994), 55–57.

22. The number of victims, as Philip Jenkins demonstrates, is wildly exaggerated. See Jenkins, *Using Murder*, 60–66. For an example of the description of serial killing as "epidemic," see Starr et al., "The Random Killers" *Newsweek*, November 26, 1984. Tellingly, the Freudian paradise depicted in *Rose Garden*, Chestnut Lodge, was sued by a patient in 1982 for only using psychotherapy and not drug therapies.

23. Thomas Harris, *Red Dragon* (New York, NY: G. P. Putnam's Sons, 1981), 137.

24. Harris, *Red Dragon*, 53, 54, 77–78.

25. Harris, *Red Dragon*, 219.

26. Harris, *Red Dragon* 115, 116.

27. Special Features, *Manhunter* directed by Michael Mann (Anchor Bay, 2000). See also Tony Williams, "From *Red Dragon* to *Manhunter*" in *Dissecting Hannibal Lecter: Essays on the Novels of Thomas Harris*, ed. Benjamin Szumskyj (Jefferson, NC: McFarland Publishing, 2008), 102–17. For a detailed discussion of *Manhunter*, see Daniel O'Brien, *The Hannibal Files: The Unauthorized Guide to the Hannibal Lecter Trilogy* (London, UK: Reynolds and Hearn, 2001), 13–63.

28. Thomas Harris, *The Silence of the Lambs* (New York, NY: St. Martin's Press, 1988), 322, 357–58.

29. Harris, *The Silence of the Lambs*, 59–60; *The Silence of the Lambs*, directed by Jonathan Demme (1991).

30. Harris, *The Silence of the Lambs*, 144, 199. Also see https://rhystranter.com /2015/08/03/hannibal-lecter-sherlock-holmes-dracula-david-sexton/, accessed February 15, 2018. Thomas Harris, *Hannibal* (New York, NY: Delacorte Press, 1999), 136–37, 156, 427.

31. Documentary on *The Silence of the Lambs Collector's Edition*, directed by Jonathan Demme (Beverly Hills, CA: MGM Home Entertainment, 2007). Hopkins quoted in Quentin Falk, *Anthony Hopkins: The Authorized Biography* (Brooklyn, NY: Interlink Publishing Group, 1994), 176.

32. Documentary on *The Silence of the Lambs Collector's Edition*, directed by Jonathan Demme (2007; Beverly Hills, CA: Twentieth Century Fox Home Entertainment), DVD.

33. Harris, *Hannibal*, 291.

34. Harris, *Hannibal*, 72, 93.

35. Harris, *Hannibal*, 70–71.

36. Thomas Harris, *Hannibal Rising* (New York, NY: Delacorte Press, 2006), 76, 283.

37. Roger Cohen, "Bret Easton Ellis Answers Critics of 'American Psycho,'" *New York Times*, March 6, 1991; Bret Easton Ellis, *American Psycho* (New York, NY: Vintage Books, 1991), 194.

38. Ellis, *American Psycho*, 6.

CHAPTER 10. STANDARDIZATION

1. *Changeling*, directed by Clint Eastwood (2008; Netflix, 2017). This seems to be a level up from "based on a true story."

2. Rachel Abramowitz, "'Changeling' Revisits a Crime that Riveted L.A.," *Los Angeles Times*, October 18, 2008; Andrew Geoff, "Clint Eastwood: The Quiet American," *Sight and Sound* 18, no. 9 (September 2008), 14–16, 19–22; Daniel Egan, "Changeling," *Film International Journal* 111, no. 12 (December 2008), 75; Ryan Gilbey, "Motherhood, Madness and Melodrama," *New Statesman* (December 1, 2008), 45.

3. *The Escaped Lunatic*, directed by Wallace McCutcheon (1904); *Maniac Chase*, directed by Edwin Porter (1904; USA: Edison Manufacturing); *The Woman in White (The Unfortunate Marriage)*, directed by Ernest C. Warde (1917; USA: Pathé Exchange).

4. Neal Gabler, *Life: The Movie; How Entertainment Conquered Reality* (New York, NY: Alfred A. Knopf, 1999), 233.

5. Daphne Scholinski with Jane Meredith Adams, *The Last Time I Wore a Dress* (New York, NY: Riverhead Books, 1997), 163.

6. Lynn Gamwell and Nancy Tomes, *Madness in America: Cultural and Medical Perceptions of Mental Illness before 1914* (New York, NY: Cornell University Press, 1995).

7. *Girl, Interrupted*, directed by James Mangold (1999; Culver City, CA: Columbia TriStar Home, 2007), DVD; *Manhunter*, directed by Michael Mann (1986); *Brain Dead*, directed by Adam Simon (1990; Los Angeles, CA: New Concorde, 2007), DVD; *In the Mouth of Madness*, directed by John Carpenter (1994; USA: New Line Home Video, 2005), DVD; *The Fisher King*, directed by Terry Gilliam (1991, USA: Columbia TriStar, 2010), DVD.

8. Commentary, *Don't Say a Word*, directed by Gary Fleder (2001; Beverly Hills, CA: Twentieth Century Fox Home Entertainment, 2001), DVD.

9. *Shine*, directed by Scott Hicks (1996; New York, NY: New Line Home Video, 1997), DVD; *Quills*, directed by Philip Kaufman (2000; Beverly Hills, CA: Twentieth Century Fox Home Entertainment, 2001), DVD.

10. *A Beautiful Mind*, directed by Ron Howard (2001; Universal City, CA: Universal, 2002), DVD. Alex Von Tunzelmann, "A Beautiful Mind Hides Ugly Truths," *The Guardian*, December 19, 2012, https://www.theguardian.com/film/filmblog/2012/dec/19/a-beautiful-mind-john-nash, accessed November 18, 2018.

11. *Terminator 2: Judgement Day Extreme DVD Edition*, directed by James Cameron (1991; Santa Monica, CA: Artisan Home Entertainment, 2003), DVD.

12. *Don Juan DeMarco*, directed by Jeremy Levin (1994; USA: New Line Home Video, 1998), DVD; *K-PAX*, directed by Iain Softley (2001; Universal City, CA: Universal, 2002), DVD. One might also consider *Ghostbusters II*, in which the paranormal trio are locked up in the Parkview Psychiatric Hospital after they try to warn the mayor about a river of slime running underneath Manhattan. *Ghostbusters II*, directed by Ivan Reitman (1989; Culver City, CA: TriStar Home Video, 1999), DVD. Despite *K-PAX*'s clichés, the director explained later that he did not want to make an asylum "message" movie. See Director Commentary, *K-PAX*, directed by Iain Softley (DVD, 2002).

13. In another example of the deserving incarcerated, in Milos Forman's *Amadeus* the villain Salieri is locked up in an asylum after a suicide attempt, regretting how he killed Mozart. The plot flows from his asylum confession to a priest. *Amadeus*, directed by Milos Forman (1984; Burbank, CA: Warner Home Video, 2009), DVD.

14. *Willowbrook: The Last Great Disgrace*, directed by Geraldo Rivera (1972). Willowbrook was called a "snake pit" as early as 1965. See David J. Rothman and Sheila M. Rothman, *The Willowbrook Wars* (New York, NY: Harper and Row, 1984). For an earlier 1960s exposé, see Burton Blatt and Fred Kaplan, *A Christmas in Purgatory: A Photographic Essay on Mental Retardation* (Boston, MA: Allyn and Bacon, 1966).

15. *Death Wish II*, directed by Michael Winner (1982; Santa Monica, CA: MGM Home Entertainment, 2004), DVD.

16. *High Anxiety*, directed by Mel Brooks (1977; Beverly Hills, CA: Twentieth Century Fox Home Entertainment, 2006), DVD. Brooks, interestingly, was at this time trying to get Frances Farmer's story made into a film with his production company. Ken Kesey, *One Flew Over the Cuckoo's Nest: Text and Criticism*, ed. John C. Pratt (New York, NY: Viking Press, 1977), 5–6.

17. *The Pink Panther Strikes Again*, directed by Blake Edwards (1976; Santa Monica, CA: MGM Home Entertainment, 1999), DVD; *Annie*, directed by John Huston (1982; Culver City, CA: Sony Pictures Home Entertainment, 2015), DVD; *Airplane II: The Sequel*, directed Ken Finkleman (1982; Hollywood, CA: Paramount, 2000), DVD; *Good Burger*, directed by Brian Robbins (1997; Hollywood, CA: Paramount, 2000), DVD.

18. *Crazy People*, directed by Tony Bill and Mitch Markowitz (1990; Hollywood, CA: Paramount, 2000), DVD.

19. *The Exorcist*, directed by William Friedkin (1973; Burbank, CA: Warner Home Video, 2010), DVD; *The Amityville Horror*, directed by Stuart Rosenberg (1979; Santa Monica, CA: MGM Home Entertainment, 1999), DVD; *The Princess Bride* directed by Rob Reiner (1987; Santa Monica, CA: MGM Home Entertainment, 2001), DVD; *A Nightmare on Elm Street*, directed by Wes Craven (1984; Los Angeles, CA: New Line, 2010), DVD.

20. In *Asylum* (1997), the room is bright and cluttered with patients. In *Gothika* (2003), it is dark gray. In *The Ring* (1999, is it an unsettling, bilious green. See *Asylum*, directed by James Seale (1997); Santa Monica, CA: Genius Entertainment, 1997), DVD; *Gothika*, directed by Mathieu Kassovitz (2003; Burbank, CA: Warner Home Video, 2004), DVD; *The Ring*, directed by Gore Verbinski (2002; Universal City, CA: DreamWorks Home Entertainment, 2004), DVD. *Unsane*, directed by Stephen Soderbergh (2018; Amazon Prime Video).

21. *12 Monkeys*, directed by Terry Gilliam (1995; Universal City, CA: Universal Studios Home Entertainment, 2005), DVD.

22. *Shock Corridor*, directed by Sam Fuller (1963; Paris, Wild Side Films, 2005), DVD.

23. *The Shining*, directed by Stanley Kubrick (1980; Burbank, CA: Warner Home Video, 2010), DVD, digitally remastered version.

24. *Possessed*, directed by Curtis Bernhardt (1947; Burbank, CA: Warner Home Video, 2005), DVD; *The Caretakers*, directed by Hall Bartlett (1963; Santa Monica,

CA: MGM Home Video, 2005), DVD; *Brain Dead*, directed by Adam Simon (1990); *Candyman*, directed by Bernard Rose (1992; Netflix).

25. *Psycho*, directed by Alfred Hitchcock (1960; Universal City, CA: Universal Studios Home Entertainment, 1998), DVD Collector's Edition.

26. *The Boston Strangler*, directed by Richard Fleischer (1968; Beverly Hills, CA: Twentieth Century Fox Home Entertainment, 2004), DVD. Sticking the psycho in the white room at the end, see *The Dentist*, directed by Brian Yuzna (1996; California: Trimark Home Video, 2000), DVD.

27. On a related note, in "Let's Go Crazy," Prince says to "Look for the purple banana / Until they put us in a truck."

28. Metallica, "Welcome Home (Sanitarium)," *Master of Puppets* (1986).

29. *E.T. The Extra-Terrestrial*, directed by Steven Spielberg (1982; Universal City, CA: Universal Studios Home Entertainment, 2012), DVD.

30. *The Return of the Pink Panther*, directed by Blake Edwards (1975; Santa Monica, CA: Artisan Home Entertainment, 1999), DVD; *Brazil*, directed by Terry Gilliam (1985; Universal City, CA: Universal Studios Home Entertainment, 1998), DVD; *Dracula*, directed by John Badham (1979; Universal City, CA: Universal Studios Home Entertainment, 2004), DVD.

31. *Final Destination 2*, directed by David R. Ellis (2003; Burbank, CA: Warner Home Video, 2003), DVD.

32. *In the Mouth of Madness*, directed by John Carpenter (1994); *The Green Mile*, directed by Frank Darabont (1999; Burbank, CA: Warner Home Video, 2000), DVD; *Beauty and the Beast*, directed by Bill Condon (2017; Burbank, CA: Buena Vista Home Entertainment, 2017), DVD.

33. *Return to Oz*, directed by Walter Murch (1985; Burbank, CA: Buena Vista Home Entertainment, 2004), DVD.

34. In *The Jacket*, directed by John Maybury (2005; Burbank, CA: Warner Home Video, 2005), DVD, a child gets ECT as a last ditch attempt to save him from catatonia. The hand wringing by the doctor and the sequence itself highlights the horror. Andrew McDonald and Gerry Walter, "The Portrayal of ECT in American Movies," *Journal of ECT* 17, no. 4 (December 2001), 271; B. Kalayam and M. J. Steinhart, "A Survey of the Attitudes on the use of Electroconvulsive Therapy," *Hospital and Community Psychiatry* 32, no. 3 (March 1981), 185–88.

35. *Requiem for a Dream*, directed by Darren Aronofsky (2000; Santa Monica, CA: Artisan Home Entertainment, 2001), DVD.

36. A rare exception, *Side Effects*, directed by Stephen Soderbergh (2013; Netflix, 2017), shows a woman receiving ECT under sedation. In this case, we watch in horror as a woman is threatened with similar treatment if she does not confess to her crime (he tells her "it damages the memory"). "What Happens during an ECT Procedure?," http://www.hopkinsmedicine.org/psychiatry/specialty_areas/brain_stimulation/ect/faq_ect.html, accessed May 30, 2017. Explain McDonald and Walter of *The House on Haunted Hill*, this is "7 years before Cerletti performed the first ECT," and yet this hospital has "no less than 18 ECT suites." In McDonald and Walter, "The Portrayal of ECT in American Movies," 270.

37. Commentary, *A Beautiful Mind*, directed by Ron Howard (Universal DVD, 2002).

38. *Session 9*, directed by Brad Anderson (2001; Universal City, CA: Universal Studios Home Entertainment, 2002), DVD; *Insanitarium*, directed by Jeff Buhler (2008; Culver City, CA: Sony Pictures Home Entertainment, 2008), DVD; *Cheech and Chong's Nice Dreams*, directed by Thomas Chong (1981; Culver City, CA: Columbia Pictures, 2006), DVD; "The Quiet Room," *The Incredible Hulk*, directed by Reza S. Badiyi (1979).

39. Commentary, *From Hell* directed by Hughes Brothers (Beverly Hills, CA: Twentieth Century Fox Home Entertainment, 2002), DVD. In the graphic novel, there is no lobotomy. See Alan Moore and Eddie Campbell, *From Hell* (Marietta, GA: Top Shelf Productions, 2006).

40. *The Jacket*, directed by John Maybury (2005). Another contender for originality is The Harvester, a demon who works in an asylum basement and sucks out your soul through your eyes, in *Asylum of the Damned*, directed by Phillip J. Jones (2003; Culver City, CA: Columbia TriStar Home Entertainment, 2004), DVD. Surprisingly, the director of *The Jacket* argued that he didn't want "too many clichés." Commentary, *The Jacket* (Warner Home Video, 2005).

41. *Girl, Interrupted*, directed by James Mangold (1999).

42. Commentary, *Girl, Interrupted*, directed by James Mangold (Columbia TriStar Home Video, 2007).

43. "HBO First Look: The Making-Of *Girl, Interrupted*," *Girl, Interrupted* (Columbia TriStar Home Video, 1999).

44. James Mangold Commentary, *Girl, Interrupted* (Columbia TriStar Home Video, 2007).

45. Alan A. Stone, "Split Personality," *Boston Review* 25, no. 3 (July 1, 2000), 48; Alice Cross, "Girl, Interrupted," *Cineaste* (June 1, 2000), 49; Stephen Holden, "Get Over It, Little Girl. Stop Your Whining," *New York Times*, December 21, 1999.

CHAPTER 11. RETURN OF THE GOTHIC

1. Mark Edmundson, *Nightmare on Main Street: Angels, Sadomasochism, and the Culture of Gothic* (Cambridge, MA: Harvard University Press, 1997).

2. *Shutter Island*, directed by Martin Scorsese (2010; Hollywood, CA: Paramount, 2010), DVD.

3. Walter C. Metz, "Adapting Dachau: Intertextuality and Martin Scorsese's *Shutter Island*," in *The Adaptation of History: Essays on Ways of Telling the Past*, ed. Laurence Raw and Defne Ersin Tutan (Jefferson, NC: McFarland Publishing, 2013), 51. Also see "Shutter Island: Movie Review," *The Christian Science Monitor*, February 19, 2010.

4. *Gothika*, directed by Mathieu Kassovitz (2003; Burbank, CA: Warner Home Video, 2004), DVD.

5. In the Director's Commentary on the DVD, Mathieu Kassovitz says of Nurse Irene that she is playing "Nurse Ratched, yeah, in, a, *One Flew Over a Cuckoo's Nest* [sic]." In *Gothika* (2004), DVD.

6. Much of *Gothika* was filmed on location in Quebec at the Saint-Vincent-de-Paul Penitentiary, an imposing brick building closed in 1989. Commentary, *Gothika* (2004), DVD.

7. Superintendent quoted in Diane L. Goeres-Gardner, *Inside Oregon State Hospital: A History of Tragedy and Triumph* (Charleston, SC: History Press, 2013), 295. *House of Dust*, directed by A. D. Calvo (2013; Beverly Hills, CA: Anchor Bay Entertainment, 2014), DVD.

8. *Shutter Island*, directed by Martin Scorsese (2010).

9. *Session 9*, directed by Brad Anderson (2001; Universal City, CA: Universal Studios Home Entertainment, 2002), DVD.

10. *The Ward*, directed by John Carpenter (2010; Santa Monica, CA: Arc Entertainment, 2011), DVD.

11. "Eastern State Hospital" *Washington State Department of Social and Health Services.* https://www.dshs.wa.gov/fsa/office-capital-programs/eastern-state-hospital, accessed November 27, 2018.

12. *Stonehearst Asylum*, directed by Brad Anderson (2014; Netflix, 2016).

13. Lisa Carey, *Love in the Asylum* (New York, NY: HarperCollins, 2004), 1–2, 51, 181, 248–49, 270.

14. Carey, *Love in the Asylum*, 3.

15. Madeleine Roux, *Asylum* (New York: HarperCollins, 2013). Also see Katie Alender, *The Dead Girls of Hysteria Hall* (New York, NY: Scholastic, 2015).

16. Mark Voger, *The Dark Age: Grim, Great, and Gimmicky Postmodern Comics* (Raleigh, NC: TwoMorrows Publishing, 2006), 5. For another possible strand of inheritance, note that Julius Schwartz, who had known Lovecraft, was also editor of DC during this period.

17. S. T. Joshi, *I Am Providence: The Life and Times of H. P. Lovecraft*, vol. 1 (New York, NY: Hippocampus Press, 2013), 25, 130, 390. For a discussion, see Troy Rondinone, "Tentacles in the Madhouse: The Role of the Asylum in the Fiction of H. P. Lovecraft," *Lovecraftian Proceedings* 2 (August 2017): 93–108.

18. H. P. Lovecraft, "The Thing on the Doorstep," *The New Annotated H. P. Lovecraft*, 703, 704. Arkham is also known as the Elizabeth Arkham Asylum for the Criminally Insane.

19. Frank Miller, *Batman: The Dark Knight Returns* (New York, NY: DC Comics, 1996); Grant Morrison, Dave McKean, and Gaspar Saladino, *Arkham Asylum: A Serious House on Serious Earth* (New York, NY: DC Comics, 2004); Alan Grant, Norm Breyfogle, and Bob Kane, *Batman: The Last Arkham* (London, UK: Titan Books, 1996).

20. *Batman Forever*, directed by Joel Schumacher (1995; Burbank, CA: Warner Home Video, 1997), DVD; *Batman & Robin*, directed by Joel Schumacher (1997; Burbank, CA: Warner Home Video, 2008), DVD; *Batman Begins*, directed by Christopher Nolan (2005; Netflix, 2017).

21. On the haunted house trope in American fiction, see Dale Bailey, *American Nightmares: The Haunted House Formula in American Popular Fiction* (Bowling Green, OH: Bowling Green State University Popular Press, 2007). Shirley Jackson, *The Haunting of Hill House* (New York, NY: Viking, 1959), 3, 34–35.

22. *Doom Asylum*, directed by Richard Friedman (1987; USA: Film World Productions, 2006), DVD.

23. *A Nightmare on Elm Street 5: The Dream Child*, directed by Stephen Hopkins (1989; Burbank, CA: Warner Home Video, 2008), DVD.

24. John Saul, *The Blackstone Chronicles: 6 Novels in 1 Volume* (New York, NY: Fawcett, 1997), 13–14, 5, 260, 135.

25. *Session 9*, directed by Brad Anderson (2001).

26. See, for example, *Doom Asylum, Crazy Eights, Grave Encounters 1 and 2, The House on Haunted Hill, House of Dust, Boo, American Horror Story: Asylum*, and *Death Tunnel*.

27. A. O. Scott, "Well, Here They Are, Wherever This May Be," *New York Times*, March 24, 2011.

28. Christina Radish, "Ryan Murphy Talks American Horror Story," *Collider*, January 13, 2013, http://collider.com/american-horror-story-asylum-season-finale-ryan-murphy-interview/, accessed August 28, 2017.

EPILOGUE

1. Colby Itkowitz, "Halloween Attractions Use Mental Illness to Scare Us: Here's Why Advocates Say It Must Stop," *Washington Post*, October 25, 2016; John Goodwin, "The Horror of Stigma: Psychosis and Mental Health Care Environments in Twenty-First Century Horror Film (Part II)" *Perspectives in Psychiatric Care* (October 1, 2014), 230. "Language Matters in Mental Health," http://hogg.utexas.edu/news-resources/language-matters-in-mental-health, accessed October 26, 2017.

2. Carrie Fisher, *Shockaholic* (New York, NY: Simon and Schuster, 2011), 4; Jane Perkis et al., "On-Screen Portrayals of Mental Illness: Extent, Nature, and Impacts," *Journal of Health Communication* 11 (2006), 536.

3. João Biehl, *Vita: Life in a Zone of Social Abandonment* (Berkeley, CA: University of California Press, 2013), 2, 8, 52, 65; Andrew Scull, *Madness in Civilization: A Cultural History of Insanity from the Bible to Freud, from the Madhouse to Modern Medicine* (Princeton, NJ: Princeton University Press, 2016), 14; Ron Powers, *No One Cares about Crazy People: The Chaos and Heartbreak of Mental Health in America* (New York, NY: Hachette Books, 2017). Art Levin, *Mental Health, Inc.: How Corruption, Lax Oversight and Failed Reforms Endanger Our Most Vulnerable Citizens* (New York, NY: Overlook Press, 2017), 32.

4. Jonathan M. Metzl, *The Protest Psychosis: How Schizophrenia Became a Black Disease* (Boston, MA: Beacon Press, 2009).

INDEX